STRAINED MERCY

The Economics of Canadian Health Care

STRAINED MERCY

The Economics of Canadian Health Care

by

Robert G. Evans

Professor of Economics
University of British Columbia

BUTTERWORTHS
TORONTO

Strained Mercy: The Economics of Canadian Health Care

© 1984 Butterworth & Co. (Canada) Ltd.

Printed and bound in Canada.

Sponsoring Editor—Janet Turner
Supervisory Editor—Linda Kee
Editor—Maura Brown
Cover—Gord Sadlier
Production—Jim Shepherd

The Butterworth Group of Companies

Canada:
Butterworth & Co. (Canada) Ltd., Toronto and Vancouver
United Kingdom:
Butterworth & Co. (Publishers) Ltd., London
Australia:
Butterworths Pty Ltd., Sydney, Melbourne, Brisbane, Adelaide and Perth
New Zealand:
Butterworths of New Zealand Ltd., Wellington and Auckland
Singapore:
Butterworth & Co. (Asia) Pte. Ltd., Singapore
South Africa:
Butterworth Publishers (Pty) Ltd., Durban and Pretoria
United States:
Butterworth Legal Publishers, Boston, Seattle, Austin and St. Paul
D & S Publishers, Clearwater

Canadian Cataloguing in Publication Data

Evans, Robert G.,
    Strained mercy : the economics of Canadian health care

Bibliography: p.
Includes index.
ISBN 0-409-82945-5

1. Medical economics.   2. Medical economics – Canada.   I. Title.

RA410.55.C3E96 1984   338.4'73621   C84-099459-1

PREFACE

Cliff Lloyd once said that anyone writing a textbook makes a simultaneous confession of arrogance, incompetence, and greed. In all fairness, I think a Canadian is guilty of only two out of three. At the end of the process, however, it is all too obvious how much has been left undone, or done inadequately. There are also, no doubt, parts that are overdone.

The end product is the result of a series of painful compromises among several different books with different purposes—such as providing a comprehensive survey of health economics, impressing one's professional colleagues, serving as a text for courses in health economics, and demonstrating the application of economics to health care services in a way that would be most interesting and useful to the people actually on the line in organizing, delivering, and funding health care—in Canada or elsewhere. This book tries to do a bit of each. But it is primarily intended for two specific audiences which are only partially overlapping.

In the first place, it is a text for courses in health economics, as part of university programs in health planning and administration, economics, or public administration. The formal economic analysis which is explicit in the text presupposes that the reader has as background a one-term course in micro-economic theory, and remembers and understands it. The concept of optimal resource allocation, and the strengths and weaknesses of price and market systems, supply and demand, in that process, as well as the basic theory of the firm, would normally be covered at that level. Some of the footnotes are used to deal with theoretical points which the text sweeps under the rug, or to cover the author's professional flanks; the reader who finds them incomprehensible can ignore them without loss.

There is, however, a much larger group of health professionals—administrators, clinical practitioners, planners, "bureaucrats" of various sorts—with a considerable interest in and knowledge about health care organization and delivery, "at the coalface," as the British say. Their work inevitably has an economic dimension, whether explicit or implicit. But their acquaintance with formal economic analysis may be variable, remote, or unsatisfactory, and they may find abstract graphic or algebraic demonstrations unhelpful at best.

Accordingly, I have tried to make the presentation self-contained in two respects. First, the economic concepts and tools of analysis which do emerge explicitly are defined and explained at each point, so that previous economic background is not essential. This is not wholly satisfactory, as the definition of a tool or concept, however complete, is not a substitute for previous experience in working with it. But it does mean that the reader can work through any part of the text without previous economic training. Some parts may require a bit of determination.

Secondly, the formal parts are in chunks which are not critical to the flow of the text. The reader who is prepared to take the demonstrations on faith can skip over them without loss of continuity. Nothing is presented which is not also described in words, so that those who find formalisms highly allergenic will not lose any of the main points. This comment applies in particular to the brief outline of the von Neumann-Morgenstern approach to utility and risk in chapter 2, the discussion of externalities and demand curves in chapter 3, and the application of Lerner's Rule in chapter 6. A considerable amount of theory is lurking behind chapters 7 and 8 as well, but it does not emerge formally. The presentation of a Leontief-type fixed coefficients manpower planning model in chapter 13 may also require a certain amount of concentration. But, in fact, everyone who thinks about health care (or anything else) at all systematically has been engaged in "modelling," usually in a similar form, just as she has always been speaking prose. The conversion to a formal language makes the process explicit, but does not introduce a new activity.

This then raises a question as to why the graphs and algebra are there at all, other than to demonstrate that the author is, indeed, an economist. Why not simply present an extended "policy analysis" study of health care, with the formal economics out of sight, if not out of mind?

The question is a serious one, because it seems to me that the insights and generalizations of experienced and thoughtful health care people are often much more reliable guides to understanding how health care systems "work" than are patterns of thought derived from off-the-shelf economic analyses of idealized "consumers," "firms," and "markets." The hospital administrator's adage that "a built bed is a filled bed," for example, or the physician's comment that "the sickness in a community must be sufficient to support the practitioners in that community," are not always and everywhere true. But they express important empirical regularities, and point to even more important underlying patterns of incentives and behaviour. A simple-minded "demand-and-supply" story, by contrast, which treats health care services as commodities analytically indistinguishable from litres of milk, is worse than useless. It obscures and diverts attention from the most interesting and important problems of health care delivery, which literally cannot be expressed in such a framework, and even for the phenomena it purports to explain it gets the empirical facts wrong. Universal "free" care, for example, does not in fact lead to overutilization and cost escalation; the whole process is a good deal more subtle and interesting than that.

But certain characteristic confusions over objectives or motives, and failures of consistency and logic, arise from the non-analytic approach. A limited amount of economic formalism can serve as a powerful check on such mistakes. There *are* a number of basic ideas and thought patterns which economists have worked out, and use routinely, such as opportunity costs, the distinction between resource costs and wealth transfers, partial versus general equilibrium or "what happens next," which non-economists are frequently unaware of, or ignore. And they go wrong as a result. Economic analysis does tend to encourage "well-ordered thoughts," while great practical experience and insight is quite consistent with surprising intellectual muddles.

Further, formal analysis not only identifies the limitations of inference from experience, it may also serve to underpin and reinforce such experience against criticisms drawn from incomplete and half-baked "pop" economics. As Joan Robinson put it, "We study economics, not to understand the economy, but to avoid being deceived by economists." And some additional understanding does come, as well. When the health care people in a policy debate are roughly right, and off-the-shelf economic analysis is precisely wrong, as may occur for example in discussions of "needs" versus "demands," the "conversation of the deaf" *can* be resolved by a more complete formal analysis. This book tries to provide that more complete analysis, and to demonstrate its resolving power.

The concentration in the text on developing and presenting an analytic framework for health economics means that it could not hope also to provide a comprehensive description, much less historical analysis, of the Canadian health care system. Canadian institutions are outlined, and a number of data series are assembled which show some aspects of its evolution over the last thirty-five years. The Canadian experience motivates and illustrates the analysis, as does the partly parallel and partly contrasting United States experience.

But the analytic framework is intended to be much more general, to be useful to people trying to understand the economics of health care through whatever national system it might be expressed. A good deal of abstract economic analysis is presented in the health economics literature as if it were fully general and free of specific institutional content, yet on closer examination it turns out to presuppose the existence of particular institutions or patterns of transactions—usually those of the United States. I have probably done the same, but I have tried to make the interaction, the "unity of theory and practice," explicit. The theory arises as inferences from our experience—where else could it come from?—but I do not think the book is only about Canada.

The work is thus complementary to more complete descriptive studies which would tell the reader what the Canadian health insurance and health care systems are like—who does what and with which and to whom. The extended essay by Maurice LeClair in *National Health Insurance: Can We Learn from Canada?* (S. Andreopoulos, ed., New York: John Wiley, 1975), Lee Soderstrom's *The Canadian Health System* (London: Croom Helm, 1978), Gordon Hatcher's *Universal Free Health Care in Canada, 1947-77* (Washington, D.C.: D.H.H.S., 1981), or Malcolm Taylor's *Health Insurance and Canadian Public Policy* (Montreal: McGill-Queen's, 1978), are all sources for a more complete description of where we are and how we got here. This book tries to contribute an interpretation of why we got here, how we might go about evaluating the situation, and where we might go next.

A preface is also an opportunity to try to thank all those whose ideas and efforts were exploited in the work. There were a lot. Morris Barer and Greg Stoddart read and commented on several chapters, to the considerable benefit of the book, as well as collaborating on a number of research projects which are reflected here in one way or another. The work shared over the decade with Geoff Robinson also made a major contribution, helping me to understand a little bit about medicine, and a bit more about medical people. The outline of the book was developed during a most exciting year at the University of Toronto as a Health and Welfare Visiting National Health Scientist—Alan Wolfson, Gene Vayda, Carolyn Tuohy, and the others in Health Administration helped to shape my thinking there. My understanding of how professions function has been greatly assisted by them and by Bill Stanbury and Michael Trebilcock. The impact of Tony Culyer's work, particularly on externality issues, will be obvious by the references, while Uwe Reinhardt and Ted Marmor have, from different perspectives, contributed a North American context which highlights the strengths and weaknesses of the Canadian system. And Brenda Lundman has, among other things, tried to keep me up to date, and more or less straight, about some of the finer (and politically crucial) points of the federal-provincial health care relationship.

These and a number of other people have provided both ideas and, perhaps as important, moral support in encouraging me to get the book written. Glen Beck, André-Pierre Contandriopoulos, John Horne, Sidney Lee, Daniel Le Touzé, Pran Manga, Dick Plain, Lee Soderstrom, and Hugh Walker, among others, have not only been sources and sounding boards, but have suggested strongly that they thought the enterprise might be worthwhile. I hope it was. My colleagues at the University of British Columbia have done likewise. Though not themselves primarily interested in health care, they have always encouraged my peculiar tastes; and I am indebted to david donaldson in particular on aspects of insurance and theoretical welfare economics. In addition, many people in Health and

Welfare Canada and Statistics Canada, and in several provincial health ministries, have been very generous with their time and data before and while this book was being written.

Much of the actual writing was done during a sabbatical year supported by U.B.C. and by a grant from the SSHRC. But the structure and content of the book have evolved over a much longer period. Successive groups of students in Economics 384 in the U.B.C. Health Services Planning program have provided an interactive experimental environment for this process, as have participants in the Banff Centre's Senior Health Administrators Program. I am grateful for their reactions and input, and like all those named above they enjoy the usual blanket absolution for remaining errors, obscurities, and inadequacies.

The writing of a book is, of course, only one stage in the production process. Margaret Francis at Population Paediatrics, U.B.C. converted the rather dubious handwriting to word processor with remarkable patience and good humour.

Finally, my family has put up with the seemingly endless process, and all the lost weekends and weeks, which inevitably go with a book. Meg's attitude has been the practical one of well, get on with it. If you have to do it, do it. Charley wanted to know if it would make any money. But my wife, Susanne, in the end, has to bear a considerable share of responsibility for the final product. If she had not been nursing at MGH when I was in graduate school, I would never have begun to work in health economics in the first place.

Robert G. Evans
Vancouver, B.C.

May 1984

TABLE OF CONTENTS

Part 2
The Provision of Health Care

Part 3
The Governance of Health Care

PART 1

THE UTILIZATION OF HEALTH CARE

CHAPTER 1

HEALTH AND THE USE OF HEALTH CARE

INTRODUCTION: THE SCOPE OF HEALTH CARE ECONOMICS

The health of people, individually and in groups, is influenced by a very wide range of factors, of which health care is only one. Moreover, while health care may be decisive for the health of a particular individual in particular circumstances, it is generally accepted that for most people, most of the time, health status is primarily dependent on sanitation, diet, shelter—the complex of factors summarized in the federal White Paper of 1974 (Lalonde) as "lifestyle" and "environmental." And the great historical improvements in mortality and morbidity, life expectancy and health status experienced in now-developed countries appear to owe much more to improvements in these areas than to the progress of health care narrowly defined. "Tell me how a people die, and I will tell you how they live."

The economics of health, which Culyer (1981) defines as the application of the discipline and tools of economics to the subject matter of health, accordingly encompasses the full range of two-way causal relations between the health status of individuals and groups and their economic activities—production, distribution, and exchange. This might include, for example, the study of the impact of unemployment and bankruptcy rates on anxiety and mental health, or of anti-malarial campaigns on agricultural labour productivity, or of the interaction between patterns of income or wealth distribution and health status.

The economics of health *care*, which is the subject of this book, is only a part of this much broader field. It restricts attention to a particular set of goods and services which have somehow been identified as having a special relationship to health status, and to the activities associated with their production and consumption. Like any other branch of economics, it studies the processes and institutions which govern the allocation of scarce social resources to these activities, the choice of techniques of production and mix of outputs, and the distribution of health care among the end users—consumers or patients.

But unless this special relationship, and health status itself, are defined narrowly, the economics of health care can easily become the economics of everything. The famous World Health Organization definition of health, "a state of complete physical, mental, and social well-being," not "merely the absence of disease or infirmity," is a splendid call to arms, but bears a striking resemblance to the economist's concept of utility or welfare. The only difference is that utility is unbounded, being constrained only by the resources available in particular circumstances. Health, on the other hand, is implicitly bounded by some state of "complete . . . well-being," beyond which one cannot go; but we are not, in fact, expected to reach that limit, in this life at least.

But if "health" is equated with welfare or well-being, then clearly there is no sphere of human activity and, in particular, no form of economic activity which does not have health as its principal concern. Economics is frequently defined as the study of the allocation of scarce resources among competing wants so as to "maximize" (in a way left undefined) the satisfaction of those wants. But if all wants are encompassed in health, then all economics is health economics.

The attractions of disciplinary imperialism are tempered by awareness of the dental and digestive problems which result from biting off more than one can chew. Accordingly, insofar as they have considered it at all, health economists have generally accepted, explicitly or implicitly, a narrower conception of health status as "absence of disease or infirmity." This restriction, however, does not suffice to identify health care as a set of commodities, or activities, which are uniquely related to health. Since sanitation, food, home and work environment, activity levels, play at least as important a role as health care in influencing the absence of disease or infirmity, it is clearly impossible to define health care as all activities or commodities influencing health, even narrowly defined, without slipping back into the "economics of everything."

The economic literature appears to display two different responses to this difficulty. One approach is simply to sidestep the definitional issue, and to accept as the proper content of health care economics whatever conventional usage has come to label health care—hospitals, doctors, drugs, and all that. Health care economics studies the behaviour of health care providers and users, whoever those may be. The development of a sub-discipline differentiated from economics in general then presumably rests on certain characteristics peculiar to the processes of resource allocation in the production and distribution of these commodities. But there is no explicit recognition of any special relationship of health care to health.

The weakness of this approach, apart from the problems of identifying boundaries which are common to any definition, is that it tends to blur important distinctions between health care and commodities in general. It thus provides no logical grounding for the characteristics which make health care "different" and which motivate not only a special sub-discipline of economics but also, in almost every society, the very special set of institutions which govern and regulate its production and distribution. Why are some activities health care, and others not, and why are the former treated differently?

The alternative, which is followed in this book, is to define health care as that set of goods and services which consumer/patients use solely or primarily because of their anticipated (positive) impact on health status. It is health, as a status, rather than health care, as a commodity, which is of value to its users. Indeed, the direct effects of most, if not all, health services on their users' well-being, independent of their anticipated health effects, is negative. Dentistry, drugs, diagnostic and therapeutic interventions, hospital stays, are frequently uncomfortable or frightening in and of themselves. Few, indeed, would choose to purchase them in the absence of an expected health benefit. And those who do—drug addicts, say, or sufferers from Münchausen's Syndrome, who derive pleasure from medical care and counterfeit illness to get it, are generally regarded as unwell. Anyone who seeks care when he is not sick, is sick.[1]

This formulation does not, of course, exclude preventive services from health care. Users of such services may be healthy at present, but they are obviously contemplating a possibility of some future deterioration in their health status. Preventive care must be believed to reduce the probability or severity of such deterioration, or it is not preventive care. Nor do we exclude the obvious variations in amenity levels surrounding various forms of care, from spartan to luxurious, assembly-line to humane and personal. There are different degrees of satisfaction or dissatisfaction associated with health care, *given* that one is ill (or more generally believes that a particular form of health care is needed to maintain or improve health). What our formulation implies is that faced with a choice between illness plus any level of associated care, and not being ill at all, the representative consumer prefers not to be ill. Further, if ill, she regards health care which is not expected to improve health (*e.g.*, interventions for teaching purposes) as a "bad," not a good. And amenities for which this is not true—colour T.V. sets or steak-and-champagne dinners in hospitals with low occupancy rates—are not health care.

---

[1] In technical terms, we define the consumer's utility function U as extending over a set of commodities X_i, including health care (HC), and also over health status HS. But health care enters positively via its presumed positive effect on HS, its direct effects are negative. Thus:

$$U = U[X_i, --- X_n, HC, HS (HC)]$$

where $\partial U/\partial HS > 0$, $dHS/dHC \geq 0$ in the relevant range (although $dHS/dHC < 0$ is technically possible), and $\partial U/\partial HC < 0$. This formulation differs from the characteristics approach to consumer theory in that HS is a characteristic of the consumer, not the commodity; and the contribution of care to health, dHS/dHC, depends on the status of the user and is not intrinsic to the commodity (Evans and Wolfson 1980).

Health care is thus clearly demarcated from other commodities which influence health, but which are consumed for their perceived direct satisfactions rather than their health effects. Nutritional value may be a consideration in food purchasing, but if it were the only or the predominant consideration we would eat much more skim milk powder and beans, and much less steak. Indeed some foods, and particularly such substances as tobacco and alcohol, are consumed despite their known harmful effects on health.[2] But anyone using health care which she believed to be harmful to health would be thought irrational, to say the least.

Explicit recognition of the role of health status in the definition of health care will provide significant assistance in our understanding of why health care as a commodity is "different," and why societies develop peculiar types of institutions for directing its production and distribution. Moreover, health status, unlike utility or well-being, is identifiable and to a degree at least measurable by observers external to the consumption process. It thus provides a standpoint and a source of additional information for the evaluation of resource allocation processes in health care, which is lacking in economic analysis in general. The economic analysis of health care can draw on the rich medical literature on efficacy and effectiveness which focusses on the relation between health care and health status. We shall show, throughout this book, that such a linkage powerfully extends the range of economic analysis and permits it to grasp important dimensions and issues of health care policy and institutional design which are inexplicable, and ignored, in a framework which treats health care as similar to any other commodity, assumed to bear directly (and positively) on the user's utility or well-being without the necessity of any mediating concept of health status.

In particular, explicit recognition of the mediating role of health status enables us to come to grips with the concepts of over- and under-utilization, which play an important role in the medical literature and in health policy discussions. These are defined in terms of the relation between health care and health status for particular consumer/patients. Use of amounts or types of care which an informed provider might reasonably expect to do a patient no good, or even harm, clearly represents overutilization, from a medical standpoint. So, as we shall show below, is care with an expected payoff in terms of the user's health status, which is positive but too small (on some cut-off criterion which must be supplied externally) to justify its cost. Under-utilization, by contrast, implies that some amounts or types of care are not being supplied and used, which could increase the health status of some patient(s) by enough to justify

---

[2] These harmful effects are presumably outweighed by the direct satisfactions of consumption, though in the case of addictive substances like tobacco this presumption may be invalid.

their cost. Inappropriate care can involve simultaneous over- and under-utilization—too much of some forms of care, not enough of others—again in terms of expected effects on the user's health status.

These rather obvious, but very important, concepts cannot even be expressed in the standard economic framework which treats health care itself as the elementary object of choice for consumer/patients, and then goes further to impose the standard non-satiation postulate that "more is always better."[3] There *is* a concept of "over-utilization" in this framework, but it is defined as a level such that the (assumed positive) benefits of care at the margin, defined in terms not of health increment but of consumer satisfaction, fall short of its resource cost. This is in general unrelated to "over-utilization" or "under-utilization" as discussed in the medical literature, except under very special circumstances. The semantic confusion between the two, particularly in the United States, has led not only to imperfect communication between economists and other health-care analysts, but also to some rather serious confusion in health policy and the design of health insurance systems.

The relationship between health status and health care also plays a central role as an organizing concept in the analysis of the regulation of health care providers. Such regulation derives its principal *raison d'être* from the fact that the provider of health care, as individual or organization, is expected not merely, or even primarily, to satisfy her customers. She is required to seek specific outcomes, in terms of improvements in patient health status, and access to professionalized occupations or markets is conditional upon demonstrated ability and willingness to behave in ways believed consistent with these objectives.

On yet another level, the whole field of cost-benefit or cost-effectiveness analysis applied to public projects in health care is focussed on health status outcomes. The question which must be answered for any such program or intervention, before any economic analysis can be carried out, is does it work? Is it efficacious and effective for the purposes claimed? (Sackett 1980). If the program yields no improvement in anyone's health status, it is not worth buying at any (positive) price. The same is true, on our definition, for any other form of health care.

---

[3] The non-satiation postulate is preserved in our framework, but it is attached to health status, not health care. More health is always better. Nor need this imply unbounded health; "perfect" health may be approached asymptotically. But the relationship between health and health care is not necessarily monotonic. Analyses of the demand for "health" as opposed to health care (*e.g.*, Grossman 1970) which assume that the marginal health productivity of health care is always positive (even constant returns to scale production functions!) are cut off by this counterfactual from the consideration of over-utilization in the sense above. Moreover, the concept of "health status" which is implicit in such analyses is only loosely related to the term as conventionally used.

THE HEALTH CARE "INDUSTRY" IN CANADA:
A BRIEF SKETCH

The collection of diverse organizations which assemble resources and produce and distribute health care is referred to as the "health care industry." The label often strikes practitioners or non-economist students of health care as odd, or even offensive; but in fact it carries no presumptions as to motivations or forms of organization, no necessary implication of belching chimneys, assembly lines, or concentration on "the bottom line." The health care industry does include privately owned, strictly for-profit corporations, of course, but it also includes professional practices, non-profit organizations such as hospitals and voluntary societies, and government departments and agencies. The range of motivations, forms of organization, and technologies (in a broad sense) is very wide; but all use up scarce resources of human time and skills, services of capital (buildings and machines), and raw material to produce or distribute goods and services whose sole or primary purpose is the improvement or maintenance of someone's health.

The structure and evolution of the Canadian health care industry is displayed at a very aggregate level in Table 1-1, which shows total expenditure on health care by category over the post-war period both in dollars and relative to Gross National Product. These expenditures are frequently referred to as "health care costs" and are alleged at various times to "spiral," to be "explosive," or to do other peculiar things. From another perspective, however, these data describe the sales of the health care industry to Canadians, by product line. They are total revenues, not costs of production. This dual nature, with each expenditure item being simultaneously a revenue item to someone else, has important implications for both interpretation and policy. Health care "expenditures" are costs to the rest of Canadian society, not to health care providers—to the providers they are income.

As the table indicates, these expenditures rose rapidly, both in dollar terms and as a percentage of total national expenditure, during the quarter century from 1946 to 1971. Expenditures on hospital care made up the largest share of the total, and also showed the most rapid growth, but physicians and prescription drug expenditures also made substantial gains. Overall, health care more than doubled its share of a national "pie" which was itself growing very rapidly during this period. Real national product (adjusted for price change) per capita rose 87.6 percent from 1946 to 1971, or 2.55 percent per year.

During the 1970s, rapid growth of health spending continued in dollar terms, but its share of national expenditure fluctuated in a range between 7 percent and $7^1/_2$ percent. The large numbers involved supported perceptions of "spiralling" costs, but like all economic measures, these

TABLE 1-1

Expenditures on Health Care in Canada, 1946-82, by Major Component ($Mn) and as Percentage of Gross National Product (Bracketed Figures)

	Hospitals	Physicians' Services	Dental Services	Prescribed Drugs	Personal Health Care*	National Health Expenditures
1946	150.7	86.7	36.3	26.8	300.5	n.a.
	(1.27)	(0.73)	(0.31)	(0.23)	(2.53)	
1951	326.4	153.0	51.0	42.9	573.3	n.a.
	(1.51)	(0.71)	(0.24)	(0.20)	(2.65)	
1956	541.5	240.1	81.5	71.8	934.9	n.a.
	(1.69)	(0.75)	(0.25)	(0.22)	(2.92)	
1961	949.0	388.3	116.7	135.8	1589.9	2375.5
	(2.39)	(0.98)	(0.29)	(0.34)	(4.01)	(6.0)
1966	1668.8	605.2	176.4	232.0	2682.3	3837.5
	(2.70)	(0.98)	(0.29)	(0.38)	(4.34)	(6.2)
1971	3152.8	1250.4	311.5	402.5	5117.2	7122.3
	(3.33)	(1.32)	(0.33)	(0.43)	(5.41)	(7.5)
1976	6571.5	2103.2	699.8	667.1	10041.6	14158.7
	(3.42)	(1.10)	(0.37)	(0.35)	(5.24)	(7.4)
1977	6928.3	2309.0	827.6	746.0	10810.9	15532.6
	(3.30)	(1.11)	(0.40)	(0.35)	(5.15)	(7.4)
1978	7483.5	2544.0	954.1	822.2	11803.8	17094.1
	(3.23)	(1.10)	(0.42)	(0.35)	(5.10)	(7.4)
1979	8239.5	2843.5	1106.0	918.2	13107.2	19067.2
	(3.12)	(1.08)	(0.42)	(0.35)	(4.96)	(7.2)
1980	9484.7	3284.7	1288.0	1011.2	15068.6	22178.6
	(3.20)	(1.11)	(0.43)	(0.34)	(5.08)	(7.5)
1981	10724.4	3741.0	1482.9	1205.0	17153.3	25769.3
	(3.16)	(1.10)	(0.44)	(0.36)	(5.06)	(7.6)
1982	12470.0	4414.3	1682.6	1473.4	20040.3	30087.7
	(3.50)	(1.24)	(0.47)	(0.41)	(5.62)	(8.4)

SOURCES: See Data Sources Appendix.

*"Personal Health Care" is the sum of the first four columns: — hospitals, physicians' and dental services, and prescribed drugs. The more inclusive series of National Health Expenditures adds to these expenditures for other forms of (health-related) institutional care, services of other self-employed professionals, non-prescribed drugs, eyeglasses and other appliances, and costs of public health, research, capital investment, education, and administration of prepayment plans. The more comprehensive data were not compiled prior to 1960.

were distorted by the inflation of the 1970s. It is clear that after 1971, the first year of complete nation-wide public insurance coverage, the trend in health care expenditures/health industry sales changed from growth in share of national output to a roughly stable share. Hospital care and dental service costs increased their shares somewhat during the first half of the decade, while physician and drug expenditure shares fell back

FIGURE 1–1

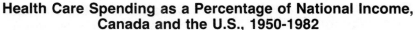

**Health Care Spending as a Percentage of National Income,
Canada and the U.S., 1950-1982**

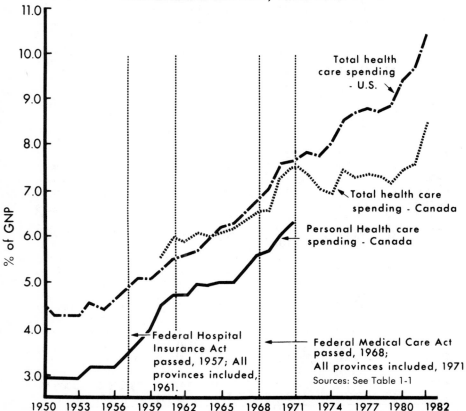

significantly. In the late seventies, hospital spending rose more slowly than GNP, while dentistry continued to expand its share, and the other two sectors were stable. But the share of health costs outside these areas began to grow, reflecting the expansion of public nursing homes and long-term care. This sector is likely to show continued growth, and substitutes to some extent for hospital services.

The significant effects of the public hospital and medical insurance programs on this cost experience are clearly shown in Figure 1-1, which displays health costs relative to GNP for both Canada and the United States from 1950 to 1982. It appears that costs escalated during the actual introduction of each program, but that the completion of universal public coverage in 1971 initiated a period of stability, in sharp contrast to previous Canadian or concurrent United States experience. Data for the early

1980s show a resurgence of growth in the health care share of GNP in both countries, though less pronounced in Canada. Deep recession in the general economy in 1982 has sharply accentuated this trend. The outlook for the 1980s, however, is a more appropriate topic for the end of this book than for the beginning.

Although the data in Table 1-1 are useful as background information about where we are and where we have come from, there is actually much less to them than meets the eye. The same data can be, and have been, used to support arguments by the Canadian Medical Association to the Parliamentary Task Force on Fiscal Arrangements (Canadian Medical Association 1981) (and elsewhere) that the health care system is "underfunded," and by various provincial Ministers of Health, that costs are "spiralling out of control." By themselves, they say nothing about whether the share of national resources devoted to health care is too high or too low, whether the mix of different types of health care services is appropriate, whether production is technically efficient or wasteful, or whether the services produced go to the right people—whoever they are. In fact, in the absence of price information, the data of Table 1-1 do not necessarily tell us about quantities of health services at all.

As noted above, health care "costs" as usually defined are total industry sales, and total incomes earned from health services production. This identity relationship, displayed in Figure 1-2, is merely a sub-component of the overall national income accounting identity which equates Gross National Income, Expenditure, and Product. Sales or expenditures are in turn the product of the total number of items produced, goods and services, represented as a vector or a "shopping list" of quantities of different kinds of items, multiplied by their respective prices. And total incomes are the product of the numbers of different types of persons drawing incomes from health services provision, multiplied by their average incomes (from this industry). Thus:

$$P_1Q_1 + \text{---} \, P_iQ_i + \text{---} \, P_nQ_n \equiv N_1Y_1 + \text{---} \, N_jY_j + \text{---} \, N_mY_m$$

where Q_i is the quantity of health care of type i produced in a given time period, office visits, say, or appendectomies, MOD restorations or aspirin tablets, and P_i is its average price. N_j is the number of people of a particular type drawing incomes from health care, and Y_j is the average income earned.[4]

---

[4] It should be kept in mind that "incomes" are more than salaries, wages, and professional fees, and "people earning incomes" is broader than health care workers per se. Since most branches of health care are labour-intensive and employ specialized and distinctive personnel, much of expenditure is identifiable as incomes of doctors, nurses, dentists, technicians, etc. But expenditures on commodities, drugs, equipment, or buildings, say, generate wages, profits, "rent interest and dividends," in the associated

FIGURE 1–2

The Health Care Sector Income-Expenditure Identity

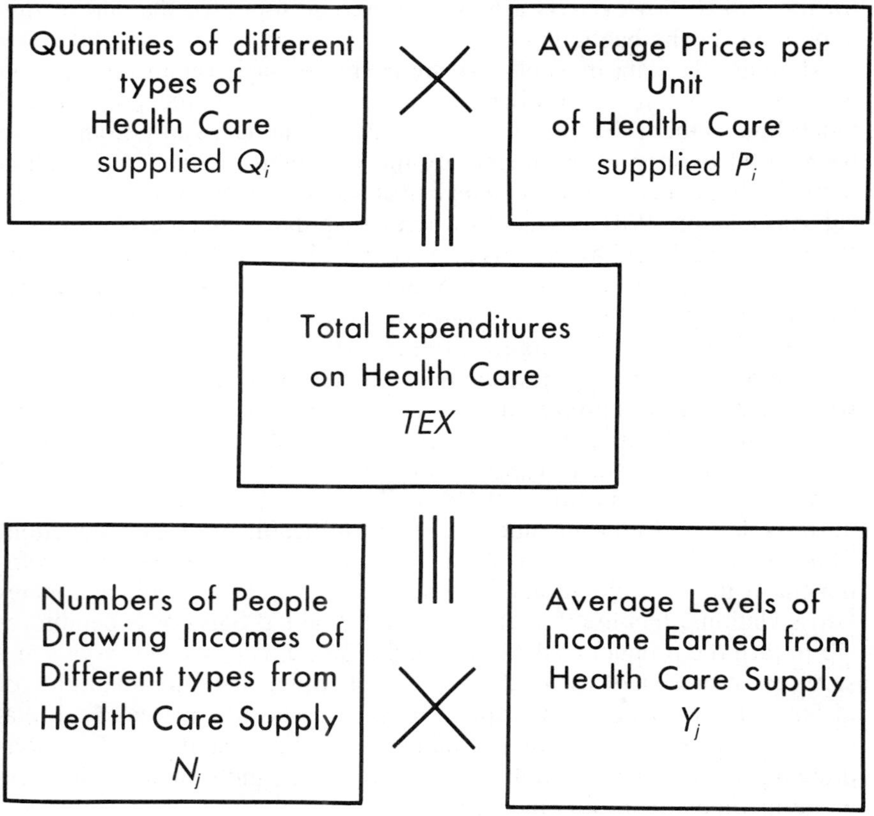

Quantities of different types of Health Care supplied Q_i	$\times$	Average Prices per Unit of Health Care supplied P_i

$|||$

Total Expenditures
on Health Care
TEX

$|||$

Numbers of People Drawing Incomes of Different types from Health Care Supply N_j	$\times$	Average Levels of Income Earned from Health Care Supply Y_j

$$\sum_i P_i \cdot Q_i \equiv TEX \equiv \sum_j N_j \cdot Y_j$$

These incomes are earned by supplying resources—labour, capital, raw materials—to health care production, and it is these resources which are the true "costs of production" of health care. They also give rise to "opportunity costs," in that resources (by definition) have alternative uses in the production of other commodities or services of value, and are scarce, insufficient to serve all the alternative valued uses to which they

---

manufacturing sectors. Not only drug- or equipment-company shareholders, but in the United States, owners of hospital bonds, form part of the set M of income earners, and analyses (or policies) which ignore their participation will be incomplete (will probably fail).

might be put. Thus the opportunity cost of health care, or of anything else, is the foregone opportunities, the other things which might have been, but were not, done with the same resources of human time and skill, bricks and mortar, equipment and raw materials.

Seen from this perspective, an increase in health care expenditures which was the result of, say, a 50 percent increase in all prices of all health care, goods and services, which in turn raised all incomes in that sector by 50 percent, but which left resource flows into (principally people working in) the industry and commodity production from it unchanged, would *not* raise the cost of health care to Canadian society as a whole. No more other things—shoes or ships or sealingwax—would be given up to produce more health care. Of course, the *distribution* of the total social product would change, with a larger share going to health care workers or other resource suppliers, and a smaller going to everyone else. A variety of secondary effects might follow from that, as more people tried to enter health care jobs, governments raised taxes, borrowed, or cut expenditures to meet the new costs, private insurers raised premiums, or patients reacted to higher out-of-pocket costs. But in the first instance, if one assumes a time before any such reactions had occurred, what would be recorded as a 50 percent rise in "health costs" would be merely a transfer of wealth from one group of Canadians to another (with some foreign participation through corporations).

The economist's focus on real resources is, of course, paralleled by the health care analyst's interest in real outputs. The increase in "health costs" from the 50 percent price/income hike has no effect on the volume and mix of health care produced either. Unless one is prepared to speculate on a placebo effect from high-priced care, it follows that the increased expenditures will have no effects on anyone's health status. Again, of course, a variety of secondary effects (patients unable to pay increased prices, new suppliers attracted into the industry) could lead to changes in the pattern of the Q_i and N_j which did have health effects. But there is no automatic link between changes in health "costs" as currently measured, and health care. Accordingly, an "underfunding" argument, unless merely a statement about relative incomes, must focus on the flow of new resources into health care and resulting larger volumes of output.

That this is not merely an abstract or theoretical issue is demonstrated by Table 1-2, which assembles some data on real outputs of the different components of health care over the post-war period. Ideally, we would like consistent, long-term sector-specific price indices to deflate the figures in Table 1-1 to constant-dollar values. But with the available data, only rather imperfect indices can be developed, particularly for earlier years, and work in this area is still incomplete (Barer and Evans 1983). But the Table 1-2 data do indicate some sharp divergences between trends in health care "costs," and in service flows.

TABLE 1-2

Hospital Utilization and Wages; Physician Availability and Incomes, Canada, 1946-1982
(Bracketed figures are average annual percent growth since last figure.)

	Hospital Inpatient Days per 1000 pop.	Index of Hospital Services per Patient Day	Hospital Relative Wages Index	Physicians per 1000 Population	Physician Relative Incomes
1946	1334.7	48.8	n.a.	1.044	3.26*
1951	1418.9	53.4	63.1	1.023	3.14
	(1.23)	(1.82)		(−0.41)	(−0.93)
1956	1578.1	58.9	70.6	1.111	3.54
	(2.15)	(1.98)	(2.27)	(1.66)	(2.43)
1961	1639.5	69.2	85.2	1.167	3.94
	(0.77)	(3.28)	(3.83)	(0.99)	(2.16)
1966	1793.9	85.3	93.2	1.325	4.83
	(1.82)	(4.27)	(1.81)	(2.57)	(4.16)
1971	1896.6	100.0	100.0	1.517	5.57
	(1.12)	(3.23)	(1.42)	(2.74)	(2.89)
1976	1954.7	112.0	114.9	1.733	3.83
	(0.61)	(2.29)	(2.82)	(2.70)	(−7.22)
1977	1976.6	111.8	114.6	1.767	3.68
	(1.12)	(−0.18)	(−0.26)	(1.96)	(−3.92)
1978	1996.0	n.a.	n.a.	1.786	3.43
	(−0.98)			(1.08)	(−6.79)
1979	1986.9	117.6	112.4	1.805	3.43
	(−0.46)	(2.56)	(−0.96)	(1.06)	(0.00)
1980	1986.8	119.7	116.9	1.828	3.36
	(0.00)	(1.79)	(4.00)	(1.27)	(−2.04)
1981	1972.4	122.5	119.1	1.859	3.28
	(−0.72)	(2.34)	(1.88)	(1.70)	(−2.38)
1982	1957.6	123.0	123.7	1.912	n.a.
	(-0.75)	(0.41)	(3.86)	(2.85)	
	Average Annual Growth Rates				
46-56	1.69%	1.90%		0.62%	0.92%*
56-66	1.29%	3.77%	2.82%	1.78%	3.16%
66-76	0.86%	2.63%	2.12%	2.72%	−2.29%
76-82	0.02%	1.57%	1.24%	1.65%	−3.05%**

SOURCES: See Data Sources Appendix.

*1947 data
**1976-1981 only

NOTE: Hospital days are public general and allied special; the index of hospital services per patient day is expenditures deflated by an index of input prices; hospital relative wages are an index divided by an index of average weekly wages and salaries. Physician incomes are from *Taxation Statistics*, relative to average taxpayers, all taxable returns, and may be downward-biased after 1976; see Data Sources Appendix. Relative wage data prior to 1961 are particularly shaky, being unadjusted for changes in skill mix or hours of work, and should be treated as impressionistic only.

The rapid increase in hospital costs in the 1950s, for example, was associated with increasing utilization rates (patient days per thousand population) and intensity of servicing (principally increases in person-hours per patient day, but also more highly trained personnel, and other inputs). In the 1960s, utilization increased at a slower rate, intensity of servicing per day increased rapidly, and relative earnings of hospital workers increased at a more rapid rate. In the 1970s, utilization is almost static, intensity is growing very slowly, and relative earnings, after a burst early in the decade, are almost flat after 1976.

For physicians' services, the changes are even more dramatic. In the period 1947-1971, the income of the average physician rose from 3.26 times that of the general taxpayer to 5.57 times. To some extent this could result from increasing productivity, but an improvement in relative income status requires productivity gains *faster* than the general average, which, as noted, was itself quite rapid in that period. A large part of the increase in expenditure on physicians' services from 1946 to 1971 was, in fact, a price/income phenomenon, which did not increase the "opportunity cost" of medical care or have any effect on anyone's health status, but merely transferred wealth from Canadians generally to physicians.[5] The actual increase in physicians per capita, which might be expected (apart from variations in working hours or numbers of other associated personnel) to translate into increased medical care use, is relatively slow until the 1960s, and then becomes very rapid.

In the early 1970s, numbers of physicians and medical care utilization per capita continued to increase rapidly. The federal government's *Medical Care Annual Report* (1981) indicates that from fiscal year 1971-72 to 1978–79, the average annual increases in physicians per capita and utilization per capita were 2.8 percent and 4.6 percent, respectively. "Costs" stayed stable over that period, however, because service prices and physician incomes (adjusted for inflation) were falling. Annual rates of medical fee increase are estimated at 4.9 percent, compared with the Consumer Price Index increase of 8.3 percent. The 1.7 percent annual increase of utilization per physician still left revenues per physician falling in real terms, and falling even more sharply relative to other workers.

---

[5] Price indices for physicians' services based on list or reported fees rose more rapidly than the CPI over the period 1947–71, at 3.6 percent per year on average, compared with 3.0 percent for the CPI (Barer and Evans 1983). But such indices of list fees do not capture the increase in prices received due to improving collections ratios, which appears to have been substantial during the period of spread of private and public medical insurance. Deflation of physician incomes by listed fees leads to implausibly high "productivity" gains. Efforts to estimate changes in fees actually received over the period 1947-71 suggest that fees collected rose between one and two percent per year faster than list fees, averaging over the whole period.

Table 1-2, drawing on taxation data, shows the same process in a longer-term context. The rapid increase in relative incomes of physicians started well before Medicare and, indeed, was most pronounced in the early 1960s. And the very sharp reversal of the early 1970s had moderated, but not ended, by 1981.[6] The stability of physician expenditures as a share of GNP since 1971 thus masks an increase in their real resource cost, more skilled manpower employed, as well as an increase in the real volume of services supplied. In the previous two decades, by contrast, the increase in opportunity cost and service volumes is greatly overstated by the expenditure data.

FROM DATA TO EVALUATION: HOW MUCH IS ENOUGH?

Even if our health expenditure data were "perfectly" adjusted for price change, however (sidestepping some important ambiguities in *that* process), they would still fail to answer questions about underfunding or over-utilization, about the appropriateness of care patterns, or about technical efficiency versus waste. The fundamental problems of resource allocation remain: How much of what sorts of resources to allocate, to the production of which forms of health care, how, and for whom? A common response by health care practitioners is that services should be provided to meet the "needs" of people in the community, either as expressed by people themselves, or as interpreted by practitioners.

Economists, on the other hand, conceive of allocation questions in terms of a trade-off or balance between the values people attach to the production from resources in any particular use, and the opportunity cost of such production. The "right" allocation to health care depends both on the perceived payoff to more health care and on the values attached to the other outputs foregone—roads, steak dinners, sewage plants, housing, fighter planes, symphony orchestras—because resources which could have been used to produce these things are instead used to produce health care.[7] So long as a society's preferences, however defined, are such that additional health care of some sort is valued more than its cost in terms

---

[6] Though as noted in Table 1-2, the income data are somewhat suspect after the mid-1970s. Alternative estimates prepared by Health and Welfare Canada show physician relative incomes rising after 1977, and up sharply in 1981 and 1982.

[7] The time period is a critical feature of these implicit substitution processes. Obviously, one cannot instantaneously convert paediatricians to fighter pilots or first violinists, or vice-versa, and sewage plants do not make good hospitals. But over a longer time horizon, say a decade or more, training programs for different forms of skilled manpower can be expanded or contracted to change significantly the types of people available, and the construction industry can turn out hospitals, roads, factories, or runways with the same human and material resources.

of foregone opportunities, then the output of that form of care should be increased. If, on the other hand, it is believed that at the current level of provision a reduction of care would reduce well-being by less than the gains from redeployment of the released resources in some other area of production, then the health sector (or part of it) is too large. The "right" allocation is that at which the value of additional resources is perceived to be equal, whether used in health care production or in the next best opportunity.

This rather abstract approach can be given more concrete form by postulating a relationship between resource inputs and health status, as shown in Figure 1-3. Panel (a) of that figure depicts a relationship consistent with the "meeting the needs" approach to resource allocation. More resources devoted to health care by a particular society yield substantial increases in health status for some members of the community, up to the point that all "needs" are met, N^*, after which further resources used yield no health benefits to anyone.[8]

Need is thus a technical concept, a statement about the capacity of particular resource inputs to influence the health of a particular person or group. The technical expert can legitimately claim special expertise in judging the needs of others; and, indeed, given the special circumstances of physical disability and emotional stress which frequently attend the use of health care, the external observer may have an advantage quite apart from expertise. Surgeons do not, in general, operate on members of their families, just as lawyers are advised not to handle their own cases.

It is clear that if panel (a) of Figure 1-3 accurately represented the technical relationship between health care and health status, resource inputs beyond N^* would represent overuse. But it does not follow that N^* is optimal. Health status per se, at least on its narrow definition, is not the only object of human activity or source of satisfaction. In panel (a), equal resource inputs up to N^* yield equal gains in health status, but these may well represent declining (though always positive) increments in utility or well-being. The "law" of diminishing marginal utility postulates that the benefits that a consumer/patient derives from further increments of any valued good or service fall, as the total amount possessed/

---

[8] The definition of health status for individuals, and its aggregation across individuals, are both highly problematic, and the aggregation of resource inputs to a single measure also raises numerous difficulties. Moreover, health status is a trajectory through time, and a static representation implies some way of representing and adding up expected future states. Culyer (1978) provides a discussion of the conceptual problems involved, and an application. Despite severe problems in its operationalization, however, some such concept of a resources-health relationship underlies all health policy discussion. (Nor should economists be overly critical—who ever estimated a Walrasian general equilibrium system?)

FIGURE 1–3

Alternative Representations of the Relationship Between Community Health Status, *HS*, and the Quantity of Real Resources of Manpower, Capital, and Raw Materials, *R*, Devoted to Health Care Production

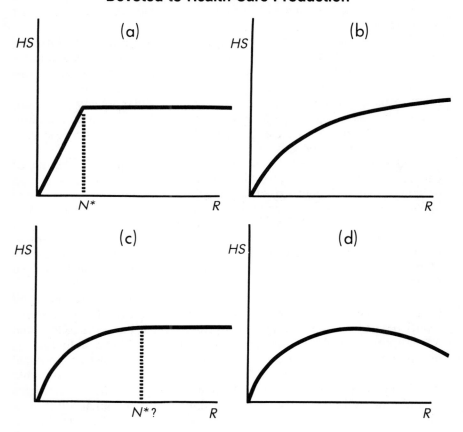

used rises. Moreover, as health care production expands, the drawing of successive increments of resources from other sectors causes them to shrink, and thus their marginal value (the opportunity cost of health care) to rise. The balancing of health status payoff and opportunity cost could occur before the health sector expanded to N^*. Some level of unmet need would then be optimal, in a broader sense.

As panel (a) is drawn, however, N^* may well be optimal. If the relation has a steep slope up to N^*—health care is highly efficacious until needs are met—and if health status is highly valued relative to other things until "perfect health" (or at least the limit of the capacity of health care to improve health) is reached, then the kink at N^* will ensure that the marginal value of health care exceeds its opportunity cost everywhere below N^*. The practitioner's focus on meeting needs is thus justified as economically efficient.

Panel (b), on the other hand, presents a more troublesome case. If the curve never flattens out, then "needs" can never be met. There is always something more which could be done. This need not imply an unbounded concept of health status; the curve could be asymptotic to a horizontal "perfect health" line. But if its slope is everywhere positive, then in a world of finite resources, unmet needs are inevitable. Every society will have to develop some institutional mechanism for deciding where and how to limit the resources devoted to health care. And this decision is *not* a technical judgement (Williams 1978). The "expert," the practitioner or researcher, may legitimately claim superior competence in identifying and describing the shape of the resource-health relationship. But the ultimate choice of where to stop is a collective and social one. The institutions evolved in different societies may give practitioners a special role in this decision process, but the decision itself cannot be based on technical considerations. Societies may also, through market mechanisms, give more or less weight to the choices of individual patients, but since the resources used are almost entirely collective resources, whether raised through public programs or private insurance, again the decision is ultimately a collective one.

Panels (c) and (d) represent additional possibilities for the resource-health relationship. In (c), "flat-of-the-curve medicine" (Enthoven 1980) is the collection of activities which have, in fact, no health payoff. Unlike panel (a), however, the flat-of-the-curve is not reached discontinuously at a well-defined "need" point. There is some point at which the slope of the curve goes to zero, but this may be very difficult to identify in practice. And the problem does not present itself to individual decision-makers, clinicians, or patients in the form of Figure 1–3, but rather as a very specific decision in an individual case. The pressures to "do something" may be intense, while information about expected payoffs may be imperfect or simply unavailable. Hence the possibility that the health industry in aggregate, or specific sub-components of it, may extend resource use well beyond the point at which interventions cease to be effective. Yet each participant may act, under imperfect information, with the best of intentions, and thus be highly resistant to the suggestion that the curve is flat in her vicinity. The aggregate curves of Figure 1–3 represent probabilistic abstractions in a world of uncertainty—health care is not an exact science.

In panel (d) is depicted the relationship described by Illich (1975): health care is hazardous to health. There is a range of output over which health care yields positive benefit; but past some point actual harm develops. It is important to stress this possibility because, for particular forms of diagnosis or therapy, it is well established that overuse leads to harm. More is most emphatically *not* better. Indiscriminate use of antibiotics, surgery on healthy organs, excessive diagnostic radiography, are obvious examples. In other areas—Caesarian section for example, or tonsillectomy—there is considerable expert concern that current levels of provision are in the downward-sloping range. Even screening can lead to interventions which endanger health. In general, for every particular form of health care, there is some point at which excess does harm. For some forms, in some places, there is evidence suggesting that point has been reached. Whether it is being approached on average or in aggregate is not clear.

Panels (c) and (d) enable us to represent overuse in health care, as well as economic, terms. Operation on the flat-of-the-curve, or *a fortiori* on the negative slope, is clearly medical overuse.[9] In panel (b), on the other hand, more is always better from a health standpoint and global over– or underuse can only be defined economically. (Particular forms of care, however, can be overprovided in health terms; in panel (b) this would imply production below the curve). Panel (a) represents the possibility of a happy coincidence of health and economic criteria which may hold in particular settings, but seems implausible in general.

In each panel the issue of technical efficiency is side-stepped by the assumption that a society's health system is operating on the curve, not below it. The curve represents the maximum health status attainable with a given resource commitment, under the constraints of present knowledge. It may of course shift, as knowledge changes. But it is always possible to be inefficient, and attain less than the maximum possible health status with given resources. Maintenance of efficient production is a problem logically separate from that of deciding how large the health sector should be, although both are "solved" by the particular set of institutions which a society establishes to operate its health care system. Moreover, one's judgements as to whether to expand or contract the resources available to health care may well depend on how efficiently one believes the system is using resources at present, or would use more.

Economic analysis tends to focus on questions of resource allocation,

---

[9] It is not *necessarily* economic overuse. Economists who treat health care as an argument in the utility function, or a valued object in and of itself, sometimes argue that "unnecessary" operations, *e.g.*, are justified if (informed) patients are willing to accept them, even if they confer no health benefit. This sounds very much like Münchausen's Syndrome again. By defining health status, not health care, as the relevant object of value, and assigning health care per se negative weight, we close off this rather peculiar argument and gain in realism.

rather than technical efficiency, on the ground that in the private sector, where production is carried on by for-profit firms, the incentive of profit maximization will ensure that costs of production are minimized and resources are not wasted. But most health care production, including as we shall see that in professional practices, is not carried on with the objective of profit maximization.[10] Accordingly, issues of technical efficiency and appropriate institutional design assume great importance in the economics of health care.

MODELLING THE HEALTH CARE UTILIZATION PROCESS

Despite the central importance of health status to the organization and delivery of health care, its investigation on a societal or system-wide basis receives remarkably little attention. *The Canadian Sickness Survey* of 1950–51 (Canada, Department of National Health and Welfare and Dominion Bureau of Statistics 1960) provided a baseline for the initial development of public hospital and medical insurance programs, but this initiative was not followed up. Almost thirty years later, the Canada Health Survey was developed for inclusion with the monthly Labour Force Survey, but what was originally intended as a continuing source of new information was converted, for budgetary reasons, to a one-time effort. We are left with a "snap-shot" at a single point in time. (Abelson et al. 1983; Canada, Health and Welfare Canada and Statistics Canada 1981). Thus Canadians now spend over $30 billion annually (1982) to improve their health, but make no systematic effort to measure the results.

Instead, the gap between health care and health status is bridged by inference and assumption, a process with significant parallels in economic methodology. To illustrate these parallels, we outline two alternative ways of conceptualizing or modelling the process of health care delivery, each with markedly different assumptions and policy implications, but very similar structure. These we label the Naive Medico-Technical and the Naive Economic models. In their naive forms they are poles apart, but more sophisticated forms converge towards each other.

The Naive Medico-Technical model begins with utilization, which may be either observed directly or inferred from capacity measures such as the number of physicians per capita. On this is superimposed assumptions about the roles and objectives of providers and users of care. Providers are assumed to supply care in response to "needs" in a technical sense, and their perceptions of "needs" are assumed to be as accurate as possible

---

[10] Self-employed practitioners may or may not maximize *incomes*, but incomes are not profits. Failure to observe this basic theoretical distinction has muddled many discussions of practitioner behaviour.

with present knowledge. They thus control the mix and volume of care supplied, subject only to "barriers to care," economic or informational, which may prevent consumer/patients from seeking needed care or complying with a recommended regimen, or to limits on the capacity of providers as a whole to meet all the "needs." The proper role of public policy, in this framework, is to remove economic barriers to care (by providing public or mandating private insurance), to ensure that sufficient personnel and facilities are trained and established, and perhaps to launch educational campaigns to encourage care-seeking and compliance.

The behavioural concept which an economist would call "supply," that is, the amount providers wish to provide at current costs of production and rates of reimbursement, is, in the Naive Medico-Technical model, equated with the technical concept of "need," and its dependence on prices is suppressed. Utilization is in turn determined by "supply," except insofar as it is constrained by barriers or shortages.

Demand, that is the amount consumer/patients themselves might wish to consume at current levels of prices and incomes, plays no important role in this process. Consumers may not demand as much care as they need, but this is presumably due to ignorance or inability to pay. Both should be corrected by appropriate policy. Consumers might also make initial visits which, in the judgement of providers, are unnecessary or "frivolous," although frivolity at the care initiation stage presumably depends on whether a particular patient could reasonably be expected to know that the contact was unnecessary. The model is a bit fuzzy on this point; if a patient thought a visit was necessary but should have known better, is that overuse? Presumably expert providers terminate unnecessary episodes of care after one visit, and attempt to educate patients as to when to seek care, so that this qualification is unlikely to be quantitatively significant. The implicit expectation that patients will rarely seek care they know to be unnecessary is consistent with our formulation above that health *status*, not health *care*, is valued by consumer/patients. On the important issues of how to ensure technical efficiency in health care production, or how the earnings of providers will or should be determined, the model is silent.

While over-utilization, utilization exceeding needs, could in principle occur in this model, it is ruled out in practice by the assumptions that providers' decisions control use and that providers respond only to need. Health planning, and particularly manpower planning, in the context of this model is constantly responding to shortages, and unmet needs, because whatever level of provision is occurring in any part of the planning jurisdiction is, by definition, no more than enough.

The Naive Medico-Technical model is easy to criticize on a number of grounds, being in particular vulnerable to the empirical observations that apparently equally competent practitioners show wide variations in their perceptions of need and in their responses and that collective perceptions of need rise steadily over time, so as to lie always at or just beyond current levels of provision. Moreover, these perceptions of need, as reflected in utilization patterns, often bear only a tenuous relation, if any, to the available scientific evidence as to the efficacy and effectiveness of particular interventions. But the Naive Economic model is equally vulnerable, differing only in identifying observed utilization with the behaviour of a different set of actors.

In the Naive Economic model, demand plays a central role. This is the amount and mix of care consumer/patients choose to accept, in response to their own preferences and incomes, and the costs to them of care. This behavioural construct is then identified, by assumption, with utilization. Informed consumers choose which forms of care to use, in what quantities. Of course, use may fall short of demand if supplies are constrained, but cannot exceed it. Nor will a shortage persist, if prices are flexible, since the quantity consumers demand depends on the prices they pay. If prices rise in response to a shortage, demand will fall, and balance is restored. Moreover supply, what providers wish to produce, is also assumed price-dependent. If prices rise, more will be offered for sale. Thus price plays the key role of equilibrating supply and demand, and so long as prices adjust smoothly, utilization will always be equal to both demand and supply. Need, on the other hand, drops out of this framework. Consumers' demands will presumably depend *inter alia* on their perceptions of their own needs. Insofar as external experts' judgements of needs correspond to consumers' judgements, they are thus embodied in demand; insofar as they differ, they are, by assumption, irrelevant.

The models could hardly be more different in appearance, yet, in fact, both share a common structure. Both start with an observed or observable statistical datum—utilization—and then assume its correspondence to a hypothesized behavioural concept—consumers' demands or providers' preferred supply patterns. In each case observed utilization can fall short of, but not exceed, the hypothetical concepts, and such shortfalls represent some form of institutional failure (barriers to care, or sticky prices). Both make specific assumptions about the processes of care provision and consumption—informed consumers or professional providers make the utilization decisions. And both have an implicit criterion for how care ought to be allocated—to meet technically determined needs, or to respond to the preferences of consumers as expressed in willingness to pay. Finally, neither model is particularly realistic.

The Medico-Technical model, however, dominated health care planning and policy making in Canada to the end of the 1960s, and still underlies much thinking on this subject. Scratch a health care provider to any depth, and she will usually turn out to conceive of health care delivery in some such terms. Yet as noted, "meeting all the needs" is not possible if the health status curve in Figure 1–3 does not flatten, nor desirable if it flattens very slowly. Nor does the empirical evidence support the hypothesized chain from unambiguous, externally determined needs, to supply, to use.

On the other hand, critiques of the organization of the health care industry have been launched for at least a generation on the basis of the Naive Economic model—usually calling for freer entry, more competition, more reliance on prices, and less on subsidies or insurance. The adoption of such a framework as a basis for analysis necessarily imposes the strong, though implicit, assumption that the extensive and detailed structure of public and self-regulation and control which governs health care in every developed society is all a terrible mistake, the result of a nefarious conspiracy by suppliers imposed on an ignorant and gullible public, which should be dismantled as soon as possible. Though all who use the unmodified free market economic model are in fact making this assumption (or are just intellectually inconsistent), few have had the courage to follow Friedman (1962) in declaring it openly.

These general critiques have had little impact in Canada (although rather more in the United States) because they are confronted with a perception among health care providers and general population alike that health care is somehow "different," that it is a commodity to which the normal rules of the marketplace do not apply. Or put another way, the patterns of resource allocation in health care which would result from reliance on private, arm's-length market-type institutions to control its production and distribution are demonstrably inferior to more regulated alternatives. Insofar as the Naive Economic model ignores the whole issue of "differentness," and begs the question of the commodity status of health care, analyses based on it have in turn been largely ignored— and probably deservedly so.

But the market model exercises a powerful attraction, not least because of the inherent weaknesses of the Medico-Technical approach. It is the standard taken for the "normal" organization of production, distribution, and exchange, and the predominant form in industrialized "mixed capitalist" economies, because under certain conditions market mechanisms for resource allocation do have powerful advantages. Moreover, if totally unregulated free markets are inappropriate institutions to organize all resource allocation in health care, it does not follow that market mechanisms of some form have no role to play. Nor can one assume that whatever system of regulated organization may have developed in a society is necessarily optimal. The arguments for licensure of physicians do not necessarily extend to pharmacists or veterinarians, nor does a case for some form of regulation necessarily imply the forms of licensure we observe. And the justifications for public insurance of hospital costs will not all survive transplantation to dental care or eyeglasses.

Thus it is of central importance to the study of the economics of health care to understand in what ways this commodity fails to meet the conditions under which private market institutions would govern its production and allocation satisfactorily. Analysis and policy can then be firmly based on a clear linkage between nature and sources of market failure and appropriate institutional response. And the question as to why unregulated markets "fail" in health care provision is another version of the question, Why is there a separate economics of health care at all?

An early response was to try to list the features of health care which distinguish it from the standard "commodity" of the economics textbooks (*e.g.*, Klarman 1965). These lists could be extensive: uncertainty of incidence of illness, and hence variability of "demand" for care; impact of the health or health care of one person on another via, *e.g.* contagion; prevalence of non-profit and non-profit-maximizing forms of organizations supplying care; barriers to entry in the form of licensure; extensive public regulation, both direct and delegated, of providers and consumers; a mix of consumption and investment services in health care; numerous and detailed job definitions with rigid barriers between jobs; large element of personal service; health care as a "need"; illness, and to some extent, care as assault on personal integrity, physical and emotional; high level of consumer ignorance about effects of care and capability of providers; mix of care and educational elements in much of provision; many consumers (children, elderly and infirm, severely injured) incapable of directing their own consumption; and so on.

An immediate response is that every one of these "peculiarities" is characteristic of some other commodities as well, to which the rebuttal is, yes but not all of them at once. But so what? The listing approach, however accurate and complete, can never tell us which peculiarities are critical, and why, and what their implications are for appropriate institutional design.

Arrow (1963) noted the important distinction between inherent and derivative characteristics, of features intrinsic to health care itself as distinct from particular institutional responses. Thus uncertainty of illness impact is inherent; but licensure or non-profit organization are derivative, social responses to other perceived peculiarities. This enables us to pare down the list considerably.

He also identified clearly the source of the difficulties created by consumer ignorance, noting that while ignorance about production technology is pervasive—how many people know how an electronic calculator is put together? — the critical issue is knowledge of what the product will do for the user.[11] The health care consumer is generally ignorant not only

---

[11] In general, the consumer with a utility function U defined over commodities X_i is assumed to know, at least as well as anyone else, the marginal utilities $\partial U/\partial X_i$ and hence to make informed consumption decisions. In the case of health care, since it is an input to health, $U[X_i, HS\,(HC)]$ implies that the consumer needs to know not only $\partial U/\partial HS$, but also the technical production function relation, dHS/dHC.

of how the commodity is produced, but of what it will do for her. The buyer of calculators, or commodities in general, is not. Moreover, knowledge is asymmetric; the provider is generally perceived, by all concerned, to have a substantially greater degree of knowledge than the user.

Arrow referred to both the unpredictability of illness and the lack of consumer information about appropriate use (and as part of this, provider quality) as "uncertainty," but the concepts are quite different. Uncertainty is now used to refer to unpredictability, by anyone, of future illness events: Will I break my leg skiing this winter? One may (or may not) know the probabilities in advance, but cannot know of the event. Asymmetry of information refers to the present situation—is my leg now broken, and what should I do about it? — and the professional provider is usually assumed to have much better information than I on this subject.

Culyer (1971) explored in more detail the issue of interpersonal effects, demonstrating that these go far beyond contagion. The concept of "need" implies not only a technical judgement about the impact of health care on health, but also an obligation on someone, or on society generally, to respond. Similarly, the identification of illness as an assault on integrity or of ill people as unable to make appropriate consumption responses, implies a special collective response to protect consumer/patients in situations in which what is at issue is not the satisfaction the consumer may derive from bundles of goods consumed, but possible radical modifications or dissolution of the consumer herself. Thus, the concept of external effects, or of interactions between one person's consumption pattern and another person's well-being, is much broader and deeper in health care than for most other commodities.

These three intrinsic characteristics, uncertainty of illness incidence, external effects in consumption, and asymmetry of information between provider and user form the fundamental triad from which all other listed characteristics can be derived, either as variants or as social responses to them. Licensure responds to asymmetry, public subsidy or supply to externalities, insurance to uncertainty. Such things as high degree of personal service or mix of consumption and investment elements are relevant only insofar as they reinforce asymmetry of information; if consumers are fully informed, then private markets handle such problems without difficulty. "Need" and "loss of personal integrity" as sources of market failure come through external effects and informational asymmetry respectively. They are the answer, at the most basic level, to the question, Why is health care different? or equivalently, Why do we see such extensive intervention in, and supersessions of, private markets in health care?

Each of these three characteristics, however, creates different problems and has different implications for institutional design; moreover, different types of health care share these characteristics to very different degrees. Accordingly, we now proceed in the next three chapters to a more detailed examination of each.

CHAPTER 2

RISK, UNCERTAINTY, AND THE LIMITS OF INSURABILITY

INSURANCE AND THE REIMBURSEMENT OF HEALTH CARE

Illness is unpredictable. Chronic conditions, or conditions which evolve through time, may have a more or less well-defined prognosis, and individuals of varying ages, circumstances, and pre-existing conditions may face very different probabilities of different states. But in general everyone's future health status is uncertain.

It follows that one's demand, or need, for health care is likewise uncertain; one cannot map out in advance an optimal pattern of health care use for the coming year as one might budget for food. And the costs associated with an unpredictable illness go well beyond the unexpected expenditures on care to which it may give rise—being sick is uncomfortable, disabling, frightening, and sometimes fatal. Uncertainty with respect to health care expenditure is only a component, and not necessarily the most significant, of the overall uncertainty associated with illness.[1] As polar cases, both catching a cold and sudden death are unexpected events which reduce welfare, but neither generates a need for health care (though an uninformed consumer may in the first case demand it).

The institutional response to uncertainty is the development of insurance mechanisms, whereby covered individuals make regular payments to some risk-pooling agency in return for guarantees of some form of reimbursement in the event of illness. This agency might be a public body or a private firm, the payments might be premiums or taxes, and the benefits might be indemnities (fixed cash payments) varying across illness events, reimbursement of all or part of actual health care expenditures, or direct provision (public or private) of services as needed.

In practice, however, the evolution of health insurance in Canada has

---

[1] The consumer's utility function may be extended thus: $U = U[X_i, HS (HC, E)]$ maximized subject to a budget constraint. Health status HS depends on health care HC and a random variable E indicating exogenous fluctuations in health (accident, infection, etc.). If E shifts so as to lower HS, U clearly falls, and HC may rise if it is "needed" (if $\partial HS/\partial HC$ increases), at the expense of other X_i. But the consumer's problem is the fluctuation in maximum U attainable with a given budget, due to the unpredictability of E, whether or not health care expenditure is increased.

been marked not only by increasing numbers of people and types of care insured, but also by a shift from the private to the public sector. The share of health spending funded through the public sector has expanded steadily over time, with the principal jumps being the introduction of universal public hospital insurance during the late fifties, and medical insurance in the late sixties. (Dates of adoption varied by province.) These public plans built on a substantial base of private health insurance, provided both by non-profit and by for-profit insurers, which had been developing since the late 1930s (Canada, Department of National Health and Welfare 1954; Shillington 1972). In addition, some provinces had partial public service or payment programs with a long history.

Table 2-1 assembles data from various sources illustrating the development of public and private insurance coverage of health care expenditures. Hospital funding has always relied heavily on various public grants and funding programs: in 1932, when private hospital insurance was virtually non-existent, public funding already covered over half of hospital costs. Economic recovery led to increased reliance on self-paying patients; by 1940 these accounted for about 70 percent of revenues. But over the next twenty years hospital expenditures were rapidly taken over, first by private insurance, and then by the public sector.

Medical care insurance developed later and grew more slowly; in the immediate post-war period such coverage was relatively rare. By 1960, over half the population had some form of medical insurance, but the degree of comprehensiveness was variable.

By 1975, as Table 2-1 shows, about 95 percent of all hospital and medical costs in Canada were funded through the universal public insurance programs. The public sector share of total health costs, through a combination of direct provision and partial insurance, had reached 75 percent. The remaining 25 percent was primarily out-of-pocket expenses for dentistry, drugs, and uninsured institutional services; private insurance (particularly for dental care) might amount to about 5 percent of total health expenditures.

Since 1975 the public share of hospital spending has declined somewhat, probably reflecting some combination of increased "deterrent" charges by provincial governments and growing preferred accommodation differentials. In addition there has been relatively rapid growth in dental and "homes for special care" (institutional care for the elderly) costs, for which public funding is relatively lower. Accordingly the public sector share of spending had slipped somewhat by 1981. But public programs for care for the elderly have grown significantly since 1975, and private insurance coverage of dental care has also expanded over this period. Total insurance coverage or public provision of health care is probably now close to 90 percent, prescribed and non-prescribed drugs and dental care being the principal remaining exclusions. Unpublished Health and

TABLE 2-1

Measures of the Extent of Health Insurance Coverage, Canada, 1945–1981

	1945	1950	1955	1960	1965	1970	1975	1978	1981
% of Spending in Public Sector[1]									
— All Health	n.a.	n.a.	n.a.	43	51	70.2	76.6	75.7	74.2
— Hospitals	n.a.	n.a.	n.a.	72	89	93.9	94.6	92.7	90.6
— Medical Care	n.a.	n.a.	n.a.	14	18	77.4	95.1	95.6	95.7
% of Population[2] with Medical Care Insurance									
— Private Comprehensive	n.a.	14.0	27.3	36.1	45.1	0.6	—	—	—
— Private Limited	n.a.	4.8	9.6	13.8	15.5	—	—	—	—
— Public	n.a.	n.a.	n.a.	7.9	12.1	96.3	100*	100*	100*
% of Hospital Expenses Paid by Third Parties[3]	37	71	86	98	100*	100*	100*	100*	100*
% of Population With Some Medical Coverage[3]	11	20	38	50	62	95	100*	100*	100*

SOURCES: 1. Canada, Health and Welfare Canada (1979, n.d. [1984]).
2. Canada, Department of National Health and Welfare (1954, 1963b); Fraser (1983); and unpublished data provided by Heath and Welfare Canada.
3. Irazuzta (1979).

*The public programs nominally provide universal coverage, but a small proportion of the population may lose coverage through failure to pay premiums in provinces where these are still required. (*De facto*, coverage is rarely impaired.) Of the hospital expenditure not covered by the public programs, some is privately insured (preferred accommodation differentials covered by Extended Health Benefit plans), some is the responsibility of other agencies (Workers' Compensation, federal government), some is accounted for by non-residents of Canada. There remain some out-of-pocket charges, including the so-called "deterrents" in certain provinces, but these are not a truly "private sector" expenditure, being rather an alternative form of public financing levy.

Welfare Canada reports based on Statistics Canada's Urban Family Expenditure Surveys showed out-of-pocket direct health expenditures per person of $90.62 in 1978, 12.6 percent of the $719.46 per capita total health spending.

Other countries have reached similar positions via different roads. In the U.K., public insurance of health care is combined with public provision through the National Health Service or other public authorities, which account for nearly 90 percent of all health spending, while a small private insurance sector covers well under 5 percent. European countries display a wide variety of institutional arrangements, but a similar predominance of payment through public and private insurance. Even the United States, which, in form and rhetoric at least, makes heavier reliance on private markets in health care than any other society, covered (in 1982) 88 percent of hospital costs, 63 percent of physician costs, and 72 percent of total health costs through insurance or direct public provision. Private insurance plays a much larger role, 34 percent of hospital and physician costs and 26 percent of the total, but out-of-pocket payment by patients for care purchased in "markets" is the exception, not the rule, even in the United States (Gibson *et al.* 1983).

The uncertainty of incidence of illness thus introduces two quite separate questions, How should insurance respond to illness, and Why *public* insurance? Opponents of public intervention in health care finance have pointed out, quite correctly, that the existence of (unwanted) uncertainty per se may be remedied by insurance, but that there are many forms of uncertainty other than illness, and the private insurance industry deals with them, apparently reasonably adequately.

We do not have public monopolies of fire, or life, or of the various forms of commercial insurance (although it should be noted that in Canada automobile insurance is in contention between the public and the private sectors). Thus to understand why Canada, and indeed every other society, has chosen to place the health insurance function in whole or in part in the public sector, we have to explore the reasons why, and to what extent, private markets might fail in the provision of health *insurance*, as well as in that of health *care*. Before doing so, however, it is necessary to analyse the relationship of insurance to the provision of health care.

MODELLING THE BENEFITS OF INSURANCE

For expositional purposes it is convenient, and common, to begin by assuming that any illness can be expressed in terms of a monetary equivalent, so that a dollar value can be assigned to the "loss" associated with a deterioration in health. This is not always true; the "health deterioration" of sudden death may not be compensable by any finite sum of money. However, it serves as a useful starting point.[2]

This monetary loss will not, of course, be equivalent to expenditure on health care. Only if care of a specific and well-defined amount were instantly and perfectly efficacious in relieving illness could one represent

---

[2] The derivation of this money equivalent requires the explicit or implicit recognition of health status in the utility function. If a consumer's utility is a function of commodities X_i and health status HS, to which one commodity HC is an argument, then for a given exogenous vector of prices we can express (maximized) utility as a function of income or wealth and health status, $U = U(W, HS)$. If $HS°$ represents perfect health, and HS' a specific illness, then we define L such that $U(W-L, HS°) \approx U(W, HS')$, and L is the monetary equivalent loss corresponding to the health deterioration from $H°$ to H'. The same point can be expressed equivalently in terms of (health) state dependent utility functions, $U(W-L) \approx V(W)$, where U is the utility from wealth when one is healthy, and V when one is ill with the specified condition.

the consequences of illness for well-being by the dollar cost of care. In general, the money equivalent loss L of an illness will exceed any consequent (change in) health spending by some amount which allows for pain and suffering, anxiety, lost wages and/or leisure, and a risk premium for uncertainty of outcome.

We consider a consumer/patient contemplating an uncertain future in which a specific illness may or may not occur.[3] Let the probability of occurrence be q, and of non-occurrence be $1 - q$, so that there are believed to be $100q$ chances out of 100 that the illness will occur. If it does, the consequences (expense plus misery) are judged by the consumer/patient as equivalent to a loss of L dollars. Taking all other things into account, her well-being during the future period in question will be related (positively) to her wealth, which is expected in the absence of illness to be $\$W$.[4] The occurrence of the illness is thus equivalent to a reduction in wealth to $W - L$.

If we express the dependence of the consumer's well-being or utility on wealth in the form $U(W)$, then we can describe well-being over the future period as $U(W)$ with a probability of $1 - q$, and the lower level of well-being $U(W - L)$ with probability q. If, *e.g.*, $q = 0.5$, there is a 50/50 chance of illness and, accordingly, a 50/50 chance of each of the levels of well-being associated with wealth W, and $W - L$. The expected level (in the sense of the mathematical expectation) is thus one-half, or 0.5, times $U(W)$ and 0.5 times $U(W - L)$. Representing this expected level as $E(U)$, we can write for the general case:

$$E(U) = (1 - q)U(W) + qU(W - L)$$

and since $U(W) > U(W - L)$, one is better off not to be ill, it follows that expected well-being is higher, for given W, as L or q are lower. The consumer is obviously better off if the future illness is less severe or less likely.

In Figure 2-1, panel (a), we represent an individual's well-being on the vertical axis, and wealth level on the horizontal. The relationship is drawn on the important assumption of diminishing marginal utility of wealth, *i.e.*, more wealth adds to well-being, but at a decreasing rate. The curve has positive, but declining slope. (People for whom this is not true, if they exist, do not buy insurance. They gamble a lot).[5]

An insurance contract offers a payment, say L, in the event that illness

---

[3] The analysis generalizes easily to a range of illness possibilities, but becomes more involved.

[4] Income is sometimes used here instead of wealth, but losses may exceed income in any one period. Moreover, the same income translates into very different levels of well-being for people at different wealth levels.

[5] Shoenmaker (1982) surveys the theoretical and empirical underpinnings of this analysis.

FIGURE 2-1

The Welfare Gain From Insurance Coverage—Diagrammatic Exposition

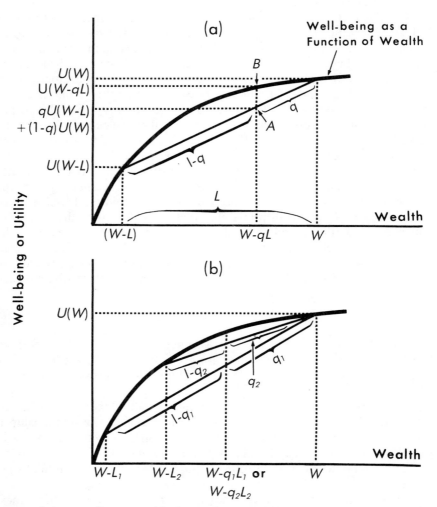

occurs, in return for a specified premium p which must be paid in either case. If the contract is actuarially fair, *i.e.*, the insurance agency makes no profit and is costless to run, then its payments over a large number of contracts will equal its receipts. The expected payment to any one insured will be the loss L multiplied by its probability of occurrence, or qL, and this will equal the premium p. Thus, the insured individual will face a wealth level $W - p$ or $W - qL$, and associated well-being $U(W - qL)$, with certainty, rather than the uncertainty of $U(W)$ or $U(W-L)$. She is certain to be out of pocket the amount p, but certain to be reimbursed the loss L, if it occurs.

As can be seen from Figure 2-1(a), however, while the expected *wealth* level is the same with or without insurance, $q(W-L) + (1-q)W = W - qL$, the expected level of well-being is greater with insurance. $U(W-qL) > qU(W-L) + (1-q)U(W)$, so long as $U(W)$ has the concave shape displayed, which for most people it appears to have. The gain in utility which results from complete insurance, coverage of the whole amount L, is the vertical distance from point A, the weighted average of the two possible uninsured utilities, to B, the certain utility when insured.

Panel (b) of Figure 2-1 represents two alternative losses, L_1 and L_2, such that $L_1 > L_2$ but the associated $q_1 < q_2$ and $q_1L_1 = q_2L_2$. These represent a low-probability event with large loss, and a higher-probability event with smaller loss, such as a rare but severe illness with hospitalization and extensive care, and a more common minor illness involving one or two physician visits and a prescription. The expected loss in each case, size of loss multiplied by probability of occurrence, is the same. An actuarially fair insurance contract would charge the same amount to cover either loss, a premium equal to the expected loss qL in each case, and sellers of such contracts would then break even, on average, over a large number of contracts.

As Figure 2-1(b) illustrates, however, the benefit to the buyer of insurance, in terms of the gain in well-being from exchanging a risky situation for a riskless one, is substantially greater in the case of the large, low-probability loss than in that of the small, more probable one. And by extension of Figure 2-1(b), we can see that in the limit, if q goes to either zero or one, or if L goes to zero, the gain from insurance becomes zero, which is as it should be. If there is no risk (whether or not there is loss) there can be no gain from insurance. If the event is certain, a fair premium will equal the loss.

As Figure 2-1 demonstrates, at this level of abstraction there is benefit from insuring fully all risky events, however small the loss or close to zero or one the probability. Moreover, if insurance is to compensate for the loss associated with illness, it must pay amounts substantially larger than the cost of health care associated with illness. Since it is obvious that patients are not in general indifferent between a state of health, with no health care, and a state of illness with all necessary care fully reimbursed, it follows that even full coverage of health care expenditures would fall well short of compensating for the loss L.[6]

---

[6] Optimal insurance for an expected-utility-maximizing consumer might not, however, be fully compensating. In Figure 2-1 we assume not only that $U(W, HS') \approx U(W-L,$

PRIVATE HEALTH INSURANCE IN PRACTICE:
DEVELOPMENT AND LIMITATIONS

In the real world, however, full compensation of all risks is neither possible nor optimal. In the first place, the size of loss L can only be known by the sufferer; it is not directly observable by an external observer. Indeed, the illness itself is rarely monitored by the insurer; while possible in principle, it is usually costly and impractical. Expenditures on health care are taken as a signal that the illness has occurred. But insurance which compensated for L would then create incentives for false signalling. Patients would be encouraged to use unnecessary care, *i.e.*, care having no or even harmful effects on health, in order to collect the compensation for putative suffering which did not in fact occur. Accordingly, health insurance typically covers only actual health care expenditures, rather than losses due to illness,[7] and in this sense all health insurance is partial and incomplete coverage.

This "moral hazard" problem, of changes in behaviour such that (real or apparent) losses rise in response to the existence of insurance, is a result of imperfect information about, or costly monitoring of, the true state of the world. An analogous problem would arise for the marketer of fire insurance if it were impossible to know how much damage a fire has done, or even if it has occurred. The insurer might then pay claims for construction services, relying on the contractor's statement that fire damage did in fact occur. The incentive problem is obvious.

Secondly, the actual process of providing insurance coverage is itself costly. Insurance agencies need staff, equipment, and buildings in order to set rates, write contracts, and adjudicate and pay claims. Competitive private companies must also allow for marketing expenses, and if for-profit, must, on average, earn a profit. Thus "actuarially fair" insurance contracts cannot exist. Premiums (or their equivalent in taxes or other payments) collected must exceed claims paid by some load factor large enough to meet the costs of the insurance function itself.

Consequently, insurance per se must add to the cost of the phenomenon being insured. The size of the load factor will vary, however, depending

---

$HS°$) (see note 2, *supra*) but also that $\partial U/\partial W$ at (W, HS') is equal to $\partial U/\partial W$ at $(W - L, HS°)$, which latter is (given diminishing marginal utility of wealth) greater than $\partial U/\partial W$ at $(W, HS°)$. This assumption, though common, is nonetheless somewhat suspect, and the expected-utility-maximizing consumer, trying to allocate her wealth so as to equalize across states the ratio of expected utility of wealth to its "price", might choose to over– or under-compensate L. But this consideration raises issues well beyond the present discussion; Dionne (1982) and Evans (1983) provide more detail.

[7]   Disability insurance goes farther, to cover part of lost income, in situations where the loss is significant enough to justify the necessary monitoring costs.

on how the insurance function is organized and marketed. It may run from under 5 percent of premiums for programs on the Canadian model, to 100 percent or more in the case of heavily marketed indemnity plans with very limited benefits. These mark-ups must be added to the actual cost of care for the insured group as a whole.

Later we shall see that the cost of health care for the insured group, both prices paid for care and amounts used, will itself vary, depending on the structure of the insurance system. The much higher cost of health care in the United States compared with Canada can be traced primarily to differences in their respective insurance systems. The overall relationship between health care costs and insurance coverage is rather complex. But an individual or small group contemplating buying health care insurance, and believing (rightly or wrongly) that the decision will not affect either prices of care or their own utilization rates, must trade off the proportion of the premium which is load factor, cost of insurance per se, against the gain in well-being from reduced uncertainty, as displayed in Figure 2-1. For small gains and/or large load factors, insurance is not worth buying.

In this trade-off, it will obviously be more advantageous to insure large and unlikely losses, because for a given premium, the gains in well-being are greater and (since few claims are processed) load factors will be smaller. Thus health insurance began historically with hospital care. Apart from public programs for the indigent or other special groups, private hospital insurance was introduced in Canada in the 1930s and spread rapidly during the 1940s and 1950s. A universal public program was first introduced in Saskatchewan in 1946, but most provinces waited until after the federal cost-sharing legislation of 1957. By 1961, every province provided universal public hospital insurance.

Medical care followed the same sequence, but somewhat later. Coverage for in-hospital surgical services, again the larger, less frequent claims, had the most rapid initial growth, but by 1960 medical and surgical coverage both reached about half the population. In 1962, Saskatchewan introduced universal public coverage of all medical expenses. By 1971, following the federal cost-sharing legislation of 1966, all provinces had universal public medical care insurance (Canada, Royal Commission on Health Services (Hall Commission) 1964, ch. 10; Le Clair, 1975).

It is important to note, however, that by the late 1950s private insurance companies were offering "major medical" policies whose market was growing very rapidly, from 228,700 persons covered in 1955, to 1,998,238 in 1961 (Canada, Department of National Health and Welfare 1963*b*). These plans reimbursed only expenditures per time period above a ceiling level or deductible. Small losses were thus not covered, unless associated in time with some larger loss. On pure insurance principles, major medical or high deductible policies appear to be a superior way of purchasing protection from significant risks without the cost of processing large numbers of small claims. Moreover their relatively rapid growth in the 1950s suggested that they represented what consumers really wanted to buy.

Yet the Hall Commission, after reviewing the question of universal "first dollar" coverage of all medical claims versus "high deductible" coverage of expenses above some ceiling, and despite energetic advocacy of the latter by the private insurance industry and representatives of organized medicine, recommended full, first-dollar, universal coverage. Further, the Commission recommended public administration of insurance by a single agency in each province, rather than a division of the market between a number of private plans with public programs for those excluded from private coverage. There were good reasons for this decision, but they are not reasons based on insurance principles. If the only purpose to be served by a health insurance system, public or private, were optimal risk-bearing (and if health care expenditures were the only losses associated with illness), then the analysis thus far suggests that the major medical advocates were right. The continued advocacy of this form of health insurance by analysts in the United States reflects the same point.

But the argument for privately marketed, high deductible insurance is seriously incomplete. As pointed out in chapter 1, uncertainty of illness incidence is only one of a number of sources of market failure, intrinsic and institutionally induced, in health care services. The argument for high deductible coverage ignores these further complications and assumes, implicitly or explicitly, that health care is a "normal" commodity whose production and distribution not only can be, but *is* governed by conventional private markets. When proper account is taken of the other forms of market failure, the argument from insurance principles loses its force, as we shall see below, and the Hall Commission conclusion (and present Canadian policy) are supported (Evans 1983).

The evolution of dental and pharmaceutical insurance in Canada contrasts with hospital and medical, reflecting the point illustrated in Figure 2-1. Dental expenses tend to be predictable and controllable, more in the nature of maintenance costs than unexpected events. While they may be high in any one year, this is usually the result of accumulated need. Moreover, while often uncomfortably large, dental expenses are not ruinous in the way hospital and medical care can be. And very expensive dental work is generally to a significant degree cosmetic, not a response to a life-threatening or disabling condition. Expenditures for prescription drugs are likewise common and small, while in-hospital drug use is already covered by hospital insurance. Extensive use of prescription drugs on an ambulatory basis is generally confined to a well-identified group of the chronically ill. Such a group may deserve subsidy, but they are not "at risk"—their condition is known.

Thus, the benefits of dental and drug insurance are relatively small, and private coverage has been relatively slow to develop (Evans and Williamson 1978). Traditionally, dentistry has been described as "uninsurable," reflecting its association with regular, small, predictable, and controllable "losses." Public programs have been established at the provincial level to cover particular groups, but these are more subsidy than risk-spreading programs.

The rapid spread of private dental insurance in the 1970s, on the other hand, would seem to belie its "uninsurability." But there are alternative explanations. One, heavily emphasized in the United States, is that the income tax system, which allows employer-paid health insurance premiums for employees as an expense deductible from the employer's taxable income, but does not tax them in the hands of the employee, encourages excessive insurance purchase (Mitchell and Vogel 1973). The argument applies to all health insurance in the United States; in Canada hospital and medical insurance premiums (where they exist) are, if employer-paid, taxable in the hands of the employee. In November 1981, employer-paid private health insurance premiums in Canada were also made taxable to the employee, and insurers expressed concern for their markets, but this provision was reversed in October 1982. A critical "experiment" on tax effects was thus lost.

Alternatively, the dynamics of collective bargaining may be such as to encourage the spread of insurance, even though its benefits to the "representative employee" are minimal or non-existent. The bargaining process does not always model the behaviour of a fully informed rational fringe-benefit purchaser: it reflects political as well as economic motives. And individual buyers may be purchasing, through insurance, budgeting services and relief from uncomfortable consumption decisions. They do not want the anxiety of balancing prices and benefits at point of service (Evans and Williamson 1978; Conrad and Marmor 1980). Furthermore, there is evidence that even individual purchases of insurance in an open market are none too rational (Eisner and Strotz 1961).

SOURCES OF "FAILURE" IN PRIVATE INSURANCE MARKETS

The historical development of health insurance, with full coverage, first of hospital care, then of medical, and lagging coverage of dental care and pharmaceuticals is thus readily explicable in terms of differential trade-offs between benefits from pure risk-reduction, and load factor costs. What is *not* explained, as emphasized, is why Canadian coverage is universal, first-dollar, and public, rather than voluntary (universal in practice implies compulsory), high deductible, and private.

The sources of failure in private insurance markets, to which public insurance is a response, can be grouped under four heads:

   (i) economies of scale,
  (ii) insufficient information for rate-making,
 (iii) adverse selection,
 (iv) moral hazard.

Of these, the latter two have been the more intensively studied by economists, and seem to have the greatest theoretical interest.

(i) Economies of Scale

As noted above, the load factor component of premiums, the cost of operating the insurance program itself, varies greatly across different programs. It is very low in the Canadian public system, while in certain private for-profit plans the load factor may significantly exceed the actual claims paid. Overall, prepayment and administration costs represent 1.5 percent of health care costs in Canada, and 2.5 percent of the hospital and medical care costs which form most of the insurance load (Canada, Health and Welfare Canada 1979). Corresponding American proportions are 5.2 percent and 9.0 percent, but these include public Medicare and Medicaid programs, as well as self-payment. Private sector prepayment and administration costs are 13.4 percent of total private sector health care reimbursement (net of out-of-pocket and public sector payment), and 19.1 percent of private hospital and medical care reimbursement (Gibson *et al.* 1983). Load factors for private insurance plans in Ontario are in the 10 - 20 percent range (Ontario, Ministry of Treasury and Economics 1981).

These discrepancies are significant: an increase in Canadian load factors from 1.5 percent to 5 percent would raise health costs by over a billion dollars in 1982. Private sector load factors, based on American or Canadian experience, would imply extra costs of several billions. But the explanation of such discrepancies involves a number of factors: they cannot be interpreted as simply differences in efficiency, or profit versus non-profit.

One source of difference is that the insurance function is subject to inherent economies of scale. While some costs — claims payment, contract administration—depend on the volume of business done, others, such as information assembly and rate-setting, are the same regardless of the number of people insured. In general load factors will be lower for large insurers than for small. But this creates a classic public utility problem. If a large number of private insurers share a market, so as to maintain the discipline of competition to restrain costs and profits, the technical costs of doing business will be higher than necessary for each. But if a small number of private firms (or one) dominate (monopolize) the market, monopolistic exploitation is to be expected. In a market of 200 million people, like the United States, there may be room for numerous competitors of efficient scale, but in a Canadian province, the trade-off between efficiency and competition would be severe. A response to this, as to the similar problem of electricity generation, is public takeover.

Such a public utility approach creates its own problems of monitoring the public agency and holding it accountable to the public; these must be compared with those of scrutinizing private monopolies or oligopolies. But it has two additional advantages. First, multiplicity of carriers generates hidden diseconomies in the form of compliance costs for providers—the administrative and clerical problems of dealing with dozens or hundreds of different insurers—which add an indeterminate but allegedly significant amount to the costs of care itself. Part of reported hospital and medical care costs in the United States are indirect insurance costs; thus the United States-Canada discrepancy in insurance costs is even larger than reported. Second, a substantial part of private administrative costs are marketing expenses and agents' commissions, generated in the process of extending and competing for markets. These costs, too, are eliminated by the public universal system. "Premium collections" are piggybacked onto general tax collections; claims payments and data handling are centralized, and costs are much lower.[8]

Economies of scale in insurance provision are not only a source of additional costs in a competitive environment, they may lead also to "failure" of private insurance markets. A consumer might wish to buy insurance if it were available at a premium reflecting risk status (the actuarially fair premium) plus a load factor corresponding to technically efficient insurance administration. But if the only contracts available embody load factors inflated by the costs of inefficient small-scale operation and marketing expense, or supernormal profit from monopoly power, such a buyer might quite rationally choose not to buy private insurance, and yet to vote for a universal public program.

---

[8] There is a question as to whether the "scale economies" may not mask a loss to consumers from the reduced range of contracts available; the higher cost private system also provides a richer menu of choices of premiums and coverage. This issue cannot be dealt with adequately until after the discussion of adverse selection and moral hazard, below.

(ii) Insufficient Information for Rate-Making

The second source of private market failure, insufficient information for rate-making, arises in the case of health problems with a long time-horizon, such as occupational illnesses. In principle, it would be quite possible for employers or employees to purchase private insurance coverage which remained in force, at least for certain conditions, after the employee left or retired. Thus, the future health consequences of exposure to present hazardous conditions or substances would be insured by current premiums. In practice, the difficulty of determining risks and assigning responsibilities for future illness states is such that these private contracts are not offered. Unless redress can be gained through the courts, a dubious and costly process, the worker or the state must bear these risks. If the risks of such future health costs are to be pooled at all, then, they are pooled through public programs. In a universal public program this happens automatically; in a private system it may occur through a public program for the elderly, or through some form of categorical assistance.

(iii) Adverse Selection

Market failure due to adverse selection is also a problem of imperfect information, arising from asymmetry of information between buyer and seller of insurance. The buyer of insurance may have better information about her risk status than the seller. In the extreme, if sellers were unable to discriminate among buyers at all, they might offer a single type of contract whose premium equalled the expected per capita loss averaged over the community as a whole, say, qL. But if the n potential buyers are distributed along a continuum of expected loss, such that:

$$q_1 L_1 < q_2 L_2 < \ldots < q_n L_n$$

where L_1 is the loss contemplated by the ith potential buyer, and q_1 is the (buyer specific) probability of its occurrence, then all low-risk buyers, at the left end, are being overcharged, paying more than an actuarially fair premium (plus appropriate load factor). They are subsidizing high-risk buyers toward the right end, who pay less than their expected loss.

The practice of charging everyone in the community the same premium is known as "community rating," and was common among the early not-for-profit plans in Canada, as well as Blue Cross and Blue Shield in the United States. It has the effect of redistributing wealth from low– to high-risk individuals *ex ante*. An "ideal" insurance program, which charged each buyer a premium equal to her own risk status $q_i L_i$, would still redistribute *ex post* to those who actually experienced the losses L_i from those who did not—all insurance redistributes after the fact. But "ideal" insurance does not redistribute *ex ante*; before the future is known it leaves each buyer's expected wealth unaffected (except for load factors) and merely relieves her of uncertainty. Community rating embodies an *ex ante* expected transfer of $q_iL_i - qL$ to each buyer, which will be positive or negative, depending on whether the individual's risk is above or below average. Whether or not such redistribution is socially desirable on other grounds, it is clearly unrelated to optimal risk-bearing.[9]

If buyers do not know their own risk status either, then community rating can persist. But if they do know it, either perfectly or to a sufficiently close approximation, then low-risk buyers at the left-hand end may conclude that the subsidy they are paying to high-risk buyers more than outweighs the benefits they gain from risk-pooling. If they do, and drop out of the market (self-insuring), then the insurer will find that average losses for the remaining insured group exceed average losses for the community as a whole. She faces adverse selection by buyers. Premiums will have to rise above qL. Depending on the pattern of the q_iL_i, and the shape of buyers' marginal utility of wealth curves, this can trigger further exits, until eventually the whole market disappears.

In practice, of course, adverse selection does not extinguish private insurance. It does, however, lead to the erosion of community rating, and to a level of coverage which falls well short of universality and comprehensiveness. Private insurance markets tend to evolve towards experience-rated group coverage, and to "major medical"—high deductible—and/or patient cost-sharing policies for individuals or groups.

The advantages of selling coverage to employee groups, conditional upon all or most of the group accepting coverage, are several. Administration costs are lower. The working population are generally healthier than the non-working. But most importantly, individuals cannot select into or out of coverage on the basis of their perceived risk status—unless they are prepared to change jobs. So the insurer need not fear that she will be covering only the bad risks.

Furthermore, group experience can be monitored over time, and premium rates adjusted to that experience and to the group characteristics associated with it. But this in turn encourages competition by insurers to identify and "cream off" low-risk groups, offering lower premiums, with the result that coverage for high-risk groups becomes more expensive. Individuals not in employee groups, who are likely to be less healthy on average anyway, and of whom the less healthy are most likely to want to buy coverage, may be priced out of the market entirely.

---

[9] A tax-financed system will also transfer from high-income to low-income people within each risk category, as well as from low-risk to high-risk people within each income category. If well-being depends on income *and* risk status, such a two-indicator redistribution system may have much to commend it. But it cannot be justified on risk-pooling grounds per se; see chapter 3.

Moreover, insurers will offer less complete coverage, in order to induce buyers to self-select into groups with differing risk status. Cost-sharing by patients, in the form of deductibles and/or coinsurance, are characteristic of the private, for-profit plans. Such features can be explained on the basis of pure insurance principles; the undesirability, in a world of positive load factors, of insuring small and/or frequent claims. But such contracts also serve to induce self-selection, as it can be shown theoretically that low-risk buyers will be more likely to purchase contracts with deductibles and coinsurance, whereas high-risk buyers will prefer more complete coverage. Accordingly, lower premia can be offered for less comprehensive contracts, not only because less is covered, but also because buyers of such contracts will, on average, be a lower-risk group.[10]

One cannot, therefore, infer preferences from purchases. A low-risk buyer or group might prefer full first-dollar coverage, *if* she could buy it at an actuarially fair premium (plus appropriate load). But if premiums for all such contracts are inflated to cover the claims of high-risk individuals, she may, as a second-best, choose a partial-coverage policy with out-of-pocket charges large enough to screen out high-risk buyers. Indeed, a low-risk buyer might be willing to buy full coverage at the community average rate, *i.e.*, one based on all low– as well as high-risk people. But under competition and adverse selection, that cannot be offered by private firms.

Competitive marketing of private insurance thus leads to a wide range of different rates, offered to groups on the basis of their own estimated expected loss. This rate differentiation is not in any sense a market "failure," rather it represents a reversal of the *ex ante* wealth redistribution from low to high risks which occurs under community rating. That reversal is costly in terms of information assembly, rate-making, and marketing. Whether or not one regards the resources as well spent depends on ones' distributional priorities, and is not a risk-pooling issue.

As identifiable good risks are creamed off, however, some of the remaining buyers will be priced out of the market. Of these, some will be simply unable to pay an actuarially fair premium because their expected risk is too large for their resources: these do not represent any failure of insurance markets per se. Their plight may be a social problem on other grounds, to be discussed in chapter 3 below, but their inability to buy insurance reflects an inability to afford the underlying (expected) care use and has nothing to do with uncertainty of incidence. They cannot afford Mercedes-Benz's either, but that is no failure of automobile markets.

---

[10] No equilibrium contract structure may exist in such markets, however; and if it does, it will not in general be Pareto-optimal. The theoretical analysis is developed from Akerlof (1970) by Rothschild and Stiglitz (1976) and Wilson (1977).

The market does fail, however, with respect to lower risk individuals who *are* able and willing to pay a premium appropriate to their risk status, but who cannot communicate that status to an insurer. Lost amid the non-group pool, which includes the chronically ill and the elderly, they can buy coverage only at a premium price well above their own expected losses, if at all. (Private insurers may simply withdraw from the individual market, to avoid the administrative and political problems of the high-risk group as a whole[11]). The position of such individuals is analogous to that of low-risk buyers who choose partial over full coverage as a second-best policy which screens out high-risk buyers. In both cases, buyers and sellers of insurance would be willing to enter into mutually advantageous full-coverage contracts, but incomplete and asymmetric information, leading to adverse selection, makes it impossible to offer such contracts without drawing in high-risk buyers who cannot be identified in advance.

Such failure of private markets raises the possibility that compulsory public insurance could extend risk pooling in a welfare-improving way, if private individuals would prefer to buy comprehensive coverage but private markets cannot offer it at a fair price. And, in fact, one of the principal arguments used by advocates of a public program was the observation that the growth of private coverage in Canada seemed to have stopped well short of 100 percent of the population, and was in the late 1950s beginning to shift towards partial and away from full, first-dollar coverage. The Hall Commission concluded that the private voluntary insurance market was incapable of extending coverage to the whole population and, in particular, tended to exclude the poorest and least healthy groups in the population. On the assumption that universal and complete coverage was an appropriate objective, the Commission recommended a universal public plan. In the United States, the same observation about inherent limitations on the coverage of private insurance led to the creation of partial public insurance programs—for the aged (Medicare), the poor (Medicaid), and for specific illnesses. While such partial or backstop programs supplement the private market significantly, they are apparently incapable of covering the whole population or of covering against all costs. About 10 percent of the United States population still has no health insurance coverage; out-of-pocket payments are about one-third of medical and 10 percent of hospital costs: and "catastrophic" expenses still strike some families who have limited or no coverage (Aday *et al.* 1980; Birnbaum *et al.* 1977). If health insurance for everyone is an appropriate

---

[11] "Of the eleven largest medical-care schemes under the sponsorship of medical groups, nine follow the same practice that is in effect in Windsor. Individual subscribers are not accepted (Associated Medical Services is one of the exceptions and that explains its higher overhead)." (Katz 1952).

social objective, then contrasting American and Canadian experiences suggest that partial public programs to supplement private markets are not an effective substitute for a universal public program.

Considerations of optimal risk pooling, however, do not necessarily imply universal first-dollar coverage as a social objective. Its advocates viewed such coverage as a way of promoting greater use of "needed" health care, and of redistributing wealth *ex ante* from those of lower to those of higher health risk status, a transfer which in general was from high to low income as well. A significant part of the population uninsured by the private sector were simply too poor to afford fair coverage. If their consequent inability to purchase health care was viewed as a social problem, and it was, that view had to be based on considerations other than incompleteness in risk-bearing markets.

Market failure due to adverse selection justifies public intervention only insofar as the uninsured or incompletely insured are willing and able to pay for additional actuarially fair coverage, but unable to buy it. We do not know how large a proportion of those excluded from or limited in private coverage in Canada prior to the public hospital and medical plans, or in the United States, then and now, fell into this category. But adverse selection considerations and current United States experience (Aday *et al*. 1980) suggest that such a group existed. And the converse implication of adverse selection is perhaps of greater importance. As noted above, the fact that people or groups buy limited (or no) private coverage does *not* indicate that they prefer this to full coverage at appropriate premium rates. Buying such partial private coverage but voting for full public coverage may be perfectly rational.

(iv) Moral Hazard

The last source of market failure in markets for private health insurance has received the most attention from economists. Moral hazard refers to a tendency for the existence of insurance coverage of any form to raise the expected losses insured against, as a result of either or both of greater loss or increased probability of occurrence. Since health insurance compensates, not for loss of health status, but for expenditure on health care services, the moral hazard problem in this context refers to a tendency for such expenditures to be larger *ceteris paribus* if a given individual or group is insured.[12] A seller of insurance contracts would thus have to

---

[12] It was pointed out above that insurance compensates for expenditures on health care, not for all losses due to illness, because of the difficulty of monitoring such losses and the incentives for false signalling. Moral hazard in the context of health care use arises from the same problem of imperfect information about actual health status. If illness events and consequent health care "needs" were easily identified, moral hazard would not arise, because insurance payments could be based on the event, not the cost of care.

set the premium above the expected loss qL for the uninsured individual or group by an amount large enough to cover this increase in loss (plus appropriate load factor), and the insurance buyer's wealth after premium payment, $W - p$, will be less than his expected wealth if uninsured, $W - qL$.

Moral hazard is quite distinct from adverse selection, although both may have similar implications for a private seller of insurance contracts who has a small share of the market. Moral hazard arises because the size of loss varies with coverage—someone's behaviour changes—and over the society as a whole total losses are increased by insurance coverage. It can occur in an insured group, all of the same risk status. Adverse selection, however, arises because people of different risk status are more or less likely to buy insurance. Over the society as a whole, adverse selection will lead to expected losses being redistributed by insurance, but total losses will not be increased.

Moral hazard may lead to market failure if potential insurance buyers predict that the rise in expected losses due to insurance coverage will more than offset the gains from insurance. If it were possible to purchase coverage *without* a change in losses, they would choose to do so, but such contracts are unavailable. One might hypothesize, for example, that dental insurance will lead dentists to raise their prices and/or patients to utilize more dental care, such that the necessary premium would substantially exceed one's current expected expenditures. Since the risk associated with dental care use is relatively small, moral hazard effects might make purchase of coverage on such terms economically irrational.[13]

THE "WELFARE BURDEN" OF HEALTH INSURANCE

The existence of moral hazard, the appropriate response by the private insurance market, and the possibility of its amelioration by public intervention in private insurance markets, all depend critically on how the "market" for health care is believed to function. Many economic analyses of this question impose, either explicitly or implicitly, the assumption that health care is a "normal" commodity, supplied by competitive profit-maximizing firms and purchased by informed buyers whose demand is a well-defined function of price, and which just happens to be insured. If one thus assumes away the intrinsic peculiarities of health care as a commodity, as well as the extensive institutional structure, other than insurance, which modifies or supplants market institutions in organizing the production and distribution of health care, then "moral hazard" becomes identifiable with elasticity of demand. Insurance coverage which reimburses health care expenditures lowers the effective price of care to consumers, and they respond to this by increasing their consumption.

---

[13] Though it might still occur, for several other reasons noted above.

Depending on conditions on the supply side of the health care "market-place," this increase in demand may drive up prices as well, but the critical behavioural response to insurance is assumed to be that of buyers. Suppliers of care play a purely passive role, responding to the market.

The result is the so-called "welfare burden" of health insurance (Pauly 1969; Feldstein 1973), illustrated in Figure 2-2. In Panel (a) of Figure 2-2, health care is assumed to be produced by a perfectly competitive, profit-maximizing, constant cost industry, supplying care at a price equal to its (long-run) marginal cost. This price accurately reflects the resource cost of an additional unit of care, in terms of the foregone opportunities, the "other things" which could have been produced with those resources, and is assumed for simplicity to be the same at each health care output level. Consumer/patients are assumed to have a well-defined demand for health care, derived from some process of utility maximization under budget constraint, such that they choose how much care to purchase and use at each price level. The demand curve *DD* represents the amount *Q* they will choose to buy at any given price *P*. Being fully (or at least adequately) informed, they make this choice on the basis of their own preferences and income/wealth constraints, and relative prices, but *not* professional advice.[14]

In Figure 2-2a, *P°* and *Q°* represent the market equilibrium price and quantity of health care, pre-insurance. At this level of output, each unit of health care bought/utilized is valued by buyers as worth more than (or no less than) its resource cost. The vertical distance to the demand curve at any level of output *Q* can be interpreted as the value, in terms of willingness-to-pay, placed on the *Q*th unit of health care by the consumer who values it most highly. If one thinks of units of care as being produced and offered sequentially to users, the first unit(s) offered are highly valued, while successive additional units are assumed to be of less and less value. The last unit bought, at any given price, is valued at that price; additional units, being valued less, are not bought. And since buyers are informed, their judgements of the value of care are assumed to define the appropriate level of care provision (the consumer sovereignty assumption).[15]

---

[14] Professional advice can be admitted if the professional is a perfect agent of the buyer (see chapter 4), but apart from the unrealism of this Hippocratic assumption, it completely undercuts the perfectly competitive profit-maximizing supply side, or indeed any other model of supply based on self-regarding transactors. The suppliers would have to be Lange-Lerner bureaucrats with rather complex instructions!

[15] Of course, the distribution of wealth in the society will affect the shape of the demand curve, as well as who gets what. All positive welfare economics depends on a prior judgement about the social acceptability of the income/wealth distribution. Furthermore, the interpretation of the demand curve as representing the marginal utility of care at each consumption level requires certain very specific restrictions on the form of the consumer's utility function.

FIGURE 2-2

The "Welfare Burden" and Wealth Transfer Effects of Health Insurance

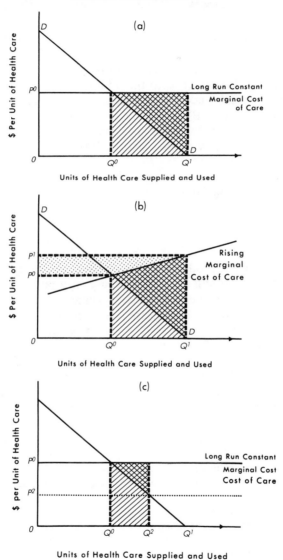

If, on the other hand, an insurance program (public or private) were brought in which reimbursed all costs of care, then according to the demand curve in 2-2a, utilization would increase to Q'—the point of utilization desired by consumers at zero prices.[16] At Q', the marginal or last unit of care bought/used is valued by consumers at very close to zero, but the resource cost, the foregone opportunities for other production, represented by that last unit, is still $P°$. Thus, resources worth $P°$ are converted to health care worth (almost) nothing—a clear misallocation and loss of welfare.

If we divide the distance between $Q°$ and Q' into incremental units of care, the demand curve implies that some user values the $Q°+1$ unit at almost $P°$. But the $Q°+2$ unit is worth less, and so on, down to the Q' unit. The total value attached to the additional output after insurance is thus the striped triangle under the demand curve whose area is $\frac{1}{2}P°(Q'-Q°)$. But its resource cost is $P°(Q'-Q°)$. Thus, the total loss of welfare, the value of opportunities foregone less that of new care received, is the cross-hatched triangle with area also $\frac{1}{2}P°(Q'-Q°)$.[17] Total health care expenditures rise from $P°Q°$ to $P°Q'$.

In Figure 2-2b, the same analysis is carried out on the assumption of a rising supply curve. Higher prices are required to induce present providers to increase output and/or to draw new providers into the market. Insurance induces an increase in quantity demanded, which drives up price to P'. Total health expenditures increase by $P'Q' - P°Q°$, but now part of the increase is a wealth transfer to suppliers who were willing to supply their services/products at $P°$, or some price between $P°$ and P', and are in fact receiving P'. The increase in total expenditures divides into the value (to consumers) of increased care, $\frac{1}{2}P°(Q' - Q°)$ (striped), the welfare burden of increased care (resource cost less value to consumers) (cross-hatched) $\frac{1}{2}P'(Q' - Q°)$, and the wealth transfer to suppliers, $\frac{1}{2}(Q° + Q')(P' - P°)$ (shaded).

The "welfare burden" of resources misallocated away from their most valuable use[18] can be mitigated by limiting the extent of coverage. Figure 2-2c demonstrates the effect of an insurance program paying 50 percent of all health care costs, in the context of prices equal to constant unit

---

[16] The non-satiation postulate of demand analysis would have utilization go to infinity at zero price, which, of course, it does not. One can remedy this by introducing time and access costs, which are not insured, but the resulting analysis gets progressively messier without providing further enlightenment. The more elaborate applications of neoclassical demand theory are, however, thus protected from refutation by reliance on unobserved quantities.

[17] This analysis neglects the premium payment, which would lower wealth and, hence, might shift DD to the left. Q' would be reduced, as would the welfare burden. It also neglects a number of other complexities surrounding the application of consumer surplus, in the belief that these would add confusion, rather than enlightenment, without changing the basic story.

[18] As judged by consumers, given a particular pattern of income/wealth distribution and of illness experience.

costs of production. From the buyer's viewpoint, this lowers the price of care to P^2, or $\frac{1}{2} P°$. Quantity demanded, or utilization, will rise to Q^2, where (if the demand curve is linear) $Q^2 = \frac{1}{2}(Q° + Q')$. Now the value of new health care output to consumers is $\frac{1}{2}(P° + P^2)(Q^2 - Q°)$ (striped) and its resource cost is as before $P°(Q^2 - Q°)$, so the welfare burden is $\frac{1}{2}(P° - P^2)(Q^2 - Q°)$ (cross-hatched). But since $P^2 = \frac{1}{2}P°$ and $Q^2 = \frac{1}{2}(Q° + Q')$, it is easy to show algebraically that the welfare burden in Figure 2-2c is only $\frac{1}{8} P°(Q' - Q°)$ or one-quarter of that under full insurance.

INADEQUACIES OF THE "WELFARE BURDEN" ANALYSIS

It is even easier, however, to show that the welfare burden is minimized when there is no insurance at all. This result contrasts sharply with the earlier demonstration (Figure 2-1) that welfare was increased by the insurance of all risky events, no matter how small. To reconcile these, recall that the former analysis focussed on an uncertain event whose expected loss qL was independent of whether or not one was insured, and which occurred to a transactor with diminishing marginal utility of wealth. The "moral hazard" analysis of Figure 2-2 in fact embodies no uncertainty at all; the transactor is in full control of her consumption patterns, and risk, loss, or changing utility of wealth play no role. The "welfare burden" of insurance does, of course, vary with elasticity of demand; if demand is wholly unresponsive to price (if DD in Figure 2-2 were vertical) then there is no welfare burden from insurance. But there is no benefit either. In the absence of risk, it should not be surprising that insurance is not worth buying.

But both analyses also leave out of account, as emphasized above, any other peculiarities, intrinsic or derived, of the commodity "health care" itself. The pure insurance argument focusses on a "loss" which has a monetary equivalent, but leaves the relation between this loss and health care expenditures unspecified. The "moral hazard" as elasticity of demand approach sidesteps the whole issue of loss in a general sense, restricting the cost of illness to its subcomponent, the cost of health care. That in turn is treated as an ordinary commodity, supplied under perfectly competitive conditions to informed consumers, whose tastes for that commodity have, for some unexplained reason, a random component.

In this framework, which underlies a large part of the formal economic analysis of health insurance, the design of optimal insurance policies or programs is treated as a problem of trading off benefits from risk reduction, as in Figure 2-1, against costs from "excessive" utilization, as in Figure 2-2. Since utilization is assumed to be a result of decisions by informed consumers, the mechanisms usually suggested are various forms of direct charges to consumers—deductibles, coinsurance, specific charges, which serve to lower the ''welfare burden'' as in Figure 2-2c. And since the only form of failure in insurance markets recognized by this analysis is that of ''moral hazard'' in this very narrow sense, there is no particular argument for public as against private insurance. Optimal coverage by either agency would require some form of cost-sharing.

The ''excessive utilization'' underlying the welfare burden argument bears a superficial resemblance to the ''frivolous use'' which is often alleged by physician advocates of direct charges to patients. But they are, in fact, quite different. ''Frivolous use'' refers to care which is unnecessary, in the sense that it does not contribute to health status; in the welfare burden case consumers are using care which they value at less than its true resource cost. Presumably, if they were fully informed, their values would reflect needs, but they may reflect other things as well, and particularly, incomes. Use of unnecessary care is medically frivolous, regardless of the income status of the user. But it is not ''excessive utilization'' in the sense of Figure 2-2, if it was used by someone who, for whatever reason, was willing to pay its true resource cost. On the other hand, effective care, which contributed significantly to the user's health status, would represent excessive use (in the sense of the ''welfare burden'' argument of Figure 2-2) if received by a poor person who could not buy it in the absence of insurance. It would be appropriate use if received by a wealthy person willing to pay its full price.

The distinction between health status and health care introduced in chapter 1 enables us to avoid these semantic confusions. If consumers value health care for its contribution to improved health status, then *informed* consumers will not buy ineffective care. If paying for care out of pocket, they will balance effectiveness against cost, and the medical concept of frivolous or unnecessary care will match[19] the economic concept of excessive utilization. But the fact that health status depends, in a technical way, on health care, simultaneously demolishes the basis for the assumption that consumers are, in fact, informed. If they are not, and their ignorance is remedied by provider-supplied information, then the demand curve *DD* in Figure 2-2 may not exist as a stable, negative relationship between prices paid by users and quantities consumed. And even if it does exist, it loses its normative significance as a guide to ''appropriate'' resource allocation.

Both the concept of moral hazard, and the analysis of health insurance generally, become richer and more complex when they are extended to take account of the external effects and asymmetry of information aspects of health care utilization, as well as the resulting extensive regulatory framework governing its production and distribution. The potential sources

[19] More or less—there are some additional sources of slippage.

of "moral hazard" in response to insurance coverage include independent forms of supplier behaviour—raising prices or changing recommendations about care use. The assumptions of perfectly informed consumers and perfectly competitive suppliers ruled out such responses except as a result of prior shifts in consumer behaviour; all effects of insurance were restricted to flow through the single channel of the consumer's utilization decision. In the real world, however, suppliers of health care are neither perfectly competitive nor profit-maximizers, and they exercise considerable independent power over both prices and quantities utilized in a "private" health care market. Consumers may control the initial decision to seek care for a particular problem, and in this decision their perceptions of, *inter alia*, costs to them of care may play the role envisioned in the demand curve of Figure 2-2. Thus, as Stoddart and Barer (1981) have shown, the demand for *episodes* of care may respond to prices in the conventional way. But the service content per episode is strongly influenced by providers, with greater control the more inherently costly (severe) the episode. And the most expensive forms of care are for chronic conditions in which the patient's entire remaining life becomes one episode. Possessing the (necessary and appropriate) power to influence patients' utilization patterns directly, providers can, and do, shift the demand curve, and vary utilization quite independently of prices paid by patients. As we shall see in chapter 4, this is the primary reason for the special regulatory framework surrounding health care supply.

Insofar as "moral hazard" arises from independent supplier behaviour, it is difficult or impossible to control directly in a framework of competitive, private insurance plans dealing with suppliers at arm's length. Attempts by American insurers, even those with apparently significant market power, to influence supplier behaviour have thus far been unsuccessful. Consumer/patient cost sharing, or incomplete insurance coverage, seems to have had some effect in the short run as an indirect mode of control over suppliers, though at significant cost in terms both of exposure of consumers to risk and of limiting the redistribution of cost burdens from ill to well. But it is not clear whether incomplete insurance serves to control overall levels of utilization and cost, or merely to redistribute care from more to less price-sensitive (usually poorer to richer) users. In any case, the longer term health care cost experience of the United States over the past thirty years suggests that present levels of insurance coverage in that country (coverage of about two-thirds of all health costs) are sufficient to permit "moral hazard" on the supply side to generate steadily escalating prices and levels of utilization.

By contrast, the public programs in Canada have, as shown in chapter 1, been quite successful in controlling utilization, and particularly price escalation, during the 1970s, without any significant exposure of consumers to cost-sharing. In effect, monopolizing the insurance function permits the control of moral hazard with comprehensive coverage; competitive insurance does not. It is sometimes claimed that much more extensive patient cost-sharing, *i.e.*, much less insurance, would eventually limit moral hazard in the United States setting. But the theoretical framework of such arguments is essentially that of Figure 2-2, so one cannot be too optimistic. It is also suggested that integration of the insurance and care delivery functions, either insurers opening clinics or providers selling insurance in the form of capitation-based reimbursement, will limit "moral hazard" on the supply side. There is some evidence for this, but its generalizability is still questionable. We will return to these issues below.

In Canada the debates over public versus private health insurance were (and are) over much more than alternative mechanisms for pooling of risks. Universal public health insurance may in some respects be superior to private forms of risk-bearing, as discussed above, but it is even more important as a framework for policy intervention in the "market for" or resource allocation process of, health care itself. Such programs are a response to market failure in that market as well as, or far more than, in the market for risk-bearing. Accordingly, issues of risk-bearing per se provide only a very limited explanation for the public role in health insurance which we observe in every developed society (although limited is not non-existent). Analyses of health insurance which focus only on these issues, and which are frequently used to support private sector provision of insurance with significant patient cost-sharing, are seriously incomplete and, consequently, frequently misleading. If uncertainty were the only characteristic of health care which distinguished it from other commodities, there would be no justification for the extensive structure of licensure, regulation, subsidy, and public or non-profit provision which characterizes the supply of health care. But it is not, and there is. Whether the justification is adequate, or the structure appropriate, is a more difficult question.

CHAPTER 3

MY SISTER'S KEEPER:
THE COMMUNITY INTEREST IN HEALTH CARE

THE SOCIAL SIGNIFICANCE OF INDIVIDUAL HEALTH STATUS

The common description of health care as a "need"—as different from ordinary commodities for which there are wants that, when backed by willingness to pay, become demands—conveys information about two of its characteristics. As noted in chapter 1, need refers to a special technical relationship between care and health status, accessible to an external observer. An expert evaluation of A's health status by B gives rise to B's judgement that A "needs" care, that utilization of specific forms of care would raise A's health status, and while this judgement may not command universal agreement, it is in a form communicable to C, D, and so on. Nor does its validity depend on A's agreement. By contrast, the value to A of commodities in general, or health status in particular, is knowledge privileged to A which B and others, however expert, can only infer by observing A's statements or actions, or by analogy from their own or others' experience in similar situations.

But "need" also carries significant ethical overtones; its allegation asserts an obligation on others. The statement that A needs care, which gains credibility if made by an expert and disinterested B, implies that A, or someone in A's family, or A's community, *ought* to do something. A's want for a particular commodity is, by contrast, neutral. The statement "Oh Lord, I *need* a Mercedes-Benz!" is a joke. "Oh Lord, I need a coronary artery by-pass graft!" is not.

But this more general social significance of health care utilization depends on its being needed in the technical sense as well. Only care which is perceived as effective in preventing or restoring deteriorations in someone's health status is a "need" in the second, obligational sense. If A asserts a desire for care which expert B judges unnecessary in the technical sense, then C, D, *et al.* will not, in general, feel any obligation to respond.

The health status of an individual thus takes on a special importance to the rest of the community beyond that of her consumption in general, but similar to that of political or judicial status. "One person, one vote"

53

is a firmly established principle, and while no one denies that money buys political influence, it is not lawful actually to buy and sell votes. Indeed in some societies exercise of the vote is a legal duty. Similarly access to justice is supposed to be available to all, regardless of ability to pay. "To no man will we sell, deny, or delay justice," it is said in Magna Carta. And though, again, the courts respond to the long purse, there is a fundamental principle that justice is not a commodity to be bought and sold like any other. When it is, it is not justice.

Such special status derives from a general perception that life, health, and freedom are not ordinary commodities, but are prerequisites to the enjoyment of all others. Maximizing one's utility across a consumption bundle remains possible if one is in hospital or prison, or disabled (though not, presumably, if dead), but there is a marked shift in the whole quality of life, a sharp discontinuity in the domain of the maximand. And since, as Colonel Rainborough put it, "The poorest he that is in England hath a life to live as the greatest he," assurance of the preconditions of living this life becomes a basic right. When threatened, such preconditions are normally defended, not in the market, but in the political arena, and not infrequently by force of arms.[1]

MODELLING THE INTERPERSONAL RELATIONSHIP

This aspect of the concept of need can be brought within economic analysis through the concept of external effects, or externalities, in consumption. The use of a commodity, in this case health care, by one individual may have positive or negative effects on the well-being of some other or others. In such a situation, private market mechanisms of resource allocation fail in the sense that they lead to under– or over-provision of the commodity in question. There is no market in which those affected by the primary consumer's consumption can register their preferences.[2]

The resulting underprovision, in the case of positive externalities, is shown for the case of two individuals in Figure 3-1, panel (a) (Culyer

---

[1] Of course, in extreme situations, food, shelter, and other necessities of life take on similar significance, as in the case of rationing under siege. It may be that the prevalence of violence and crime in the U.S. can be interpreted as a disorganized form of taking up arms in defense of perceived preconditions of life.

[2] If such a market could be developed, then conceivably bargaining between the parties concerned could lead to an "efficient" level of consumption by all concerned. But the informational conditions under which this is possible are so severe as to make this theoretical possibility irrelevant in general (Cooter 1982).

FIGURE 3-1
Market, and Optimal, Levels of Provision of Care to an Individual in the Presence of Consumption Externalities

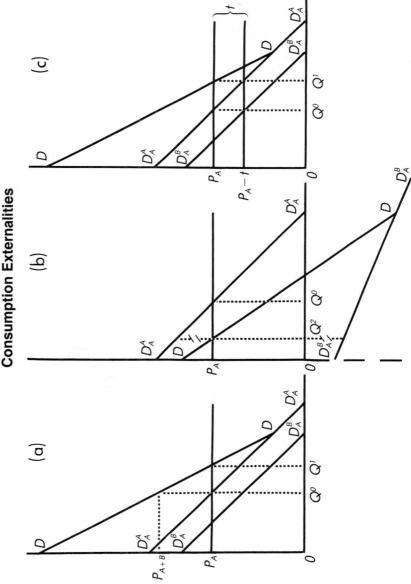

1971). A particular commodity Q, say health care, is valued by A; $D_A^A D_A^A$ represents her demand for it. If the price charged to her is P_A, then she will choose to buy Q° units of care. But B also has an interest in A's use of care, represented by $D_A^B D_A^B$. This represents B's willingness to pay for care *for* A, not B's own demand for care. Thus, the total value to A and B together of care for A is represented by the vertical sum of $D_A^A D_A^A$ and $D_A^B D_A^B$, or DD. If A makes her decisions as to care consumption without reference to B's interests, then at price P_A and output Q°, the value of the last unit purchased of Q to A is equal to or greater than P_A, and of the next (not purchased) is less than P_A. But its total value to society (A and B) is P_{A+B}. Assuming P_A represents the real resource cost of producing care, its opportunity cost in terms of other things foregone, then at Q° the value of one more unit of Q to society exceeds its resource cost. Its production should be expanded, to Q', at which point the value to A and B together of the last unit of care used by A just equals its resource cost.

If, on the other hand, care received by A were viewed negatively by B, then B would require compensation for A's receipt of care. Care to A would involve both resource costs and the cost of loss of welfare to B.[3]

This possibility is shown in panel (b) of Figure 3-1, where $D_A^B D_A^B$ lies below the zero-price axis. The sum DD now lies inside $D_A^A D_A^A$, and the socially optimal level of provision of care for A is now Q^2 where the value which A places on her last unit of consumption just balances its opportunity cost in resources used up, *plus* the additional distress it causes B. The private market will lead to an excessive supply to, and utilization of, care by A.

Economists studying health care have traditionally assumed a priori that the external effects involved were positive, pointing particularly to contagious diseases and immunization. It is quite clear that A's decision to seek immunization, or to accept care and isolation if ill with a contagious disease, reduces B's probability of becoming ill. There has been rather less attention given to the negative externalities associated with, *e.g.*, extensive use of antibiotics; A's use raising the probability of B's encountering a resistant strain.[4]

---

[3] For convenience, we assume marginal utilities of income constant in the relevant ranges.

[4] This form of externality arises because A's activity has a direct effect on B's well-being. In the presence of either public or private health care insurance, A's activity also has financial implications for B. A's bills are paid from B's premiums/taxes. This problem does not arise in a "pure" insurance system, in which each participant pays according to her risk status and is unable to affect her own expected loss. In reality insurance plans *do* build in cross-subsidies, in part, as we shall suggest below, in response to direct external effects of the sort described here. And as a result of imperfect risk rating and "moral hazard," B's well-being will indeed be reduced by A's use of care/generation of expense. If the care is effective, however, and if B has an interest in A's health, the net effect may be positive. But A's use of ineffective care harms B as well.

This may be because the conventional response to the private market underprovision of a commodity with positive externalities is some form of subsidy[5] to reduce the price paid by users below its resource cost. Panel (c), Figure 3-1, replicates panel (a), and includes a public subsidy of t per unit (raised through taxes) paid to buyers of care. A now confronts a price in the market of $P_A - t$. At this price, she will choose to consume Q', which is just the amount at which the marginal resource cost of care equals its value to both A and B. The information required to determine the optimal t yielding this result may be substantial. In particular, however, the optimal t need not equal $P°$. Externalities do not necessarily justify "free" care; the optimal subsidy might be less than $P°$, as it is in Figure 3-1c. Or it could be greater. Abstracting from problems of false reporting, we might in the presence of strong externalities (many and/or strongly concerned B's) not only provide "free" care, but pay A to use it.

In the case of activities with negative externalities, however, the subsidy becomes a tax. If antibiotic use raises the rate of development of resistant strains, imposing costs on others, then optimal use achieved through the market mechanism requires a tax of t per unit on antibiotics such that A's consumption decisions will reflect the costs imposed on B. The average non-economist, confronted with the proposition that efficient resource allocation requires such a tax, would have strong reservations about the validity of the analysis. And rightly so, because the treatment of external effects in this framework, while technically correct, is seriously incomplete.

EXTENDING THE RANGE OF EXTERNALITIES

In the first place, the contagion issue is now a relatively minor part of health care activity. That is not to say it is unimportant in the broader scheme of things. Control of contagious diseases through improvements in sanitation, nutrition, and health care have clearly added enormously to our well-being, lengthening and improving the quality of life. But they no longer account for a major share of the resources of the health care industry, at least in developed countries. In 1981-82, for example, infectious and parasitic diseases in British Columbia accounted for 1.4 percent of cases separated from hospitals, and 1.3 percent of patient-days. Another 8.8 percent of cases and 6.3 percent of days were for diseases of the respiratory system, many but by no means all contagious (British Columbia, Ministry of Health n.d. (*i.e.* 1983)). In total, contagious illness probably accounts for about 5 percent of hospital use and

---

[5] In the two-person case, of course, B could subsidize A directly or A could compensate B, depending on the prior legal assignment of property rights. But if the relevant B's are numerous and difficult to identify, this may be impossible. A tax-financed subsidy of the price for care paid by A achieves the desired result.

significantly less than 5 percent of costs. Its share of ambulatory medical costs may be somewhat higher, of in-hospital medical costs, substantially lower. Thus an explanation of the present structure of health care delivery and financing as a response to the external effects of contagion represents the tail wagging the dog.

Of course, historically, contagion has been a much more important phenomenon. But it has been dealt with directly through public health services, by a combination of regulation and direct public sector delivery, not through the general medical care system. Rather than subsidizing A's acceptance of immunization, most societies provide it free, on a mass basis in schools or public health clinics, and in certain circumstances (sensitive occupations, foreign travel) require it by law. Formerly, if A became ill, quarantine enforced isolation (with or without other care) to protect B, and was backed up by legal penalties, not taxes or subsidies. Sanitation likewise is enforced by regulation: "The Common Law of England does not recognize a prescriptive right to remain dirty."

The boundaries between public health services and the general health care system are currently rather contentious, and may well be in flux, for reasons which we will address below. The point to recognize, however, is that such boundaries do exist. The primary social response to the external effects of contagion, and the associated needs for prevention or care, has been public provision and regulation for that particular sector alone.

The social or public interest in health care, however, goes well beyond contagion. As reflected in public discussions of health care delivery, it emphasizes access to care for those in need as an end in itself, not merely as a way of protecting the rest of the community. The public health insurance program was intended not only to spread the economic burden of care more equitably, to transfer financial resources from low to high users of care or from low-risk to high-risk buyers of insurance, but also to lower the barriers to ("needed") care. Health care use was subsidized in order to increase utilization by some, at least, of the population. The general social interest in use of health care by private individuals was strong enough that the community were prepared to tax themselves to subsidize this use.

But public insurance is only one of several forms of subsidy to health care. Public funds contribute extensively to capital formation, both human and non-human, in this industry. The costs of training health care personnel are largely borne by government; this is true of all post-secondary education, but since health care personnel are more expensive to train, the size of the subsidy per trainee is larger than for post-secondary students generally. Hospital capital—buildings and equipment—is predominantly financed by government, as is a large share of health care research. And private voluntary organizations mobilize collective resources to fund individual treatments of particular types.

All such subsidies, whether to increase the capacity of the health care system—people and facilities—or to lower the costs faced by users, can be described as efforts to improve access to services, rather than providing for their direct delivery or mandating their use. Access in the positive sense is rather difficult to define or measure, but in the negative sense, barriers to access are readily identifiable and of many different forms. Economic barriers, direct charges to users of care at point of service or otherwise related to use, are the most obvious; it is these which are reduced or eliminated by universal public insurance. But geographic or social distance between provider and user, rigidities in the organization of supply, or simple capacity inadequate to meet needs, all represent additional barriers which are addressed by other types of public policy, usually including some form of subsidy (Evans 1978). The whole area of educational and manpower planning for health care, and the concomitant public concern for an appropriate geographic distribution of services, are evidence of the sense of a social or public responsibility to assure access. And this concern is separate from the public insurance program itself, as is evidenced by governmental concerns over the mal-distribution of dentists, for whose services public coverage is only partial and province-specific. The same issues arise in the United States, where universal public health insurance has become a rather remote possibility, at least in the near term.

The impact of Canada's public programs on utilization patterns, as opposed to overall levels, has been significant. In the early 1950s utilization of care varied directly with income. *The Canadian Sickness Survey* showed that low-income persons experienced substantially more illness and disability than medium– and upper-income persons. They received less care, however, and the differences were particularly striking when care use was measured relative to days of disability. Low-income people received just over half as many physician visits and operations per disability day as the average person surveyed, upper-income people received about a third more. Differences in hospital use were less pronounced, but still significant (Canada, Department of National Health and Welfare and Dominion Bureau of Statistics 1960).

Studies of the introduction of public medical insurance, in particular, have shown that its effect was generally to remove the influence of income on utilization patterns, and to redistribute care from upper– to lower-income groups. Whether it also raised overall utilization levels, or whether these are more a function of overall levels of health system capacity, personnel, and facilities, is a more difficult issue which we shall try to deal with below. But the redistributive effect of public insurance seems well established. In fact there is now a clear tendency for utilization to be negatively related to income, and students of the issue have concluded that this is not the result of differences in the "price of time" or any other indirect price effects, but simply that poor people are sicker (Boulet and Henderson 1979; Broyles *et al.* 1983). Public health insurance does appear to have changed the distribution of health care utilization away from its previous relation to income, and closer to some external standard of medical need, which was its principal announced objective.

The fact that the public program was declared to have this objective, that it appears to have met it, or at least moved a great distance toward it, and that there is widespread and general satisfaction with this result, supports the proposition that the community at large feels an interest in the consumption of *needed* health care by individuals. To express this relationship in the language of external effects, we must draw some distinctions as to the nature of these effects. In making such distinctions, the relationship between health status and health care which we have emphasized throughout will be of considerable assistance.

ALTERNATIVE FORMS OF INTERPERSONAL EFFECTS

There appear to be three different types of externalities which may underlie B's interest in A's health care, the selfish, the altruistic, and the paternalistic.[6] Selfish externalities are expressed in the case of contagious diseases. In this case, B (or the rest of society) has no interest in A for her own sake, but only insofar as her status or behaviour affects B's *health*. For technical reasons, contagion, A's health status affects B's health status, and B cares about her own health. Thus insofar as A's care affects A's health status, it also affects that of B. The community interest in A's care, then, is restricted to those forms of care which are effective in improving A's health status in those particular dimensions which affect B's health. A's attitude toward the care she is to receive is of no interest to B. In fact, isolation, quarantine, or driving A out of the community might serve as well; hence the selfish aspect of the external effect relationship. As noted, the actual social response to contagion has been consistent with the existence of this sort of relationship; public health policies toward contagious disease have not historically depended solely or principally on the consent of the ill. But this form of external effect, or relationship between one person's use of health care and another's

---

[6] Formally, the utility or welfare of B, U_B, is a function of the health care received by A, HC_A. In the selfish case, $U_B = U_B\{HS_B[HS_A(HC_A)]\}$. A's health care affects A's health status, HS_A, which affects B's health status, HS_B (via contagion), which affects B's well-being. In the altruistic case, $U_B = U_B\{U_A[HS_A(HC_A)]\}$, B's welfare depends directly on A's welfare, which in turn depends *inter alia* on A's health and thereby A's health care. In the paternalistic case, B's well-being may depend directly on A's health care, but more plausibly, as discussed below, on A's health status, $U_B = U_B[HS_A(HC_A)]$, and thus on A's health care. For a more extensive discussion see Culyer and Simpson (1980).

well-being, does not serve to explain the extensive public interventions we observe in the financing of health care.

The second form of interaction, the purely altruistic, is present when B's interest in A's health care arises from a more general concern of B for A's well-being. We might postulate that B derives satisfaction from seeing A happy, and suffers along with A—Adam Smith's concept of sympathy (Collard 1978).

This framework, however, is also inadequate to explain the actual institutions and the cross-subsidies which we observe, not just in Canada, but virtually universally. The altruistic form of externality is not specific to any particular type of commodity or source of satisfactions. If B is really interested in A's well-being, however attained, she should strictly respect A's preferences, and be as willing to subsidize gin as penicillin, if that is what A wants. And the criteria for subsidy will be A's preferences, regardless of the effectiveness of the care received or the harm done by the gin (or vice-versa). Thus altruistic externalities lead to progressive income taxes and welfare or public assistance schemes, which transfer wealth to particular deserving A's but leave their use of it unrestricted. It is a standard exercise in elementary economic theory to demonstrate that any given augmentation of well-being for a recipient A can be achieved by a smaller transfer of resources if it is through an income transfer than if it is by subsidy of a particular commodity.[7] If B's interest is in A's well-being, the implication is that B should give A money. This argument underlies some advocacy of negative income taxes as a cheaper and more effective form of assistance, substituting for various categorical and commodity-specific social programs—like public health insurance.

The argument from altruistic externalities to cash transfers rather than commodity subsidies does, however, have a serious gap in the case of health insurance and health care. B's interest in A's well-being, when expressed through a program which subsidizes health care use, responds to fluctuations in A's well-being which arise from changes in health status. A general negative income tax, or cash transfer program from rich to poor, does not. Thus an altruistic society might very well choose to subsidize health care as a partial compensation for differences in well-being which arise, not from income or wealth differences, but from health status differences. Ideally, the compensation would be directly associated with health status, not linked to it indirectly through health care use. But, as noted above, it is generally impractical for a public agency or insurer to monitor health status directly. Care use is taken as a signal for poor health.

---

[7] *Ceteris paribus*, holding prices fixed, no work-leisure trade-off, and no after-markets in the commodity. Relax these assumptions, and predictions become both less secure and more complex, but the general principle is maintained.

Of course, people can always buy insurance. Thus one might argue that, if instead of subsidizing health care a society redistributes income, formerly poor people can then choose to buy health insurance, or not, as they see fit. But in the first place this presumes a more-or-less smoothly functioning insurance market, which, as we have seen above, is least likely to exist for the poor, elderly, and high-risk groups most likely to need care. Secondly, even if such a market existed, high-risk people would still have to pay higher premiums. Thus the cash transfer which expresses collective B's interest in individual A's welfare would have to be related to A's *ex ante* expectation of illness, or at least of health care use, or else significant inequalities would remain among A's at similar money income levels (after adjustment). Indeed the costs of fair insurance for some particular chronically ill A's could easily exceed the total amount which society was prepared to transfer to each individual A for income support. In the presence of large variations in expected health care use, general income transfers plus even the fairest of insurance cannot substitute for a direct subsidy program.[8]

Such a direct subsidy could, in principle, take the form of an attempt, as part of the income transfer system, to estimate each individual's risk status *ex ante* and adjust her income tax/transfer position accordingly.[9] Alternatively, and more realistically, it could be based on the risk-evaluation process in private insurance markets. Each person's premiums, for a standard form of coverage, could be determined in that market, and a tax-financed subsidy would then be paid, not necessarily contingent on actual purchase of insurance, to people in high-risk categories. In effect, such premiums would be deducted from income in computing relative income for the general redistribution program. This of course presupposes efficient and fully informed insurance markets. In practice such a system

---

[8] In practice, of course, direct subsidies have the significant additional advantage that they may in fact be provided. Those who oppose direct subsidy or provision of specific commodities on the ground that hypothetical income transfers would in principle be superior, rarely advocate such transfers with equal energy. And a *de facto* policy of "do nothing" has no a priori support.

[9] Even if a redistribution program is sufficiently sensitive to take account of differences in risk status as well as in income or wealth position, it turns out that a policy of non-paternalistic wealth redistribution plus subsequent purchase of actuarially fair insurance by perfectly informed, rational customers is still not socially optimal in general. As Hammond (1982, 1983) demonstrates, redistribution which maximizes a social welfare function defined over *ex ante* individually maximized expected utilities will not maximize the expected value of the same social welfare function defined over *ex post* individual utility outcomes, except under very restrictive and implausible conditions. *Ex ante* and *ex post* optimality conditions are simply inconsistent, and neither has ethical priority in principle. In practice, given the severe informational deficiencies of "markets" for both health insurance and health care, we find the *ex post* criteria more compelling.

would be very expensive, unreliable, and inaccurate for those who need it most. It would also be a source of substantial increases in insurance overhead costs, *i.e.*, revenues for the private insurance industry.

Finally, of course, there is the "bleeding cheat" problem (Archibald and Donaldson 1976). Income is transferred, but recipients spend it on gin, not health insurance. Some become ill, a few gravely so. If society is not prepared to let them die, then *ex post* a further subsidy will be paid. In Canada at least, and we suspect in most other developed societies, improvident A's would not be denied needed care, at least not life-saving care. Knowing this, why should A's receiving income transfers purchase insurance?

The practical inadequacies of income transfer plus insurance schemes indicate that direct subsidy of health care use could be a second-best response to purely altruistic, non-paternalistic relationships among the members of a community. The Canadian approach, of financing care costs from tax revenues plus (in some provinces) compulsory "premiums" unrelated to risk status, serves to redistribute a substantial amount of wealth from low– to high-risk persons, as well as (like any insurance program), from well to ill.[10] This transfer, which is independent of any effect of the public insurance program on levels of utilization, is consistent with the altruistic, non-paternalistic form of external effects.

But consideration of community attitudes towards gin and penicillin suggests that the externalities are in fact paternalistic, rather than altruistic. Health care is what the public finance literature calls a "merit good"— society in general feels that individuals in particular circumstances ought to use it—as opposed to alcohol, which is a demerit good, and taxed. But public responsiveness to concerns over frivolous use and unnecessary care, whatever the source of payment for such care, suggests that it is only effective, needed care which is the merit good. The social interest is in A's health status, and in her health care use only insofar as it contributes to that. Indeed, Canada's medical insurance program provides reimbursement only for "medically necessary" services.[11]

POLICY RESPONSES TO EXTERNAL EFFECTS

If society's, or other individual B's, preferences display this paternalistic (or perhaps maternalistic) characteristic, as it appears that they do,

---

[10] The trouble and cost of identifying risk status explicitly (or the unfairness of ignoring it!) in general transfer policy is saved at the cost of denying consumers free choice of insurance coverage. Most Canadians seem to think the price acceptable.

[11] In practice, a physician's submission of a claim is generally accepted as evidence of necessity, so that if the physician feels the utilization was unnecessary or "frivolous," she ought, according to the Act, to bill the patient, not the insurance program, for the full cost of the service. Therefore, any physician who argues that unnecessary and "frivolous" use is widespread, whether initiated by patients or promoted by physicians, is implicitly accusing her colleagues of (or confessing to) fraud. The provider who billed a public plan for such care thereby attested to its medical necessity.

then optimal allocation of resources to health care production and use will require some sort of social program to subsidize and expand this output beyond private market levels. The beneficiaries of such transfers may be less well off than they would be with a straight cash transfer conditional on illness (they might prefer the gin), but the payers of the subsidy will be happier.[12] The form this subsidy should take, however, is not determined by the existence of the external effects themselves. The strengths and weaknesses of alternative institutional approaches can only be analysed in the context of the other peculiarities and sources of market failure intrinsic to the commodity, health care.

The range of possible alternatives is in fact two-dimensional, running from completely public provision, to completely private, with variable degrees of public subsidy in both insurance and care markets. A completely nationalized health service, along the lines of the British National Health Service, represents public insurance and public provision; the state bears risks and delivers care. In the United States, most of both the insurance and the provision functions are in the private sector, at least superficially. But large public sector subsidies flow to different groups in many different ways. The Veterans' Administration provides both public insurance and public delivery to its eligible population. The tax system provides public subsidy to both private insurance purchase and, above a threshold, private care use, in amounts which increase with income level. Medicare for the elderly and Medicaid for the poor involve private delivery, and a mix of predominantly public with some private insurance. The functions of insurance administration are contracted to the private sector, while the public sector bears the risks and subsidizes the costs. Those who qualify for subsidy neither by age, nor by poverty, nor by special status or special illness, may receive no assistance at all.

In Canada, the insurance function is public for hospital and medical care, and part of dental and pharmaceutical. Subsidies flow through tax plus uniform premium finance of hospital and medical care, with insignificant out-of-pocket charges. Dental and pharmaceutical costs are subsidized for children, the elderly, and the poor, in amounts varying from province to province. Most provide a subsidized public insurance program for private delivery; Saskatchewan and Prince Edward Island provide direct dental care delivery for children.

In form, the hospital and medical care delivery systems are private and contract with the public insurance program to provide care at specified rates of reimbursement. In practice, however, the monopsonistic power of the

---

[12] These should not necessarily be thought of as two separate classes of people. I may well prefer complete discretion over my own care, but feel paternalistic about yours, and vice-versa.

public programs in hospital and medical care has been used to exert significant influence on the delivery system to the point that hospitals, at least, can no longer be thought of as purely private sector institutions. Unlike their American counterparts, they occupy a middle ground between public agencies and private "firms," with entrepreneurial decision-making power fragmented between hospital managements themselves, governments, and private physicians. Physicians are farther toward the private contractor end of the spectrum, and dentists even more so.

If external effects in consumption were the only source of market failure in health care, the form of the public subsidy to individual use would not be a significant issue. A health care market supplied by private, for-profit firms, competitive in pricing, with free, unlicensed entry, and unregulated as to choice of technique, would, according to conventional economic theory, be marketing its products at minimum cost. Fully informed buyers would select the care which was of most value to them, relative to the prices they were required to pay. Since private sector delivery would be both technically efficient and price-competitive, it would make care available at a price equal to its marginal resource cost ($P = MC$, as in Figure 3-1 or 2-2), so there would be no particular advantage in public sector provision. Indeed, the absence of competition, plus bureaucratic regulation, might be expected to make public sector provision more costly and less efficient. By a similar argument, and ignoring the problems of market failure in insurance markets, it would appear that the risk-bearing and premium/claims administration functions would be best carried out in the competitive and efficient private sector. The public response to externalities in consumption could then be restricted to subsidizing (partially or fully) health insurance premiums for those whose income levels and/or expected health care use were such that they could not pay for private insurance, at all, or without undue sacrifice, and to subsidizing and/or mandating the use of specific services which were of particular significance to the rest of society (immunizations, *e.g.*, or the care of children).

A few additional problems would remain, of course. In view of the "bleeding cheat" problem, minimal coverage would have to be mandatory for everyone. Secondly, the community interest only in effective care would have to be reconciled with individual interests, which might be broader. We have argued above that rational individuals attach negative value to health care per se, and value positively only its health status benefits, but care believed effective clearly also has an amenity dimension. Thus, the mandated and subsidized care would have to be restricted, insofar as possible, to the care which, when received by individual A's, was perceived by collective B's as effective and of an appropriate amenity standard.

This, however, opens up a serious issue of the moral hazard variety. Suppose the relationship of health care to health status takes the form of

Figure 1-3, panel (b). The payoff to more care is always positive, but declines as care increases. Collective B's cannot then undertake to subsidize *all* effective care for individual A's, but must somehow impose a cut-off point at which further effect is judged not worth the cost to society. Schemes for the public subsidy of private insurance and delivery envision this as taking place through more or less sophisticated systems of patient cost-sharing; the mandated and subsidized minimal insurance policy would embody such provisions to limit patient/consumer-initiated moral hazard and to ensure that the public subsidy commitment was not open-ended. Thus access to social resources (insurance funds plus public subsidy) would be conditional on individual willingness-to-pay, which, in turn, would require cost-sharing to be carefully matched to individual resources if it were not to discriminate against lower-income people, not only in utilization of care, but in access to financial subsidy as well.

A program of direct public provision, by contrast, can limit utilization by direct rationing without a structure of patient cost-sharing. The limitations on individual A's access to collective resources are imposed by refusal to provide, either directly or, more commonly, in the form of restrictions on available personnel and facilities. Both the British National Health Service and the Canadian public insurance program do this; the latter as a monopsony buyer of care can determine the terms on which suppliers will be reimbursed, as well as (for hospitals) providing capital by direct grant. The public agency thus determines the amount of hospital space and facilities available; its influence over manpower is more problematic.

SUBSIDY POLICY IN THE CONTEXT OF INFORMATIONAL ASYMMETRY

Proposals for a minimal public program, of subsidy to or supplementation of private insurance, were made by the private insurance industry and the medical associations to the Royal Commission on Health Services before the Canadian Medicare system was introduced. They were also brought forward before the United States enacted Medicare, and remain an important component of the periodic American debates over national health insurance. They have also been attractive to some Canadian provincial governments wishing to enter the dental insurance field on a small scale, and at minimum risk. The Report of the Hall Commission, and the actual health insurance programs developed in Canada, represent a decisive rejection of this approach, but proposals for modifications to the present system along such lines continue to surface regularly from the medical community, with the details rather fuzzy.

The weakness of such proposals is not that they are illogical, but that they are incomplete. They rest on the assumption that health care is in fact a commodity like any other, except for its peculiar interpersonal significance, and its uncertainty of incidence. If the supply side of the market were as described above, offering care at a price more or less corresponding to its marginal resource cost, and if buyers were sufficiently informed as to make their own consumption choices, then a good case could be made for public subsidy of private insurance, with perhaps some additional institutional modifications to deal with the problems of incompleteness in private insurance markets. Externalities per se do not support Canada's rejection of this approach; and while the universal public insurance program does respond to specific identifiable failures in private insurance markets, it is rather a massive response.

But the supply side of the health care market is not perfectly competitive. It is shot through with all sorts of institutional restrictions on entry to the market and on conduct in it. Licensure has been the traditional mode of restricting entry; to this has now been added the attainment of approval for reimbursement. Self-regulation, backed up by threat of delicensure, is used to regulate conduct, in particular competitive behaviour. Not-for-profit motivation dominates in the hospital sector. And so on. If the sole peculiarities of health care were uncertainty and external effects, *none* of the regulations on the supply side would be justified. Insurers, public or private, might still wish to use disinterested experts to certify the health status of claimants for reimbursement, and consumer/patients who felt themselves inadequately informed might also prefer care from certified suppliers.[13] But all this would be voluntary. There is no justification, in the discussion of either of the two previous chapters, for the extensive network of direct and ''self''-regulation which surrounds the supply of health care.

The existence of such a web of regulation, then, raises two types of questions. First, to what extent can it be justified, if at all, by intrinsic peculiarities of health care as a commodity? And second, to what extent is the analysis of the effects of, and appropriate responses to, uncertainty and external effects modified by either these additional peculiarities, or the very existence of the regulatory structure itself, however justified?

In this respect, some of the right-wing critiques of health care delivery in the United States are intellectually quite consistent. They argue that the regulation of the supply side is not, in fact, justified in terms of market failure, and that its effects on the delivery, and costs, of health care are harmful and profound. They then argue for massive deregulation of health care, including removal of all licensure or other restraints on entry and

---

[13] Certification is an authoritative statement, perhaps by a public body, that a provider has completed certain training or displayed certain abilities. But uncertified providers are free to offer services, if they can find a market. Licensure prohibits unlicensed providers from offering services.

conduct, along with, or before, specific (minimal) policies to deal with uncertainty or external effects. Considering the range of vested interests threatened by such a strategy, as well as the implausibility of its underlying assumptions, its political feasibility is probably minimal. But it *is* honest.

What is *not* consistent, or honest, is simply to ignore the whole question of the organization of health care delivery, and to analyse and propose policies for insurance markets and public subsidy programs as if this organization were indistinguishable from purely private, competitive industries. To assume, as in Figure 2-2 or 3-1, that the market price of health care in the absence of subsidy equals its marginal resource cost, is to assume either that the regulatory structure does not exist, or that it is without effect. Neither assumption seems defensible. Further, to assume a demand curve which defines the utilization responses of consumers to prices of care, independently of any influence by suppliers, and to use these hypothesized responses as a basis for policy evaluation, is to assume away the problem of imperfect patient/consumer information which, rightly or wrongly, forms the primary argument for regulation of the supply side.

Suppose, however, that one is unable to accept the assumptions both that imperfect information is not a serious problem for patient/consumers of health care, and that the elaborate professional/regulatory structure which purports to address this problem is either, despite appearances, not really there, or else is without influence on the prices, quantities, qualities, and types of health care offered. Then the argument for a restriction of public intervention to subsidy and supplementation of private insurance against expenditures on privately provided health care falls to the ground. Of course, a corresponding argument for either universal public health insurance or a national health service does not necessarily rise from the ruins. Rather, we must proceed to explore the implications of this imperfect information, and of the institutional responses to it, which make the organization and delivery of health care so unusual relative to other commodities. We shall find that one cannot begin to understand the utilization of health care without consideration of the conditions of its provision. The converse is also true.[14]

---

[14] What is surprising, and depressing, is that so many analyses of health care utilization, particularly by economists, have addressed problems of optimal insurance design and/ or response to externalities, in complete disregard of the structure of supply. Worse, they have brought forward the results as policy recommendations. It is quite understandable that representatives of the private insurance industry, or of medical associations, should attempt to assume away any problems of technical efficiency, of completeness, or of price formation in their respective markets. They have a well-defined economic interest in doing so. But economists should know better.

CHAPTER 4

LICENSURE, CONSUMER IGNORANCE, AND AGENCY

REGULATION OF HEALTH CARE AS PROTECTION OF UNINFORMED CONSUMERS

Public provision of health insurance is a relatively recent phenomenon in Canada, having developed almost entirely since 1945.[1] But the regulation of health care provision is much older, its basic structure having been established in most jurisdictions during the nineteenth century. In Ontario it pre-dates Confederation. The state either determines, or delegates to groups of providers power to determine, who may perform health care activities, who may provide them to the public, and how such providers must behave in the professional, economic, and often other spheres as well. There has never been a free market, or free enterprise in medical practice, in Canada, nor have private, for-profit hospitals ever played any significant role. And there has never been a serious proposal for dismantling the regulatory structure of health care provision and placing primary reliance on free competitive markets to allocate resources in this area. Only in rhetoric is there a conflict between state control and private organization of medical practice; in reality "private versus public" debates are over who shall direct the power of the state in regulating the health care market.

Present United States health care policy, by contrast, appears to take much more seriously the possibility of substituting competition for regulation in health care production and delivery, partly for ideological reasons quite separate from health care and partly because United States regulatory policies in the 1970s seem to have been much less successful than those in Canada. But it is too early to tell whether the policy rhetoric represents a real shift to competitive supply, which would require *inter alia* a dramatic reduction or elimination of the powers of the self-regulating professions, and of their influence over other providers. Alternatively, "competition" policy may serve merely as an excuse for relieving from public accountability the private organizations wielding state authority in this area (and for reduced public subsidy). So long as

---

[1] Small-scale programs of subsidy to particular providers or patients, or direct delivery of certain services, have a much longer history.

the state will prosecute those who contravene rules of market entry or conduct laid down by private organizations,[2] the industry is regulated; and references to free or private enterprise are (often deliberately) misleading.

Over the last decade there has been considerable discussion and analysis of the particular forms and extent of public and self-regulation, reflecting concerns that the balance between the interests of those regulated and of the wider society may not be appropriately struck. But the need for some forms of control over provider entry to and conduct in health care markets is (almost) universally accepted, on the ground that consumer/patients are insufficiently informed to protect their own interests. The technology of health care is sufficiently complex that consumers purchasing care in arm's-length transactions, responding only to relative prices, would make mistakes. Moreover such mistakes may be serious, and potentially irreversible—the wrong care or care of poor quality (or no care) at a critical point can have permanently damaging or fatal results. And the possibilities for learning from the experience of others, or even from one's own, are distinctly limited. In cases of chronic illness, or of well-defined and fairly common episodic illnesses, one may be guided by past, or others', experience. But the same presenting complaint or symptom may at different times or in different persons represent very different problems and require quite different responses.

In theory the consumer can always "buy" information with money or effort. But health problems may have a very significant time dimension, developing on a timetable which makes the acquisition of information not merely costly but impossible. At the same time, the mental state of the consumer may be such as to degrade sharply his capacity for information acquisition and informed choice. To characterize a person suddenly confronted with an acute abdomen or a severe fever as facing a conventional problem of optimal consumer choice subject to costly information is distinctly implausible. For the unconscious accident victim, it is bizarre.

Information is not only difficult and expensive (in time, trouble, and risk as well as money) to acquire, it is also costly to have. There is a genuine welfare loss involved in being aware of all the possibilities inherent in a situation. Most of us, if fully informed about health matters,

---

[2] The public or private status of regulatory bodies in health care is ambiguous. In medicine there is a College of Physicians and Surgeons in each province, which is formally a statutory body responsible to the provincial legislature for regulating medical practice in the public interest. The provincial medical association represents the collective interests of physicians. In practice, however, colleges appear to regard the public interest as an extension of the interests of the profession. Dentists have in some provinces simply amalgamated the two bodies, thus making explicit the "capture" of a nominally public regulatory body by a private association.

would probably hesitate to get out of bed in the morning;[3] we would certainly not ski, or ride bicycles in traffic.

ASYMMETRY OF INFORMATION BETWEEN PROVIDER AND CONSUMER

The significance of consumer ignorance for the optimum allocation of health care is not merely that it is extreme and pervasive, but that it is asymmetric. If both buyer and provider were equally ill-informed about the effects of a good or service, there would be no market failure and no case for public regulation.[4] Buyers and sellers of economic or astrological forecasts are dealing in a highly uncertain commodity, but it is doubtful that the provider has any better idea of its value (to the user) than the user. Nor is there information about the value of the commodity available elsewhere in the economy which is being left unexploited in the market transaction itself. Imperfect information in these cases is part of the state of nature.

But in the case of health care, and of professional services generally, it is perceived by buyer and seller, and by the wider society, that the seller/provider of health care services has a very large informational advantage over the buyer. This asymmetry of information leaves open the possibility (or certainty) of severe exploitation of buyers by sellers in an arms-length, *caveat emptor* market environment.[5] And private markets will "fail" in that they will give rise to a pattern of health care use—too much of some things, not enough of others—which yields a significantly lower level of consumer/patient satisfaction than could be

---

[3] Were it not for the possibilities of decubitus ulcer or thrombosis!

[4] Although there may be some justification for the banning of potentially dangerous commodities whose specific effects are unknown to both buyer and seller. Fortune-telling has at some times been banned on related grounds, though not, as far as I am aware, economic analysis.

[5] Trebilcock and Shaul (1983) point out that in most parts of Canada the provision of *mental* health services is much less tightly regulated than that of physical health services, and that the background, training, and methods of providers are correspondingly much more diverse. They ascribe this difference to the absence of asymmetry of information in this field. Providers (collectively at least) have no more information about what "works" than patients do. There is no evidence that any one form of training or set of methods achieves superior therapeutic results.

Thus they argue, consistent with our discussion, that public regulation should *not* take the traditional form of licensure of self-regulating professions, but should focus on control of dangerous or exploitative practices. Subject to such control, the "market" for mental health services should be left open to a number of different types of competing therapists and methods.

achieved by alternative resource allocations. "Quackery" to the economist is a problem of resource mis-allocation, of inefficient use of human time and skills.

Of course consumers are constantly venturing into transactions, throughout the economy, with incomplete information, and the social response is not licensure of all producers (yet). But the informational asymmetry in health care, or professional services generally, takes a rather special form. Most producers know much more than most buyers about the technology of production, and the characteristics of the commodities produced. But the buyer is better informed as to what those characteristics mean *for her* than the seller is. She knows her own needs. Moreover, insofar as there is remaining uncertainty about the capabilities and reliability of a complex product, these uncertainties are specific to that product, not to the user. The buyer can thus accumulate information by questioning sellers or other users, or various sources of product-specific information. The seller can offer warranties. Or the state can establish minimum quality standards and grading systems, as for food products. There is no need to license sellers of canned beans, only to inspect the contents periodically for insect parts or rodent faeces.

But in health care the informational asymmetry extends beyond the process of production or specific characteristics of a good or service, to what its effects will be *on the user*. How will the care used interact with the patient's condition, whatever that is? The buyer is no longer the best judge of her own interests, but must rely on the seller's advice, which in turn implies that the seller accepts some responsibility for serving the buyer's interest. Their relationship cannot be arms-length.[6]

The informational asymmetry problem is conveniently captured in the health status/health care distinction. The consumer/patient values health status per se, not health care, but health status cannot be bought. Rather she buys health care in the expectation that it will contribute to health status. The normal consumer sovereignty assumption is that the consumer

---

[6] The interaction between service and patient condition also introduces "first-mover advantages" (Williamson 1975) for the supplier, which undercut the potential competitiveness of supply. Before recommending care for a particular episode, each provider must acquire information about the patient which may be extensive and expensive. Thus patient "shopping" among providers involves substantial real costs (to patients, providers, or insurers) of replicated effort, and/or impaired effectiveness of care. Indeed the stress by providers on the desirability of a continuing relationship reflects the fact that the effectiveness of care in a particular case may be related to an extensive past history which is difficult, if not impossible, to communicate among providers. Nor, in a competitive, arms-length market, would providers have any incentive to do so— quite the contrary. "Professionalism" is at least some check on proprietary control of patient-specific information, though it can also be used to control patient access to information.

is the best judge of the value to herself of different valued commodities or states; this includes health status. But it does not extend to health care, because that is not itself of value. There is a technical relationship which is specific to each consumer and condition, by which health care affects health, and the expert provider is much better informed than the consumer/patient about the structure of this relationship.[7]

The asymmetry of information between provider and consumer is thus quite consistent with a general value postulate of consumer sovereignty as a guiding principle in the organization of economic activity. It locates the source of market failure, not in the inability of consumers to interpret the value to themselves of valued entities such as health, but in the obvious inability of consumers to be informed about the contribution of health care to the "production" of health, in specific situations. If health could be purchased directly, no difficulty would arise. Of course, patients who are unconscious, mentally disordered, in great emotional distress, or otherwise unable to protect their own interests may not be capable of making appropriate use of information even if they possess it. For these patients, who in fact account for a significant share of health care use, the application of the consumer sovereignty postulate itself is inappropriate, and someone else will have to make judgements about the value of health status as well as the efficacy of health care. It is not however obvious a priori that the same person is best equipped to make both types of decisions.

LIMITS ON THE PROFESSIONAL'S ROLE

For the consumer/patient who is not in some way disabled from making her own judgements, however, the health status/health care distinction has important implications for the limits of professional expertise. Superior information about the effects of health care does *not* imply a similar advantage with respect to the value of health per se. The dental patient may accept the dentist's expertise in deciding, on technical grounds,

---

[7] As before, $U = U[X, ..., HS(HC, ...,)]$, the consumer's level of well-being depends *inter alia* on health status. The partial impact of health status on well-being, $\partial U/\partial HS$, is (by consumer sovereignty) information privileged to the consumer. But the technical relation $\partial HS/\partial HC$ is not. The informational advantage of the provider is with respect to the structure of the functional relation $HS(HC ...)$.

There are in the literature analytical models of health care use which emphasize its relationship with health as the ultimately demanded entity, but which then assume that the consumer is fully informed (or at least as well informed as the provider) about the structure of the $HS(HC ...)$ function itself. No justification for this counter-factual assumption, other than analytical tractability, comes to mind. If it were justified, it would undercut any rationale for regulation of the supply side of health care.

which teeth should be filled, which capped, and where endodontia would be successful, as well as her definition of how such services are best performed. But the patient is the best judge of whether the resulting oral condition is worth paying for. The different levels of dental care have cosmetic and perhaps comfort and convenience implications, but crowns versus fillings has no life-threatening implications and little if any in the way of external effects. For the professional to urge a particular course of treatment on a patient who is in fact informed of the relevant outcomes, is to step beyond the bounds of professional advice and into the area of marketing.[8]

In a graver setting, the choice of surgery versus radiation therapy for certain cancers turns on the values patients attach to different outcomes—in particular to the trade-off between probabilities of short and long-term survival—and to the quality of remaining life (McNeil *et al.* 1978). Surgery may have a higher short-term fatality rate, but a better five-year survival rate. Only the patient can judge which is to be preferred. Physicians who routinely advise surgery on the basis of the five-year survival rate may be leading some patients to the wrong choice.

Thus there remains an important role for patient information and choice of therapy in conjunction with professional advice, in selecting among available outcomes and perhaps taking account *inter alia* of their cost. But the prospects for elimination or significant reduction in informational asymmetry as to the effects of health care on health appear to be very small. Patient education is not a substitute for professional regulation.[9] Indeed all of what presently passes for "health education," other than rather banal exhortations to eat a balanced diet and get more exercise and sleep, include recommendations to see one's doctor, dentist, or other provider more frequently, and to comply with their instructions. In any other context this would be easily recognized, not as education, but as marketing of professional services.

THE AGENCY RELATIONSHIP AND THE PROBLEM OF INCOMPLETENESS

The professional relationship can therefore be interpreted as a social response to situations in which the informational asymmetry between

---

[8] In chapter 1 this same distinction was discussed from the point of view of a society deciding how much to allocate to health care—again the ultimate question is not a professional one.

[9] The strong interest in information and self-care among certain groups of females in particular appears to be a response to predominantly male providers who are alleged to use expertise in the technical domain to try to impose their own preferences in the outcome domain, *i.e.*, to enforce by control of information and access to other facilities or commodities, choices which lead to the health outcomes providers think patients ought to want, whether or not they do.

parties to certain types of transactions is perceived as sufficiently pronounced that independent, arm's-length transactions would permit one party to exploit the other, and to impose severe and possibly irreversible damage.[10] Further, the mitigation of this asymmetry by other social mechanisms is viewed as impractical or impossible (Arrow 1963). Thus an occupational role is professionalized, in economic analysis, insofar as it involves a conflict of interest between acting as an economic principal, on one's own behalf, and acting as an agent, consciously and deliberately serving the interests of someone else even at the expense of one's own. The professional-as-agent assumes responsibility for directing the health care utilization of the patient, not as a profit-maximizing seller of care, but as an agent trying to choose what the patient would have chosen, had she been as well-informed as the professional. Thus the problem of asymmetrical information is to a degree at least circumvented, as the patient's "decisions" are based on the much better information available to the provider.

If this agency relationship were complete, the professional would take on entirely the patient's point of view and act as if she *were* the patient. All consumption choices made for the patient by the provider would be made so as to maximize the patient's well-being, subject to constraints imposed by income and prices. In this Hippocratic ideal case, there would be no remaining market failure due to incomplete information. The "physician-patient pair" would form the transacting unit on the demand side of the market, would be in fact the consumer, and this centaur-like creature would combine the information of the provider with the objectives and constraints of the patient. Assuming that providers were as close as is practical to fully informed, the market for health care would display no further informational problems.

It would, however, display some other problems. The perfect agent cannot at the same time be an economic principal—unless she is also a perfect schizophrenic. The provider has interests of her own—income, leisure, professional satisfaction, which are partially congruent and partly in conflict with those of the patient. The "perfect agent" would need a split brain, one half advising the patient solely in the patient's interest, the other half reacting to the patient's resulting consumption choices in a self-interested, own-welfare maximizing way. Economic analyses which assume self-interested, profit or income maximizing providers must either implicitly assume such schizophrenia as well, or else assume away the

---

[10] The Ontario Professional Organizations Committee (Trebilcock *et al.* 1979) uses a more general definition in which professionalization is intended to protect "vulnerable interests," not defended in an arm's-length transaction, whether or not they are parties to the transaction. But the significance of this extension is primarily outside health care.

asymmetry of information problem and the agency relationship entirely (thus removing any justification for regulation). Not surprisingly, such analyses rarely spell out their assumptions in detail.

In fact, however, the agency relationship is incomplete. There are several important sources of divergence between the objectives of the patient and those which will be sought by provider-agents advising or directing patient utilization. The primary public justification for regulation, particularly professional self-regulation, is to protect providers from competitive market pressures—both competition among themselves and market entry by non-professionals—which would tend to degrade or destroy the agency relationship. In the unregulated environment the consumer cannot in general tell which providers are genuinely acting in her interest and which are only pretending; and if the latter behaviour is more profitable it will prevail in the long run.[11] But protection from competitive forces does not remove all the sources of incompleteness in the agency relationship, and indeed provider regulation as currently applied in Canada generates additional forms of resource mis-allocation. Such regulation may still be preferable to none at all, but there is room for improvement.

In the first place, the provider is not trained to respond to, and cannot in fact know, the patient's more general interests. The idealized long-time family physician may have understood his patients as whole persons, but few professionals can hope, or care, to have this knowledge in the modern world. Thus the provider-as-agent will direct and provide care so as to improve his patients' health, not to maximize their well-being in a general sense. Moreover as noted above it is a frequent criticism of much health care practice that it focusses on illness not wellness, cure not prevention. This could be interpreted as saying that the professional provider seeks, not to maximize health status as such, but to provide any and all health care which will contribute to health for given levels of other activities and services.[12] The professional provider might reasonably retort that she cannot control all the other consumption choices which

---

[11] Some theoretical analyses assume that informational asymmetry disappears in the long run, that patient information about specific services, or providers, progressively improves in such a way as to drive out or at least limit quackery. But this class of assumptions lacks any support beyond analytic convenience, and loses the essence of the patient's problem. For her there may not *be* a long run!

[12] The patient's well-being $U[X_i, ... HS(HC, X_i)]$ depends on health and other things. The "perfect agent" in conjunction with the patient, would direct use of HC and all other X_i, X_j so as to maximize U (for a given budget constraint and prices, but how would perfect agents also set the prices of their own services?) The real-life provider may try to direct health care use to a point where $\partial HS/\partial HC = 0$, taking little account of the internal structure of the $HS(\ )$ function (prevention, in a general sense) or of the patient's marginal rate of substitution between HS and the various other X_i.

affect health or well-being generally; nevertheless the result will be over-provision of health care relative both to other factors affecting health status, and to other non-health sources of well-being. Costs of care, in the form of either direct disutility or other consumption opportunities foregone, are likely to be denigrated or ignored.[13]

Thus one source of incompleteness in the agency relationship is that the provider may respond to an incomplete or biased perception of the patient's interests. Related to this, the provider's perception of technical efficacy, the relationship between health care and health, may also be incomplete or biased. The "perfect agent" is assumed to be perfectly informed about health care technology and its application to a particular patient, the real life provider is not. And the combination of professional training with the perfectly natural human desire to "do good" (or more important, to have done good) for one's patients leads to an overestimate of the efficacy of interventions in general, relative to what can be scientifically substantiated. The urge to "do something" in the face of distress, and the self-limiting character of much illness, lead naturally to such bias in the clinical setting—hence the long history of popular therapies later shown ineffective (Banta *et al.* 1981).

Information is, however, more usefully considered in relative rather than absolute terms. No real-life individual or institution ever attains "perfect" information about anything. A more reasonable standard or objective for social organization is that decisions should be taken, and resources allocated, on the basis of information which is "optimal" in terms of the balance between its cost and its expected usefulness. Resources can be wasted if effort and expense are devoted to gathering information which yields little or no improvement in decision-making; one can collect too much as well as too little information.

The agency relationship could therefore be considered "complete" if the professional-as-agent bases recommendations for care use on technical information on effectiveness which is optimal in this more limited sense. The "perfect agent" is not "perfectly" informed, because that would represent an over-allocation of resources to information acquisition. A complete agency relationship would, and should, be based on some degree of incomplete information.

Unfortunately there is no a priori reason to assume that any particular organizational setting, whether competitive market or regulated environment, will generate this optimal level of information. Different forms of delivery system organization create different patterns of biases in practitioner information and behaviour. The possibilities for improving the

---

[13] This is particularly apparent in the case of insured care, when providers recommend care of limited usefulness (diagnostic testing, *e.g.*) because it is "free." It is not, however, free to consumer/patients collectively, as it must be paid for in premiums or taxes.

level of provider information, and the efficiency or effectiveness of resultant patterns of health care utilization, by modifying the organization of health care delivery, are significant policy issues for discussion below.

Public support for continuing professional education, technology assessment, and research into and particularly dissemination of information about the effectiveness of current patterns of health care practice, all address perceived imperfections in the information available to providers, and reflect a belief that there is information available in, or accessible at reasonable cost to, the wider society which would improve physician decision-making and resource allocation.

PROFESSIONALISM AS A RESPONSE TO INCOMPLETE AGENCY

But the incompleteness of the agency relationship is not solely, or even primarily, a result of the imperfect information, on either effectiveness of care or patient preferences, available to agents. Even if the professional had all the information available in the mind of God, perfect agency would also require the use of that information to direct the patient's utilization, solely in the patient's interests, at complete disregard for her own. In fact, such complete selflessness is rarely found, among professionals or anyone else. The professional's influence on the utilization decision will in general respond to some blend of the patient's and the provider's interests, with the proportions in the blend varying according to the circumstances of each. Rarely will the professional seek to influence utilization in ways which she knows to be harmful to the patient, solely in her own interests. But practical health care situations are sufficiently complex and uncertain that the provider's perceptions of patient interests can readily adjust themselves to accommodate provider interests as well.

The existence of the balance is critical. The perfect agent has no independent existence as economic principal. The non-agent, arm's-length seller, however well-informed or however complex the commodity or service, looks only after her own interests and expects the buyer to do likewise. Only the professional as real-life incomplete agent has a foot in both camps and has to wrestle with the conflict of interest resulting from being a party to both sides of the health care transaction.

Nor is this role restricted to the self-employed professions. All who provide commodities or services in an environment of asymmetric information (or a fortiori restricted or absent patient ability to make rational decisions) are in a position to exploit this asymmetry to their own advantage and the consumer/patient's detriment. Professionalization is a process of trying to mould the objectives of providers, as well as to impose specific conduct regulations on them, so as to limit their willingness to exploit such situations. The marked segregation and peculiar socialization which is traditional in professional training cannot be explained by the technical content of the training itself; in fact the process often appears inimical to education as generally conceived. But it may be understood, in part at least, as a method of changing the objectives of providers so as to enable them to balance the interests of patients against their own in a way not expected of, say, used car salesmen. The training is intended, not just to ensure competence, but to modify behaviour.[14]

In the same way much of professional self-regulation, particularly that of conduct after licensure, appears unrelated to issues of information and competence per se. Rather it is justified as discouraging conduct which would tend to break down the agency relationship. The argument is as old as Adam Smith (at least), that professionals must be protected to some degree from competitive market forces if they are to occupy positions of trust, to seek their patients'/clients' interests as well as, and sometimes at the expense of, their own.[15]

This is not, of course, to suggest that the sole or even the primary motivation for post-entry regulation, or the content of licensure requirements, is maintenance of the agency relationship in the public or consumer interest. Self-regulating professions collectively act as agents on behalf of the public generally, in assuring quality and ethical standards, in the same way as individual professionals act as agents for members of the

---

[14] There are some less idealistic interpretations, in terms of generating the collegiate loyalty necessary for a large group to function as a cartel, as well as psychological interpretations focussing on dealing with uncertainty and stress. Different interpretations are not mutually exclusive.

[15] There is in the economic literature a discussion of the "principal-agent problem" which should not be confused (as its students occasionally do) with the professional relationship and the phenomenon of incomplete agency. In the principal-agent problem, the agent performs certain acts which affect the well-being of both principal and agent. The principal cannot directly control the agent's behaviour, but can within limits influence the way in which the agent's well-being depends on the agent's acts. The principal's problem is to influence the agent's payoff such that the act(s) which most benefit the principal are also those which most benefit the agent and hence will be chosen.

In this formulation the *objectives* of principal and agent are strictly separated; each intends to serve only her own interests. What distinguishes the professional agency relation is that the professional includes part at least of the patient's/client's interests in her own objectives. If, for example, there were some act which the agent could perform which would benefit the agent at the expense of the principal, but which the principal (or anyone else) could never detect, the professional-as-perfect-agent would not do it. The professional-as-imperfect-agent might, but not always, or some would and some would not. In the usual formulation of the principal-agent problem, the agent always does it. Such an agent is not a professional and no agency relationship, as the concept is used here, exists.

public (Tuohy and Wolfson 1977, 1978). And this collective agency relation is also incomplete. There are numerous examples of self-regulatory bodies promulgating regulations whose primary or sole intent appears to be the economic or more general professional well-being of their members. Almost all students of the collective agency relationship (except for representatives of the self-governing professions themselves) have concluded that reform of the institutions of self-government is necessary to redress the balance of public and private interests served. Few, however, have suggested outright abolition.

Indeed Tuohy and Wolfson stress the parallel and mutually reinforcing nature of the individual and collective agency roles. Public perceptions of the professional-patient relationship provide the political support for self-government, just as self-government provides the institutional framework to protect the agency relation at the individual level, and they argue that neither can long persist without the other. The situation of pharmacy, whose individual agency role has largely disappeared, makes an interesting test case. Pharmacists' organizations have sought, thus far with very limited success, to recreate at least the impression of an agency role on behalf of buyers of drugs. And the self-regulatory privilege of pharmacy collectively has come under searching questioning. Nevertheless self-regulation persists.

There is yet another source of incompleteness in the agency relationship, which is for the future perhaps the most difficult of all to deal with. The perfect agent acts perfectly, but solely, on behalf of her patient or client. But when professionally directed services are collectively funded, whether by public or private insurance or public provision, the agent is simultaneously determining the level of others' resources to be devoted to the patient's well-being—a political, distributional function as well as the exercise of technical expertise. If the health status curve (Figure 1-3) displays a very small positive slope throughout the relevant range, the professional's attempts to draw on collective resources will be unbounded (or bounded only by perceptions of the negative direct effects of health care on patient well-being).

Thus the institutional responses to the first two forms of market failure, uncertainty of illness incidence and external effects, create further problems of agency. Optimal resource allocation requires the physician to act as agent, not only of her patient, but of the wider society as well. Three sets of interests, not two, are involved. Insofar as collective financing mitigates the conflict between provider and user in the economic domain, it creates a new economic conflict between both together and the paying agency, or rather those who finance it. Efforts to train "cost-conscious physicians" represent attempts to extend the agency role to respond to this public dimension, but it is hard to be optimistic about the results.

Yet the alternatives, if providers do not accept this extended agency role, appear to be only three, and in the long run only two. One can accept, for a time, ever expanding costs, as the United States has done. One can directly restrict the numbers of and facilities available to providers, as Canada has done. Or one can cut back on collective funding and ration access to services once again by ability to pay, as the United States appears to be in the process of doing.[16] There do not seem to be any other choices. But there are, as will be touched on below, a number of different ways of expressing these choices in public policy.

THE IMPLICATIONS OF INFORMATIONAL ASYMMETRY FOR ECONOMIC ANALYSIS

The asymmetry of information between user and provider of health care is its most fundamental peculiarity as a commodity, and the source of the most serious failures of market processes as resource allocators in this field. Its implications for the theoretical analysis of resource allocation in health care, as well as for the organization of its delivery and finance, are profound.

The institutional responses to asymmetry—professionalization, self-regulation, and the development of an agency relation between individual transactors and between the professions and society collectively—make the conventional economic theory of supply inapplicable to these markets. Professionals themselves, and the institutions for which they act as gate-keepers, supply goods and services in response to diverse and complex motivations, under equally diverse and complex constraints which we shall attempt to analyse in more detail in subsequent chapters. What is clear, however, is that they do not behave as, and cannot sensibly be represented as, competitive for-profit firms, at arm's-length from their customers, supplying services in response to competitively determined input and product prices.[17] A well-defined supply curve, showing amounts offered for sale by price-taking suppliers at each of a series of market prices, does not exist. Nor is the simple theory of monopoly applicable to the behaviour of large numbers of more or less co-ordinated suppliers, partly co-operating and partly competitive with each other.

Accordingly there is no tendency for market forces to lead to health care being offered at a price equal to its marginal cost. In the absence of insurance or subsidy, the monopoly power inherent in regulation will lead to prices above marginal cost, and hence *ceteris paribus* (which they

---

[16] Whether this will contain overall costs, or merely shift the pattern of care use and the distribution of economic burden within an ever growing total, remains to be seen.

[17] They can of course be so represented, and often are, but the resulting analyses are usually more misleading than enlightening. Elegance may be gained, but relevance is lost.

are not) to underprovision of health care.[18] This potential for monopoly exploitation is mitigated by the extension of the agency relation to the economic domain. Sliding-scale billing, *ex ante* anticipated uncollectable accounts, and overtly free care in the pre-insurance era indicated some provider concern for the patient's economic as well as physical well-being. But the extension of private insurance coverage led to steady increases in prices; United States unions frequently observed with some bitterness that whenever they negotiated insurance coverage for medical care, physicians' fees rose. And in Canada physician fees and incomes rose steadily relative to general levels of prices and incomes, all through the period of growth of private coverage (Barer and Evans 1983). Whether one interprets this phenomenon as direct agency behaviour—physicians raising prices because the burden of prices to (individual) patients is reduced—or indirect—exploitation of the monopoly power conferred by self-regulation which in turn rests on agency—the message is the same. Insurance coverage combined with non-competitive pricing behaviour leads to price escalation. Monopsonistic and compulsory insurance with negotiated prices can control this; private competitive insurance cannot.

Hence the asymmetry of information problem, and its associated in-stitutional responses, provide powerful support for the Canadian decision to provide health insurance directly, not just to subsidize private coverage (Evans 1983). Once the supply side of health care delivery has by reg-ulation been largely exempted from control by market forces, direct con-trol of prices and incomes through the insurance mechanism (or directly, as by Canada's Anti-Inflation Board or the United States Economic Sta-bilization Program) follows. Alternatively one must rely on a partial insurance mechanism which inflicts sufficient economic pain on users as to restrain suppliers through the agency relation itself. But a combination of self-regulation plus full or relatively generous insurance coverage with-out direct controls leaves price escalation unbounded.[19]

---

[18] The case of the supplier as perfectly price-discriminating monopolist is a bit more involved, as the marginal unit of care sold will be priced at marginal cost, and hence apparently the level of provision is optimal. But it is a *different* optimum from the competitive one. The wealth transfer which results from perfect price discrimination will shift the *MRS* between income and leisure for self-employed providers, raising the opportunity cost of own-time, which is the principal component of the cost of such firms. So, if a non-discriminating self-employed monopolist begins to discriminate, output will indeed shift to where (marginal) $P = MC$, but the whole MC curve will rise. The result could be rising or falling output. This ambiguity reflects the flabbiness of the Pareto optimality criterion, and its sensitivity to wealth distribution. The non-discriminating monopolist is producing less than (Pareto) optimal output, but when she shifts to perfect price discrimination the result is optimal output even if output falls!

[19] This conclusion would not necessarily apply in the event of a radical reconstruction of the supply side along the lines of the U.S. HMOs (Enthoven 1980), but this raises issues deferred to subsequent chapters.

Even more significant, however, are the implications of asymmetry and agency for the "demand side" of the health care utilization process. The demand curve, as drawn in Figures 2-2 or 3-1, assumes that independent consumers of care are not directly influenced by suppliers in their decisions to use care, or alternatively that if such direct influence exists, its level is determined external to the market process itself. Non-agent suppliers simply offer care at the going market price; consumer/patients decide to buy, or not, after consulting their own tastes and wealth and the price they would have to pay. Perfect agents simply supply perfect, or best available, information to buyers. But real-life incomplete or imperfect agents supply information which will depend partly on technical considerations and partly on their own (and the buyer's) economic and professional circumstances. The demand curve is shifted by the advice suppliers give.

This direct influence over demand, sometimes referred to as supplier-induced demand, is precisely what the agency relation is supposed to achieve. Ill-informed buyers are protected, by provider advice, from consumption of unnecessary or harmful services (either inappropriate or poor quality) and also from failure to consume needed services. The provider directs the use of her own services, and of co-operant hospital, drug, prosthetic, and other services. Thus the quantity of care buyers wish to purchase, at any given price to themselves, depends on the advice, direction, permission they receive from suppliers.[20]

The Naive Medico-Technical model, referred to above, recognizes this dependence, but assumes that provider advice is in turn determined by unambiguous externally set and uniform "need" standards and hence insensitive to price. Insofar as actual consumer choices are price-responsive, the reduction in use in response to prices represents "unmet need" due to compliance problems or economic barriers to care. These should be removed by subsidy or public insurance, and by consumer education. But the socially "right" level of provision is the need standard interpreted by the provider. The Naive Economic model simply ignores

---

[20] This approach to health care utilization most emphatically does *not* assume that the decision to utilize care is insensitive to price. *Ceteris paribus*, including among the *ceteris* the consumer's perceptions of health status and the effectiveness of health care, one would expect use to respond negatively to price in the conventional way, through increased reluctance to initiate episodes of care or increased questioning of/non-compliance with provider advice (though the elasticity of response is unlikely to be large overall). The critical point is that the *ceteris* are *not paribus*, since the patient's perceptions of both health status and health care efficacy are directly influenced by the provider. And these influences, in the incomplete agency framework, will depend on the providers' circumstances, economic, professional, and personal. Thus an increase in provider supply, *e.g.*, lowers average incomes and workloads, and the response is to advise increased amounts of servicing. The "demand curve" shifts laterally (Stoddart and Barer 1981; Barer, Evans, and Stoddart 1979).

the existence of need, or of the professional agency relationship, and takes as socially "right" that level of care which consumers, however informed, value (at the margin) at or above its marginal resource cost.

PROVIDER INFLUENCE OVER DEMAND: NORMATIVE AND POSITIVE IMPLICATIONS

The direct influence of providers on use, however, has both normative and positive consequences. At the normative level, willingness-to-pay can no longer be interpreted as reflecting consumer preferences. Uninformed consumers may make choices which, if fully informed, they would regret. But so may those accepting professional advice. And to define patients responding to professional advice as fully informed, so as to give their utilization normative significance—whatever the observed level of use, it must be right—is a dodge worthy only of Pangloss.[21] Even Pangloss would have a little difficulty in rationalizing the dramatic swings that we observe inter-regionally and inter-temporally in specific patterns of utilization—as for example when identifiable providers move into or out of an area. (But of course he could do it!) If providers in fact exercise significant or predominant influence over utilization levels or patterns we can no longer appeal to consumer sovereignty as a normative justification for accepting those patterns, but must instead judge them against more general criteria of what we, either collectively or as individuals, consider appropriate and are willing to pay for. In this judgement process, "need" standards have obvious appeal. The fully informed patient, whose behaviour we rarely if ever observe,[22] might reasonably be expected, as a first approximation, to value care according to its contribution to health status, adjusted for its direct disutility. Consumption of *ex ante* ineffective or harmful care is a mistake, not a representation of consumer preferences for care per se, and optimal resource allocation processes should not respond to such mistakes.[23]

At the positive level, the shifting of the "demand curve" in response

---

[21] "All is for the best, in the best of all possible worlds"—which follows from the assumption that Divine Providence is both beneficent and omnipotent. The significance of Pangloss is that, given his assumptions, he cannot be refuted. But he can be held up to ridicule, as Voltaire did.

[22] In particular we do not observe her among physicians, or their families. They are particularly vulnerable to overestimates of the efficacy of therapy, for quite apparent reasons.

[23] Of course in an uncertain world some forms of care will turn out after the fact to be useless or even harmful—some level of error is to be expected. But care which could reasonably be *forecast*, on the basis of presently available or reasonably accessible information, to be useless or harmful, clearly represents inappropriate care.

to provider advice modifies or reverses the pattern of interactions among price, quantity, and capacity data predicted by "conventional" economic analysis. For example, an exogenous expansion in the supply of physicians or of hospital beds should, if one assumes a stable demand schedule as in Figures 2-2 or 3-1, lead to a drop in prices and an increase in quantities demanded and utilized.[24] Yet it is notorious in health care studies that increases in capacity tend to translate directly into utilization increase, with or without a corresponding price decrease.

Indeed in the case of physicians, there is usually a *positive* correlation between available supply and price, which can be interpreted as the result of physicians adjusting their behaviour to seek some sort of "target" income. When average workloads and incomes fall, due to exogenous increases in supply, physicians change their practice patterns to increase utilization. But if this expansion is insufficient to maintain income "targets," prices will be increased as well.[25]

EMPIRICAL EVIDENCE OF "SUPPLIER-INDUCED DEMAND"

In the hospital sector, the direct influence of providers on use is reflected in the universal observation that bed availability is the principal determinant of bed use—"A built bed is a filled bed"—sometimes referred to as Roemer's Law (Roemer 1961). The direct effect of availability on use, long known to health care people, has also been demonstrated statistically in numerous jurisdictions, independently of price change (if any), demographic factors, or any other measured variables which might be expected to influence use. The relationship does not hold for all beds; paediatric and obstetric use in particular does not appear to respond to low observed occupancy rates. And even for medical and surgical beds, the "Law" is not literally true, additional capacity is not 100 percent occupied; and indeed statistical analyses suggest that occupancy rates do fall as capacity expands ("a built bed is only half filled"). But overall bed capacity emerges from study after study as the single most important

---

[24] Universal first dollar insurance is in theory no bar to this price adjustment; suppliers could always pay rebates, in kind if not in cash.

[25] The "target income" model is justly suspect among economists, because of its rather *ad hoc* flavour and its failure to explain the origins of targets. Further, physician real incomes are not as stable as it seems to suggest. It can, however, be recast in a more sophisticated version based on a general model of physician utility maximization (see below, chapter 7) which allows for provider discretion over both prices and quantities. Such a model predicts behaviour rather similar to the "target income" approach.

factor influencing hospital inpatient utilization, and the level of bed capacity at which use would appear to stop responding to increases is double or triple current capacity or need estimates.[26]

For facility planning purposes, this observation has the fundamental implication that there is no external "demand" standard, based on observed utilization, from which "needed" levels can be inferred. Providers will themselves determine use on the basis of, *inter alia*, available capacity. For our purposes, however, the significant point of the dependence of use on capacity is that it reflects the direct influence of providers on demand. When occupancy rates are low, physicians may find hospital access less costly to themselves, or administrators may in a variety of ways encourage use, but whatever the linkages, physicians react by admitting more patients and/or keeping them longer. And patients accept the recommendations quite independently of any price shifts.

Hospital use is of course a reflection of patterns of medical practice. But one can also examine those patterns directly, to observe the role of provider influence independently of price. There are numerous examples of dramatic shifts over time in utilization of particular procedures or services which are traceable to provider, not patient, behaviour. During the 1970s the rate of performance of tonsillectomy, for example, dropped by half to two-thirds, all across Canada. Physician training patterns and attitudes had changed, and their criteria for recommending the operation became much tighter. But there was no change in prices faced by patients, and no evidence of independent patient choice at all. The agency relationship worked as intended—new information or education led directly to new patterns of utilization without mediation by the price system.

Over a longer period, the steady reduction in frequency of house calls responded to some combination of physicians' professional concerns about providing adequate care in the home environment, and their economic concerns about the opportunity cost of travel and visit time. The exogenous demand model predicts that these concerns would lead to a rise in the relative cost of house calls, and a drop in the quantity demanded by consumers. But this did not happen. Relative prices of house calls did not increase; physicians simply refused to make them, and educated their patients not to ask for them. Yet another example, the dramatic fluctuation in hysterectomy rates in Saskatchewan in the early 1970s reported by Dyck *et al.* (1977) was apparently a response by surgeons to the threat of audit by the insurance commission—of which patients were of course unaware.

---

[26] Of course use can respond to capacity in the trivial sense that when there is a "shortage"—desired use exceeds capacity available—more capacity will permit proportionately more use. But "Roemer's Law" applies in situations of average bed occupancy from near 100 percent on down to 50 percent or below.

Further examples could be multiplied almost endlessly, of individual procedures whose rate of performance has varied significantly in response to factors affecting providers, not patients, and without price adjustment. At the aggregate level this influence appears to underlie a sort of "Roemer's Law" for physicians as well, that more capacity leads to more use. During the period 1971-72 to 1980-81, physician supply per capita in Canada rose 2.7 percent per year, insurance coverage was universal throughout, and utilization per physician not only kept pace, but rose 1.7 percent per year (Table 7-5). Taking a longer view, from 1960 to 1981 the physician to population ratio rose 63.5 percent. And while increases in collection ratios make it difficult to identify true fee levels during the 1960s, it appears that physician workloads expanded by at least 1.5 percent per year throughout that twenty-one year period, and probably over 2 percent. There were very large swings in average physician relative incomes—up very fast from 1960 to 1971, down equally fast thereafter—but these were the result of adjustments in fee levels, not workloads (Barer and Evans 1983).

There may be some point at which saturation occurs, but we have yet to find it. And inter-regional comparisons suggest that there is still plenty of room for expansion. Cross-regional studies show physician use per capita varying almost directly in proportion to physician availability, even at levels of availability well above the cross-regional average.

Nor are these patterns solely the result of Canada's universal public insurance system. Similar patterns are observed in the United States, where about one-third of physician service costs are paid out of pocket. There, too, cross-sectional studies show utilization *and price* of medical services varying positively with physician availability. And the SOSSUS study of the mid-1970s (American College of Surgeons and American Surgical Association, 1975) made the point that despite an apparent surplus of surgeons (such that operative workloads were on average so low as to lead to questions of continuing competence), overall surgeon workloads, fees, and incomes steadfastly refused to fall. If anything, prices went up.

Similar behaviour is found in dentistry in Canada, despite the predominance of self-pay and private insurance relationships. A combination of community water fluoridation, (perhaps) better diet and oral hygiene, and increases in dental manpower and capacity has led to a reduction in the prevalence of dental disease and (in some quarters) allegations of an excess supply of dentists, at least relative to what the private market will support. But this surplus, if it exists, has placed no detectable downward pressure on dental fees. Rather, fees have continued to rise relative to the general price level (Table 7-3). Instead, the profession is responding with quite explicit promotion of care which is cosmetic as much as health-oriented, as well as of greatly expanded "preventive" care of undetermined efficacy. The evidence suggests, then, that in health care markets generally, prices do not appear to adjust so as to equate supply and demand, rather both price and utilization are directly influenced by providers. Part of the influence is through agency and advice to patients, and part through the control over their collective economic and professional conduct conferred by self-regulatory power.

PROVIDER INFLUENCE AND THE MEDICO-TECHNICAL MODEL: SOME DISCREPANCIES

One might anticipate that, as in the dentistry case, the role of providers in influencing utilization would be most prominent in those services which are both provider-directed and relatively discretionary on "need" grounds, and to some extent this is true. One also might expect that the initial decision to seek care for an illness episode would be beyond the provider's influence, while well-defined conditions for which care of a particular type was mandatory would leave little room for discretion. There is also some evidence to support this view. But in fact physicians and patients educate each other about appropriate cues for initiation of an episode, so that over time changing standards of medical practice can modify patient decisions. And significant inter-regional variations in treatment patterns are often found for care which might appear mandatory.

Indeed the wide variations across regions and providers in patterns of utilization or choice of technique of care (visit rates, rates of hospital admission and lengths of stay, rates of performance of diagnostic and therapeutic interventions), without corresponding observable variations in outcome, suggest that the Medico-Technical model is also unsatisfactory as an explanation of observed utilization patterns. While it is clear that providers exert predominant influence over levels and patterns of utilization, it is not at all clear what criteria guide them in this process. But on the basis of the often weak (or non-existent) links from utilization to outcome, we may presume that some patients, at least, would if fully informed choose different patterns and levels of care. There is considerable scope for improving the completeness of the agency relationship, or supplementing it with additional information or constraints.

While the influence of providers over utilization is reinforced by the regulatory structure of health care, it does not follow that an across-the-board deregulatory policy would necessarily yield superior economic performance. Such a blunt instrument would probably lead to significantly more competition in pricing behaviour. But providers' allegations that it would also lead to significant increases in provider-generated inappropriate utilization, at least within the present structure of health care delivery, cannot be lightly dismissed. The problem of informational asymmetry is real, and the agency relationship, while it may be in some respects unsatisfactory, incomplete, and inefficient, is a real response. The problem cannot be wished away by wholesale "deregulation," much less by a phoney deregulation which would remove direct public oversight but leave the private regulatory structure of licensure and collusion intact.

Nor does the profound influence of providers on utilization imply that the result is wholly unresponsive either to economic forces or to objective "need" considerations. The fact that care patterns for similar patients vary considerably across regions, and from provider to provider, does not mean that a provider's reaction to a particular problem is arbitrary or random. The primary influence on utilization levels and patterns is obviously the provider's perception of patient health status and of the potential benefits from available diagnostic and therapeutic manoeuvres. And the degree of discretion in care permitted by prevailing best practice standards will vary greatly from one condition to another.

But there remains, particularly for diagnostic and monitoring activities, a broad zone of uncertainty in which optimal treatment and the limits of efficacy have not been scientifically established. In this zone, the provider can exercise considerable discretion before encountering ethical constraints. Economic considerations, conscious or otherwise, then can exert an effect on preferred practice patterns, and on advice to patients. Such considerations may be confounded, of course, with an ethic of "doing everything possible" for patients, subject to constraints on time and energy, so that when a physician sees fewer patients (because of a rise in the physician/population ratio, *e.g.*), she feels able to do more for each. Whether this is interpreted as more comprehensive care, or generation of utilization to maintain incomes, matters little to the outcome.

AGENCY AND THE EFFECT OF ECONOMIC FACTORS ON UTILIZATION

But patient initiative and compliance, as well as provider perceptions of patient ability to pay or comply, also affect utilization, and these too may respond to economic factors. Willingness to contact a provider, or to accept recommended treatment, is clearly related to out-of-pocket cost. The "demand curve" is not vertical. And this price sensitivity is likely to be greater for types of care about which patients feel themselves to be better informed, or less at risk of death or grave disability. Studies of ambulatory medical care use, in particular, have shown patient response to prices, although those which allow for health status differences as well usually show price responses swamped by health effects. As one might anticipate, the primary and dominant determinant of patient decisions to seek and use care, and provider decisions to recommend and provide it, is illness.

What does not follow from observed price sensitivity by individual patients, however, is either that higher out-of-pocket charges to patients will lower overall use, or that any changes in utilization which occur will be among the least needed forms of care.

On the first point, the argument from individual to group response rests on the assumption that provider recommendations will not change as patient-initiated contacts or compliance with recommendations fall. Such passivity in response to falling incomes and workloads is precisely what the incomplete agency relationship suggests will *not* occur, for any plausible formulation of provider objectives. Instead, providers will provide more care to those patients who come. As a result, overall use may not fall at all, and utilization will shift from more to less price sensitive patients or types of care. Such sensitivity is usually associated with income, and indeed studies in Canada have found that the principal effect of introducing or removing direct charges is to redirect care from poor to rich or rich to poor, whether or not the overall volume of use falls.[27]

Whatever the response of utilization to economic factors, the relationship of this use to need is an entirely separate issue. Policy analysis using demand curves and willingness-to-pay as normative criteria for determining what levels and patterns of care ought or ought not (from a broader social perspective) to be provided, rests on a positive assumption of fully, or adequately, informed consumers as well as on individualist ideology. Asymmetry of information makes this assumption untenable, unless salvaged by the equally unattractive perfect agency model of professionals. So we cannot assume a priori that the utilization which is foregone in response to economic factors is either technically least necessary, or socially least valued.

Empirically, we find evidence that illness and low income are correlated, as are price sensitivity and low income. Moreover, several studies have shown that under universal insurance, low-income people now use

---

[27] Some studies show an overall fall, others do not (Beck and Horne 1978; Enterline *et al.* 1973). The difficulty in interpretation is that an increase in physician incomes would tend *ceteris paribus* to lead to less demand generation and lower overall use. So a pure demand-side, patient response can only be measured if physician incomes are held constant in real terms. The RAND experiment in the U.S. is designed such that the effects of patient responses to charges which are felt by any one provider should be trivial or undetectable; accordingly the *ceteris paribus* assumption should apply to provider behaviour, and the estimated responses (Newhouse *et al.* 1982) should represent the slope of a stable demand curve for part at least of the population. Unfortunately, for just that reason, such results give no information at all about what the effects would be of a general program of increased charges to patients, which *would* (if it affected use) lower each provider's income and workload. The experimental results, by design, cannot be generalized.

more services per (age-adjusted) capita than average, whereas in the pre-insurance period they used less; and this use appears correlated with greater illness (Boulet and Henderson 1979; Siemiatycki *et al.* 1980; Broyles *et al.* 1983). On balance, then, it appears that unless prices faced by users are scaled proportionately to their economic resources *and* expected illness status, user charges will selectively deter low-income, not "frivolous," users. If such detailed scaling were feasible, we simply do not know whether any resulting impact on the mix or (if any) overall volume of health care use would be to increase or to reduce the proportion of "unnecessary" care.

The responsiveness of health care utilization to economic factors, as to any other, cannot be analyzed separately from provider objectives, constraints, and behaviour. To formulate models of "demand" for medical or hospital care, or pharmaceuticals, which exclude the direct influence of the physician, is to try to stage "Hamlet" without the Prince of Denmark. Equally, however, we shall see that one cannot explain the behaviour of providers without reference to at least their perceptions of patients' interests and conditions. The "supply" and "demand" sides of the health care "market" interpenetrate each other to an extent which renders invalid the traditional economic dichotomy of separate spheres of decision linked only by transactions at a given price. The fundamental importance for optimal resource allocation of the rich two-way flow of non-price information between provider and user is recognized by the extensive regulatory structure of health care delivery, which is intended *inter alia* to preserve and promote both the quantity and especially the quality of this flow. Resulting utilization patterns are neither "demand" nor "supply" in the conventional sense; thus we cannot use the conventional demand and supply apparatus in the conventional way, if at all. Asymmetry of information between provider and user, and the resulting professional agency relation, are the most fundamental sources of the "differentness" of health care as a commodity, in terms of the forms of economic analysis appropriate to its study, as well as the institutional framework which surrounds its organization and delivery. The implications of this asymmetry ramify as we shall see throughout the whole field of health care, prevention, insurance, education and training, investment and research. Absent informational asymmetry, and the uncertainty and externality problems could be dealt with by relatively limited public interventions in private markets.

CHAPTER 5

MARKET FAILURE AND THE EVOLUTION OF HEALTH CARE INSTITUTIONS: A HISTORICAL PARABLE

MARKET FAILURE, POLICY "THERAPIES," AND SIDE EFFECTS: A FIGURATIVE SUMMARY

The analysis of the previous chapters can be summarized and synthesized into an "historical parable," a very much oversimplified description of how the Canadian health care system has developed through time to reach its current state. In this "parable," institutional evolution can be represented as a challenge and response. Each set of institutions arises in response to problems with the preceding set, and in turn generates its own problems.

The general theme of the story is that the nature of health care as a commodity, its intrinsic peculiarities discussed above, leads to certain distinctive forms of "market failure." Such "failure" means that the organization of health care production and distribution through unregulated private markets—purely voluntary exchange processes—governed by the price mechanism, leads to unsatisfactory outcomes. Resources are not allocated to or used in health care production, and/or the care produced is not distributed among users, in a way which most of the members of society find acceptable. Accordingly various forms of intervention, institutional responses, arise in both the public and the private sectors, which either supplement or supplant private market relationships. These interventions—regulation, public subsidy, insurance, private charity, etc.— are anticipated to lead to patterns of resource allocation and/or output distribution in the health care sector which are more generally acceptable to the wider society.[1]

---

[1] Such improvement is not "Paretian" improvement, in the sense of leaving everyone at least as well off as in the pure voluntary exchange case. It may be "potential Paretian" in the sense that where market failure exists, idealized regulation can lead to outcomes in which gainers could compensate losers (though they probably will not do so), but that criterion has well-known problems. "Improvement" probably really means according to some more general Social Welfare Function which the analyst believes she sees revealed by a society's actual behaviour, as well as in the public pronouncements of its opinion leaders or recorders.

But these responses have the problems common to therapy in other fields—they have harmful side effects. Furthermore, multiple therapies for multiple problems result in interactions which often accentuate these side effects. Side effects give rise, in turn, to further institutional responses which have their own strengths and weaknesses, and thus the system evolves through time.

There may or may not be a "final answer," an optimal health care system. Many such have been suggested, and located in hypothetical futures or imaginary pasts, but they tend to differ radically from each other. At present it seems fair to say that if a "best" way of organizing health care delivery exists, it has yet to be found—in Canada or elsewhere.

But there do appear to be better and worse approaches to delivery system design. And while each country's experience is rooted in its own historical and cultural background, it does not appear that that background wholly determines the outcome. Reasonable people may, by taking thought and devoting effort, improve existing systems; conversely, by failure to do so, they can bring on, or permit, deterioration.[2] In making international comparisons of health care systems, Canadians tend to be rather smug, and perhaps with some justification. But reasonable satisfaction with the present is no guarantee of the future.

Looked at another way, while the intrinsic characteristics of health care analysed above may have dictated some pattern of regulatory intervention, they did not necessarily dictate the pattern we have. Nor is there any reason to believe that the pattern of regulation we have is the best which could have been established, even in Canada. Whatever is actual may indeed be rational, but is not necessarily optimal.

What does seem clear, however, is that the market failure problem and the process of institutional evolution are an interactive totality. Theoretically optimal "solutions" to the specific problems of uncertainty, externalities, or asymmetry of information, analysed in isolation from other sources of market failure whether intrinsic or derivative, provide few useful guides to policy. There is little point in controlling the patient's arthritis with a therapy which induces a bleeding stomach ulcer, or even of controlling that by contributing to kidney failure.

The process of institutional evolution may be traced out through time—hence the "historical parable"—so long as it is clearly understood that the tracing *is* a parable. The complex and messy realities of the historical record can (and will) be crammed into a preconceived analytic framework—for which no apologies are offered. But the result does not, it is hoped, do undue violence to what actually occurred in Canada, while it provides a convenient way of interpreting that experience. Moreover the

---

[2] It is, of course, true that at a deeper level this is a pure statement of faith; the Free Will/Determinism question does not appear to be resolvable, at least by the intellect.

framework is general enough that, with only a bit more violence, it can be applied to other countries as well.

Figure 5-1 presents this framework. On the left-hand side are the various intrinsic characteristics of health care as a commodity which give rise to "market failure." In the middle are the various institutional responses to these, their interactions, and their consequences. On the right are a number of potential further policy responses, which are currently being tested or are under discussion in Canada and elsewhere. These are not so much specific policies as clusters of policies, themes, or policy stances. Each is then related back through its label—A, B, . . . E—to the particular stage(s) in the analytic framework which would be its primary focal point.

THE CAUSAL STRUCTURE OF INSTITUTIONAL EVOLUTION

To the upper left of Figure 5-1 is the process of technological extension.[3] While this factor appears in the figure to be the underlying dynamic force in the whole evolutionary process, it is important to remember that it is public *perceptions* of the state of technology, not that technology itself, which give rise to social responses. Looking backward, we may believe that earlier perceptions were in error, and that many older technologies were useless or harmful. But the validity or otherwise of these perceptions, when judged against "absolute" standards of truth (*i.e.*, the perceptions of our own day), is quite separate from their institutional consequences.

Technological extension, over time, has tended to enhance all three of the intrinsic sources of market failure in health care. As the range and complexity of diagnostic and therapeutic interventions expands, and the subtleties of the human organism unfold, the information gap between provider and user of services becomes even larger. Providers specialize and sub-specialize, knowing "more and more about less and less," but, collectively, their information progressively expands relative to that of the patient. And the more powerful and specific their interventions, the more danger follows from mis-application.

By itself, such growth in provider knowledge need not lead to market failure; as noted in chapter 4, it is not the complexity of technology per se, but the difficulty for the user in determining the effects of its consumption on herself which creates problems. And one can think of specific changes in health care which have made, or could make, some forms of self-diagnosis or self-treatment more feasible. But in practice the extension of technology has been such as to accentuate asymmetry of information about the consequences of use.

---

[3] Frequently described as "technical advance," or "progress," but in the health care context a less judgemental label is called for.

FIGURE 5-1
Historical Evolution of Health Care Delivery in Canada

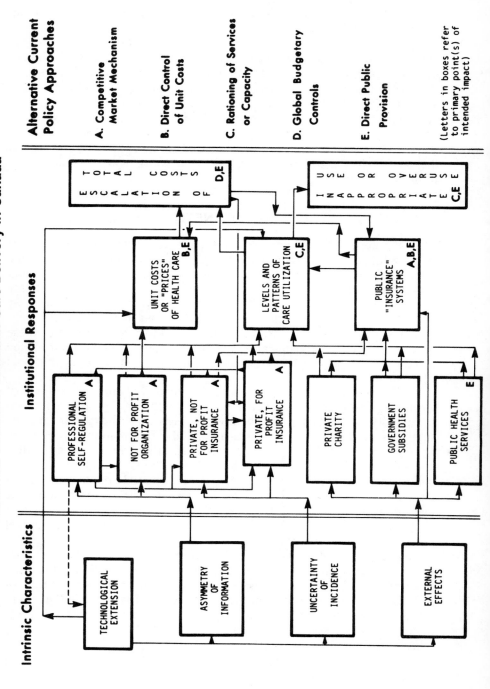

Intrinsic Characteristics

TECHNOLOGICAL EXTENSION

ASYMMETRY OF INFORMATION

UNCERTAINTY OF INCIDENCE

EXTERNAL EFFECTS

Institutional Responses

PROFESSIONAL SELF-REGULATION A

NOT FOR PROFIT ORGANIZATION A

PRIVATE, NOT FOR PROFIT INSURANCE A

PRIVATE, FOR PROFIT INSURANCE A

PRIVATE CHARITY

GOVERNMENT SUBSIDIES

PUBLIC HEALTH SERVICES E

UNIT COSTS OR "PRICES" OF HEALTH CARE B,E

LEVELS AND PATTERNS OF CARE UTILIZATION C,E

PUBLIC "INSURANCE" SYSTEMS A,B,E

TOTAL COSTS OF ESCALATION D,E

INAPPROPRIATE USE OR OVERUSE C,E

Alternative Current Policy Approaches

A. Competitive Market Mechanism

B. Direct Control of Unit Costs

C. Rationing of Services or Capacity

D. Global Budgetary Controls

E. Direct Public Provision

(Letters in boxes refer to primary point(s) of intended impact)

While the principal impact of technology is on informational asymmetry, it also bears upon uncertainty. Fluctuations in health status obviously generate corresponding fluctuations in well-being, and such uncertainties are per se undesirable. In the absence of effective interventions, however, health *care* expenditures will not show similar fluctuations. As noted above, neither colds nor sudden death represent a need for care. But as the range of possibly effective interventions expands, so does the variance of "needed" care and of expenditure. This, too, need not be so in principle; some technologies (polio vaccine, *e.g.*) may lower the variance of financial outlays. But again, the actual pattern of health technology has tended to increase such variance.

The external effects of illness may or may not be accentuated by technological change, but the policy responses to them certainly are. When effective technologies do not exist, externalities may be expressed through prayer and care, or isolation and quarantine. But their impact on health care use is small. As more is perceived to be possible, so more is "needed." Indeed, external effects may flow specifically from the discrepancy between the actual and the possible. The regret, and perhaps outrage, felt by others (as well as oneself!) over a potentially avoidable adverse consequence exceeds that over an uncontrollable "visitation of God." So "needs" are defined in large part by prevailing technology.[4]

The primary institutional responses to these characteristics are displayed in Figure 5-1. Delegation of public authority to the self-regulating professions to control both entry to occupations and service markets, and conduct of persons/firms in those markets, is a response to informational asymmetry, as is the promotion of not-for-profit modes of organization. Private insurance programs respond to uncertainty of illness/expenditure incidence, though as noted in chapter 2, the earlier private not-for-profit insurers responded also to issues of equity, and to professional objectives, in a way that the later for-profits did not. External effects lead to private charitable efforts, to public subsidies for specific individuals or organizations, and to direct public provision of services.

Each of these responses, however, leads to "side effects" (which may in some cases have been specifically intended). Self-regulation by providers confers upon them, individually and collectively, enormous power to control "markets" for their services by a very diverse collection of overt and subtle mechanisms which would be impossible and, in many cases, illegal (indeed, criminal offences) in "ordinary" industries. This

---

[4] This may even be entirely separated from efficacy, in the event that involved others wish, almost as a ritual, to ensure that "everything possible" is done—regardless of its expected payoff, if any. This raises the interesting question of how the range of "everything possible" comes to be defined, and by whom.

has tended to drive up the costs per unit of such services, in a number of different ways, and thus to enhance the incomes of their suppliers.[5]

Non-profit organization is alleged to lead to the same result, permitting "organizational slack" in management, gold-plating of production to the satisfaction of providers rather than users, and rates of wage and salary payment which are above competitive market rates. For-profit firms in a competitive environment would be more strongly motivated to hold down costs, and would be forced to hold down prices.[6]

These unit-cost-inflating tendencies are then reinforced by insurance, of whatever type, which spreads the consequences over large groups and reduces or removes the connection between provider costs and market share. The structure of the insurance contract will determine whether the link is merely attenuated, or severed entirely. Furthermore, the self-regulatory power of providers can be, and has been, used to influence insurance markets so as to encourage the spread of forms of insurance which maximize provider discretion over pricing and patterns of servicing.

But the importance of the insurance process is easily (and frequently) over-emphasized. If providers collectively use their regulatory power to suppress competition over market share, then the hypothetical significance of alternative forms of insurance for the behaviour of individual providers becomes irrelevant. What does seem clear, however, is that the total flow of resources into the health care industry is strongly affected by the level of insurance coverage. This effect shows up partly in increased utilization, but also, to a great extent, in increases in service prices/costs and provider incomes. The relative incomes of physicians and hospital workers rose dramatically throughout the 1950s and 1960s, as first private and then public hospital and medical insurance coverage extended across Canada; the growth of private dental insurance in the 1970s has done the same for dentists (see Table 7-4 below, and Barer and Evans 1983).

The interaction between self-regulation and insurance in their effects on utilization is less clear-cut, particularly since one must be careful about the choice of hypothetical alternatives against which to measure such effects. The role of providers in influencing ("inducing," "steering," "controlling") utilization is well established, and it appears that, as a result, the level and mix of health services used is more sensitive to levels

---

[5] Some argue that the income gains are all dissipated in "rent-seeking," in the long run at least. The case for full dissipation seems unsustainable, but in any case does not affect the discussion here.

[6] Neither argument, of course, extends to for-profit firms in a *non-competitive* environment. Sir John Hicks' famous dictum, "The best of all monopoly profits is the quiet life" points out that for-profit firms sheltered from competitive pressures may also let costs rise for a number of reasons; and even if they do not, a for-profit monopolist will certainly seek to elevate *prices* above costs of production (including normal profit).

of supply and to the professional and economic objectives of providers than it would be if determined by the free consumption choices of hypothetical fully informed buyers. But such buyers exist only in abstract economic models; in reality, the choice may be between professional control and for-profit control in a market of ill-informed users. As we shall develop in more detail below, both theory and experience with for-profit organization (the American clinical laboratory industry, *e.g.*, and, increasingly, the American hospital industry) suggest that professional control and not-for-profit organization may, on balance, *restrain* overall output, or at least lead to less rapid escalation, and may yield a mix more closely related to needs than does the for-profit alternative.

The institutional responses to external effects all tend to influence utilization of health care. In the short run all tend to stimulate use, though public provision of (effective) preventive services, such as immunization, may lower other forms of use in the longer run (including further prevention, as in the case of smallpox). They may also affect mix—disease-specific charities, or public provision of specific services. But general public subsidies, or later, public insurance financed from general tax revenue (whether or not including compulsory "premiums" unrelated to risk) serve merely to influence overall utilization and unit costs.[7]

Indeed, the most general utilization effects probably arise from public subsidy of the training of health personnel, of new facilities construction, and of new technology acquisition. Insofar as utilization tends to be driven by capacity—more doctors ➡ more medical care use, more beds ➡ more hospital use—such subsidies probably have a greater long-run impact on utilization than any other factor. Once again, however, different institutions interlock. If the self-regulating professions could not set very high mandatory entrance standards, entry to the industry (as opposed to particular professions) would not be as dependent on large public subsidies. And if insurance, public or private, did not exist, utilization might not be so dominated by capacity.

FEEDBACK LOOPS IN INSTITUTIONAL RESPONSES: CIRCLES VICIOUS OR OTHERWISE

These effects generate some interesting feedback loops. Both increased use and increased unit cost increase (obviously) total expenditures. This, in turn, encourages further insurance coverage. But the increased cost of such coverage also stimulates the development of private for-profit insurance, offering experience-related coverage to low-risk groups and building on the methods of the non-profits. United States history suggests (Canada

---

[7] Whether up or down depends, as we shall note later, on how they are used.

had not progressed as far down this road when we "went public") that as insurance evolves from non-profit, community-rated to for-profit, experience-rated, self-governing providers will attempt to control the form of insurance. Efforts by whatever form of private insurer to influence the content or the costs of medical practice will, as far as possible, be suppressed (Goldberg and Greenberg 1977).[8] Thus private insurance is also cost-expanding.

The combination of public subsidy programs, and private coverage which is both incomplete and progressively more expensive, creates pressure for public intervention. *Some* form of public insurance seems to follow automatically from the observation that private insurance cannot cover those most in need, or exercise any control over costs or use. At this point one can go to universal or to selective public coverage—Canada or the United States. Both seem to be, or to have been, successful in supporting provision of care for a significant proportion of the population—aged, poor, chronically ill—who would otherwise receive inadequate care or do without. The partial approach does, however, provide much less comprehensive coverage, and drops a non-trivial proportion of the population "through the cracks"—uninsurable by any public or private program (Aday *et al.* 1980).

The key difference seems to be that universal public insurance permits (though it does *not* guarantee) the collective control, both of unit costs of care, and of the overall level and mix of utilization. Thus, while all countries see themselves as facing "crises" of escalating health costs, the problem is measurably and significantly less severe in countries with a universal, sole-source-funded public insurance or delivery system (Canada, the U.K.) than in those with multiple sources of insurance and/or delivery, whether public or private (the United States, Germany).[9] Indeed, provider spokesmen in Canada claim that public insurance leads to "underfunding"—too low a level of costs—because the share of national income devoted to health care has grown more slowly in the 1970s than in previous decades, or in other countries. The impact of the *introduction* of public insurance, however, was clearly to raise service costs, provider incomes, and health expenditures, though its subsequent application has tended, at least in relative terms, to hold them down.

---

[8]   As of 1983, there is some indication in the U.S. that this generalization may be breaking down and that private insurers *will* be able to influence medical practice. But it is too soon to tell, and in any case, leadership in this process has come from the U.S. public (Medicare and Medicaid) programs.

[9]   Sweden might seem an exception, with full public funding and very high cost. The difference appears to be that in Sweden funding sources are decentralized to the regional level, and are essentially "captured" by providers. Sole source funding must be at a level of government high enough to confront provider aspirations; the "political market" must be balanced (Marmor *et al.* 1976; Marmor and Bridges 1980).

Another feedback loop of considerable interest runs from the self-regulatory process to the evolution of technology. The ability to regulate access to, and conduct in, service markets confers a powerful influence over the forms of technology which can be deployed, and therefore over the types of research effort which are likely to be profitable. As we shall see later, this has, been a factor in inducing a bias toward cost—and utilization—expanding technologies, and away from cost reduction.

The effects of the various institutional responses to market failure in the health care sector have thus tended, singly and in combination, to promote increases in both utilization and costs per unit of service. Hence the (almost) universal concern in all developed countries with the overall costs of health care and their rate of expansion. Underlying that concern, however, is the concern that the level and mix of services being provided is inappropriate—too much of the wrong things—and that the process of provision is unnecessarily costly as a result of either or both of technically inefficient production or "too high" incomes of providers. In terms of Figure 1-3, we are both too far out on the curve, and below it, and Figure 5-1 displays some of the processes which have brought us there.[10] This is not primarily a result of incompetence, stupidity, or venality; the present set of problems are a natural result of the social responses to earlier, and quite real, problems of market failure. But they are no less troubling for that.

CURRENT POSSIBILITIES FOR POLICY RESPONSE

An attempt to assess the prospects for alternative "solutions" or at least further responses, requires considerable *hubris* at any stage of discussion. It would also be quite inappropriate here because we have yet to explore the peculiar characteristics, objectives, and behaviour of the providers of health care, as well as of public programs for its regulation, subsidy, or provision. A synopsis is useful, however, because it is the institutional structure of Figure 5-1, responding to the peculiarities of health care as a commodity, which motivates the subsequent discussion. Otherwise health care providers would simply be the private for-profit firms of the micro-economic theory textbooks, or at least their real-world counterparts.

Among the policy themes or responses to the problems of cost escalation and utilization patterns which are displayed in the right-hand panel

---

[10] If this view is not accepted, it is hard to see what meaning can be given to a "cost crisis." A health sector which was expanding its share of resources because it was producing a larger and larger quantity of highly valued outputs, in a highly efficient manner—eliminating the common cold, *e.g.*, and developing ways of dissolving arterial plaques (safely)—would hardly be "in crisis," any more than is the personal computer industry, whose costs/sales are expanding much faster than those in health care.

of Figure 5-1 is a set of proposals which would lead in just that direction. The current enthusiasm in the United States for competition, and for market or market-type institutions to control the production and pricing of health care, focusses attention on the roles of public and self-regulation and of insurance in promoting cost escalation and utilization. The competitive response would be to modify or dismantle the self-regulatory powers of present providers, making entry to the market easier for a variety of alternative providers. It would also remove public subsidies (through the tax system) to particular types of insurance coverage, and would promote, or at least not restrict, the development of combined insurance/service programs.[11]

Much less complex in conception, and probably less far-reaching in effect, are the varieties of direct controls over unit costs, quantities of output, and their product, total cost. The Canadian provincial governments have a number of years of experience of direct fee bargaining with physicians, controlling prices but not (directly) quantities of services supplied. This appears to hold down overall costs, over a time horizon of several years at least, but tends to encourage increased servicing (see Table 7-5 below). American experience during the Economic Stabilization Program was similar, with an even more pronounced utilization response, possibly because measures of utilization were more open to manipulation. Experience with controls on unit costs in hospitals in some American states suggests even more difficult problems of quantity definition and control.

Direct rationing can take place by focussing on specific services—who shall or shall not receive organ transplants or immunizations, *e.g.*—or by limiting overall capacity. Canadian experience so far has been primarily with the latter; efforts have been made to slow the rate of growth of manpower (especially physicians), to lower acute bed-population ratios, and to limit the acquisition of new technology. The anticipated result is less rapid escalation of use rates, with the implicit assumption that

---

[11] The competitive approach in the U.S. is often, perhaps deliberately, confused with a pseudo-competitive alternative, which would neither modify the self-regulatory power of providers, nor promote alternatives to conventional "bill-paying" insurance, but would merely remove public subsidies to insurance and promote high-deductible, high-coinsurance rate coverage. Its proponents' objectives seem to be the removal of public oversight from a privately regulated and cartelized industry, so as to permit further cost escalation. The Canadian counterpart is a push for direct and extra billing by physicians, and "deterrent" charges in hospitals. But out-of-pocket payments by patients at point-of-service are neither necessary nor sufficient for a competitive approach. In this discussion and elsewhere, I assume that public health care policies are designed to address health care problems, not merely to limit government's liability and pass the problems back to patients. The latter interpretation is of course possible, but not very interesting.

providers will determine mix of use in an optimal or at least satisfactory manner. But little attention has been devoted to specific use patterns.

Paralleling capacity constraints, one can simply limit global budgets—overall rates of reimbursement—and let the institutions concerned allocate funds between incomes and outputs. Most effective and least demanding of information in the short run, such "freeze" policies raise questions of long-run viability.

Alternatively, governments could respond by direct takeover of some or all parts of the health services system, to run a public health care service. This would give direct control, at least in principle and subject to the complexities of management in this sector, over levels and patterns of output, and, subject to the problems of wage negotiation, over total outlays.

This last set of policy alternatives serves to highlight the underlying problem. A public health care service concentrates power and responsibility into identifiable hands, but does not tell those hands what to do. The market approach decentralizes decision-making, ostensibly to provide maximum scope for the expression of users' preferences. It will be noted that the letters indicating the intended point of application of different policy approaches in Figure 5-1 show the competitive market policies, A, influencing the farther left-hand side structural characteristics, rather than directly addressing outcomes. The assumption is that a "right" or "best" structure can be found which will automatically induce appropriate outcomes. But just as market failure undermines the appeal of competitive policies, and forces their (serious) advocates to seek other institutional mechanisms to shore up the market, so the imperfections of the political process generate concerns about a totally centralized scheme, both for users and for governments. It is no accident that Canadian provincial governments, while exercising great powers over hospitals, have so far refrained from direct takeover of their boards. The direct restriction alternatives provide greater scope for the more or less independent providers of care to work with the public sector—or against it.

This discussion of the institutional evolution of health care has attempted to trace out the processes whereby cost escalation and utilization problems have emerged in Canada. Most other countries have reached the same set of problems and concerns, although some by rather different roads. Levels of expenditure seem to vary considerably across countries, depending on the road chosen. But in every country the conflict over share of national resources is being fought out between the health system and the rest of society, regardless of the level or share of resources currently devoted to health care. As Figure 5-1 suggests, there is no mechanism within the health care system itself to balance the pressures for expansion. "Equilibrium" or an "appropriate" funding level is viewed by that system as a share of national income which is expanding at each point in time—always a bit more than we now have. The reasons for this perception will be developed in our discussion of the providers of health care, but its implication at this point is that a policy of "no policy," a public decision not to confront the health care system over funding, will merely lead to persistence of relative cost expansion, and postponement of confrontation to a later, more expensive stage.

FROM POSITIVE TO NORMATIVE, OR "IS" TO "OUGHT": LERNER'S RULE

But the discussion thus far, based on Figure 5-1, is incomplete. It has concentrated on the processes whereby the intrinsic characteristics of health care have led to institutional responses, all of which in turn tend to inflate both utilization and costs, and has tried to outline a range of different policy philosophies for responding to that expansion. But it has nowhere addressed explicitly the question of "How much, and of what services, is enough?" In fact, each policy alternative addresses that question implicitly. The public service approach presumably relies on epidemiological and technical data in a bureaucratic framework to decide what is to be done. The various forms of control over prices, capacity, or budgets leave a high degree of discretion over mix of services in the hands of providers and try to limit overall costs. The market-oriented policies try to find ways of introducing consumer choices into the decision-making process in contexts which are less vulnerable to informational asymmetry. The nature of the problem faced by all such approaches, however, can be represented compactly in a framework known as Lerner's Rule (Lerner 1944).

The problem of how much of its resources a society should allocate to particular activities can be represented in marginal terms as one of equating

$$MSV = MSC \qquad (5-1)$$

the Marginal Social Value of the activity should equal its Marginal Social Cost. This is simply the balancing of benefits against opportunity costs as discussed in chapter 1, although with new labels. An expansion of health care activity, a marginal increment to care output, will, viewed by society as a whole, generate benefits labelled *MSV*, the value to that society of a marginal change in health care output. But the necessary resources, drawn from other lines of activity, have opportunity costs insofar as those other activities must be reduced in scale or scope. Other things are given up.

On the assumption that as the health care sector expands, it supplies the most valued outputs first, and then devotes additional resources to lower priority uses, the *MSV* of health care will fall as output expands (though changes in technology, needs, or preferences may cause it to shift up—or down—at any given level of activity). This is just Figure 1-3, with the health status axis replaced by "value to society," and can be described as diminishing marginal utility of health care, for technical as well as preference reasons.[12] But by the same argument, a rational society (if there are such) would withdraw the resources required from their least-valued alternative uses. Thus (for a fixed overall resource endowment) an expansion of the health care system withdraws resources from progressively more valuable alternatives. The *MSC* rises, as health care output increases. But since *MSV* is falling, and *MSC* rising, there will be some point at which they are equal, and that represents the optimal size of the health care system.[13]

Formulated at this level of abstraction, the optimal allocation of resources to health care looks like a central planner's problem of daunting complexity—but it is no different from the problem of resource allocation for goods in general. What Lerner's Rule displays is the way in which market mechanisms can be used to "solve" this problem, on a decentralized basis, but under very specific conditions. It thus enables us to pinpoint the various distortions created by market failure in the health care context, and to see their implications for optimal resource allocation in the abstract, as well as for the historical evolution of institutions and of cost and output patterns.

The market interposes between *MSV* and *MSC* a set of intermediate quantities or concepts, among which equality can be achieved by a chain of private decisions, like stepping stones.

$$MSV = MPV = P = MPC = MSC \qquad (5\text{-}2)$$

The unit price of the commodity in question (or price vector, for commodity baskets) is *P*. *MPV* and *MPC* represent marginal private valuations and costs, respectively, as experienced by the buyer/user of the last (marginal) unit produced, and by its producer/seller. The equation between *MPV* and *P* will occur if informed consumers, knowing their

---

[12] Those who are uncomfortable with an explicit representation in terms of utility are welcome to carry out the translation into the language of marginal rates of substitution. The argument goes through, but is, I believe, a good deal more opaque for non-economists.

[13] Corner solutions, with health care output equal to zero or to the whole GNP, are theoretically possible but practically uninteresting. Furthermore, this relationship addresses only the issue of real resources to be allocated to health care, not their rate of reimbursement. In an idealized market system, the one follows from the other; but in the real world the relative income status of providers represents another major set of parameters in determining the cost of health care to the rest of society.

own values, transact freely in smoothly functioning markets. It is represented by the point $P°$, $Q°$ in Figure 2-2a, where purchasers of the commodity all value it at, or above, the price they must pay for it. For the buyer who values it least, $MPV = P$; those for whom $P > MPV$ do not buy. Output and sales will be at a point where $P =$ (society-wide) MPV. On the supply side, perfectly competitive profit-maximizing firms will choose to produce levels of output such that $P = MC$. If any firm can produce additional output at an incremental cost below the current selling price, it will, in a perfectly competitive market, choose to do so— that will increase profits. So will cutting back output when its marginal cost exceeds price. Equilibrium will occur when $P = MPC$, *assuming* perfectly price-competitive markets, including free entry and exit, served by for-profit firms. The price level itself, of course, responds (in a smoothly functioning market) such that the amount buyers want to purchase always equals the amount sellers want to supply, *at the going price.* Excess demand (supply) leads immediately to rising (falling) prices.

The linkages between MSV and MPV, and MSC and MPC, require both the satisfaction of specific technical relationships—absence of external effects—and the acceptance of the particular political or philosophical value judgements embodied in the consumer sovereignty postulate. At the technical level, it is necessary that no one person's consumption activity affects another's well-being, and that no firm's production affects either another's costs, or (except for its purchases/sales) consumers' well-being. All the costs and benefits associated with an activity (other than those reflected in changes in market prices) must be borne by the party or parties whose decisions govern that activity. But further, society must be willing to accept the principle that what people want (and are willing/able to pay for) is what they ought to get. In particular their "needs," as distinct from wants, have no normative significance for themselves or anyone else. The normative case for markets is ultimately rooted in this political judgement.[14]

In the health care system, almost every condition of Lerner's Rule is violated. An extended version of equation 5-2 makes this point clear.

$$MSV \overset{?}{>} MPV' \gtrless \begin{bmatrix} MPV^U \\ MPV^A \end{bmatrix} = P^b < P^s > MPC < MSC \qquad (5\text{-}3)$$

In this framework there are two prices, P^b paid by the buyer/user of services and P^s received by the seller, and three different sources of users' valuations. The uncertainty of incidence causes MPV to fluctuate at any given use level—depending on whether or not one is ill—which would in itself make it difficult (though not, in principle, impossible) to be sure

[14] Which may have considerable appeal in our society, but is hardly "science"!

that $MPV = P$. But insurance contracts, responding to that uncertainty, drive a wedge between prices paid and prices received. The difference $P^s - P^b$, which may equal P^s if care is "free," is made up by insurance.

But the MPV concept, in a world of asymmetric information, is difficult to formulate precisely. We have suggested three concepts: MPV^I, MPV^U, and MPV^A. The first is the valuation which would be placed on care by the hypothetical fully informed consumer of the textbooks, who would know the true structure of the relationship between health care and health. Less ambitiously, she might be assumed to share the best current knowledge about that structure. But she would not be restricted to the knowledge actually in the possession of her physician or other professional provider. On the other hand, MPV^U is the uninformed judgement of the patient confronting the health care system and initiating an episode of care. The intermediate case, MPV^A, is the valuation of care felt and expressed by the patient after being advised by her professional provider-agent.

None of these equates to MSV. The political/philosophical principle of consumer sovereignty presumably attaches to MPV^I, as one can hardly think of an uninformed or misinformed person making free choices. Indeed, deliberate misinformation is as much a form of coercion as physical intervention. But $MSV \gtrless MPV^I$, because of the external effects involved; the ? is inserted to remind us that while true in general, this inequality does not apply to all forms of care, or independently of the state of health of the user.

On the other side, the patient/consumer will equate P^b to her view of MPV, subject to any direct restrictions on access. (One cannot, without professional approval, buy prescription drugs, sign oneself into a hospital, or choose to receive treatment there). The shift from $MPV^U = P^b$ to $MPV^A = P^b$ occurs as the patient interacts with the provider and is informed or directed as to care use. This is the point at which the "demand curve" of the patient, as in Figure 2-2, is shifted right or left on the basis of professional advice, and control over utilization shifts from patient to provider. In principle, $MPV^A \lessgtr MPV^U$, provider advice can either raise or lower patients' perceptions of the value of particular forms of care, as the provider will usually discourage or refuse to provide harmful or unnecessary care. But in general, $MPV^A > MPV^U$ as, for many forms of care, patients' preferences are totally undefined before they contact the care system. They are unaware of the existence of such services.

The problem of overuse then, in this framework, is that $MPV^I < MPV^A$. The agency role of the provider leads to care provision which the fully informed patient might not have chosen. In terms of costs, $MPV^I < MPV^A = P^b < P^s$ implies a dual discrepancy; the user of unnecessary care is led to overestimate its value and underestimate its price. On the other hand, the discrepancy between MPV^I and MPV^U, in detail, if not in total, is likely to be much greater. The justification for agency and profession-alism, in the context of the consumer sovereignty value framework, is that the substitution of provider for patient judgement is presumed to lead to results closer to what the patient herself would have wanted, if fully informed, and that it is the latter preferences which society wishes to respect.

But the monopoly powers conferred by self-regulation, and the non-profit environment, intended to support the agency relationship, also enable providers to hold selling prices above costs of production. This discrepancy shows up in both technically inefficient production, and above-market provider incomes. Thus $P^s > MPC$. Yet $MPC < MSC$ in general, because of the extensive system of public subsidies to private providers, as well as the possibility of negative externalities in production.

OVER TO THE SUPPLY SIDE

If the reader is left somewhat bewildered by the string of counteracting inequalities, that is as it should be. Reality is like that. While any one form of market failure (except for informational asymmetry) leads to a single inequality and a predictable bias in the $MSV = MSC$ relationship, the collection of all forms in equation 5-3 leaves us in total unable to predict, on a priori grounds alone, where we are relative to the optimum, above or below.[15] And the various equilibrium mechanisms, which in theoretical market systems tend to lead us toward optimality, are clearly absent. Consequently, the normative significance of whatever levels and patterns of utilization and processes of production happen to emerge from these relationships is wholly undercut. Even accepting consumers' sov-ereignty as a value postulate, we are unable to infer "ought" from "is," or standards of optimal resource allocation from observed behaviour.

The pervasive "failure" of markets in health care delivery, even in situations where apparently voluntary exchange of money for services persists, leaves us with two classes of problems. The price system, in a theoretical perfect market system, performs both positive and normative functions. It determines, or guides, what will be produced, how, and for whom. And it generates, or at least elicits and records, the information from which (assuming the prior consumer sovereignty postulate) criteria of performance are developed. In health care, the price system is capable of playing neither role. Accordingly, in chapter 1, we introduced health status as a proximate objective, an alternative source of criteria for good and bad performance. This, we suggested, might more closely approxi-mate what fully informed patients, and others with an interest in their

---

[15] This is *not* a justification for assuming that the status quo is satisfactory! That would be a result of purest chance, and in any case we need not rely on a priori analysis.

well-being, *would* choose as an objective. "Revealed preference" or willingness-to-use, in an environment of pervasive information failure and regulatory constraints on supply, will be an inadequate, and inaccurate, way of reflecting those hypothetical choices.

But the positive problem remains. If the market system does not govern patterns of production, delivery, and utilization in health care, or does so only to a limited extent, what fills the gap? The answer, of course, is that providers of health care have a degree of discretion, of direct influence over patterns of utilization and production of health care, which is highly unusual, if not unique, in a supposedly market-governed economy. If consumers' unaided preferences are not, and for good reason should not be, the primary data governing health care delivery, then the way is open for producers to make the key decisions—and they do. To understand and to evaluate the quality of those decisions, and of their results, we must develop an explicit analysis of the behaviour of the different classes of health care providers, their objectives, constraints, and performance. In this performance, the automatic attainment of technical efficiency and opportunity-cost pricing can no more be taken for granted than can appropriate, efficacious, or optimal output patterns. No "market" enforces these. How providers choose what to do, and how to do it, occupies the central place in health care economics. And to this we now turn.

PART 2

THE PROVISION OF HEALTH CARE

CHAPTER 6

HEALTH CARE FIRMS: PROVIDERS, PRACTICES, AND PEOPLE

THE FIRM AS ORGANIZATION: PRACTITIONERS ARE NOT PRACTICES

Health care services and commodities are produced and delivered by a wide variety of people and organizations: self-employed professional practitioners, voluntary societies, large clinics and hospitals, government departments, and small or large for-profit corporations. Those people or organizations who are actually in contact with the recipients of care are commonly referred to as providers, a usage which has been followed above.

The term tends, however, to blur the distinction between people and the organizations in which they work. This distinction is of central importance to the economic analysis of production, as well as to certain aspects of health policy and planning. The economic conceptualization of production is of a process of transforming particular inputs, productive resources, into outputs of valued goods and services. The conceptual entity which performs this transformation is called a firm, and the same label is applied to actual organizations which carry out the same process. The technical constraints which govern this transformation are summarized for economic analysis as a "production function," a general description of the minimum amounts of different inputs which are necessary to produce any specified level of output or mix of outputs. The structure of this production function will then express the extent to which different combinations of inputs can be used to produce a given output bundle, or the possibilities for substitution between different types of inputs.[1]

---

[1] In theoretical analysis this production function is usually given an analytic form, becoming a mathematical expression. But this carries with it implicit assumptions as to continuity and homogeneity of inputs, outputs, and production processes which may be quite out of place in the actual circumstances of a particular production process. Moreover, the analytic production function is usually expressed as an equality between amount(s) of input and amount(s) of output, which, while mathematically tractable, suppresses important questions of technical efficiency. The technical constraints of production are *in*equalities—waste is always possible—and the equality requires the additional behavioural postulate of cost-minimization. This again may not be appro-

The principal inputs to production in any field are human time, effort, and skills. But people obviously work with various forms of capital equipment—buildings and machinery— and use various sorts of raw materials and "intermediate" commodities. Physical capital, intermediate commodities, and raw materials are themselves produced by labour and skills applied to the natural environment, and indeed, skills themselves are acquired through time and effort and thus are often referred to as "human capital." To avoid infinite regress problems, however, it is convenient to categorize the various inputs as labour and skills, services of capital equipment, and supplies used up in production.

Health care production is characterized as highly labour-intensive, meaning that it requires a high proportion of direct labour and skills. A refinery, steel mill, or farm, by contrast, has a much higher ratio of capital or land services to direct labour input. But some amounts of other inputs are almost always needed in health care as well; only the most emergent of emergency care is provided with bare hands on a street corner.

The assembly of these inputs takes place within specific organizations, corresponding to a greater or lesser degree to the economic concept of a firm. Hospitals, for example, are obviously organizations drawing together inputs, resources of various sorts and directing their transformation into a number of specific forms of health care. So are medical or dental practices, government public health departments, or private drug or equipment firms. *But specific practitioners are not themselves firms.* A person may supply labour to a firm, working for or in it, just as she may rent space or facilities to it or lend money to it. Or a person may perform some or all of the functions of management, either by right of ownership or because hired by the owner to do so. And of course persons own firms, or firms that own firms. Ownership implies a legal right to any surplus of revenues over expenditures generated by the firm's activities (or liability for any deficit, if the firm is not a limited liability company)— residual claimant status—as well as a right to direct the organization or appoint its directors. But the owner is not the organization. Thus the firm in ambulatory care is the medical or dental practice or the pharmacy or the outpatient clinic, but not the professional persons involved.

From the point of view of the supply of health care, a particular

---

priate in firms outside perfectly competitive markets. On the whole, the production function concept is probably more useful without a strict analytic representation; it may be viewed rather as a set of rules for input combinations which might be expressed in the practice of an actual firm, the knowledge of engineers or other technical experts, a computer simulation model, or even a set of verbal statements. A formal equation, $Q = F(X)$ [Quantity of output is equal to some analytic function of quantity of input, each as scalar or vector], tends when applied to the investigation of actual firms, to conceal more than it enlightens.

professional can be thought of as a bundle of skills or capacities, a mix of types of human capital, associated with a physical person who supplies time and effort. Neither skill without effort nor effort without skill is productive. Different professional roles or definitions are made up of different skill or capacity bundles, which tend for technical and historical reasons to be associated with each other in a particular way. Intermediate-level health practitioners, paraprofessionals, represent less extensive or "smaller" skill bundles than those of the "peak" professionals (*not* "lower quality" skills! Such a person will usually be as competent at what he does as would be a professional trained in additional or more complex functions, if not more so.) Since the bundle boundaries observed in any system are to a considerable extent arbitrary, questions of jurisdiction will often arise. But the services of each are all inputs to the process of health care production, whether or not the person possessing a particular set of technical capacities also happens to own the firm which uses those capacities. It makes no difference, from the technical point of view, whether self-employed physicians or dentists own their own firms, and hire other workers, or whether nurses own practices and hire physicians, or whether both are employed in a practice owned by the Hudson's Bay Company.

Legally, however, there is a constraint. Canadian licensure laws in medicine and dentistry (and with some qualifications, in pharmacy) prohibit the ownership of any part of a practice by anyone other than a licensed member of the profession.[2] They thus define the practice of medicine, dentistry, etc., in terms not only of certain technical activities— diagnosis and treatment procedures—but also of economic functions— ownership of the organizations providing care.[3] This represents a significant extension of the licensure function; one need not, for example, be a licensed pilot to own or manage an airline or a licensed gasfitter to be a heating contractor. One must only ensure that a licensed person (pilot, gasfitter) is employed to perform the regulated functions. The public interest justification of this extension of licensure to the economic domain is presumably the preservation of the agency relationship, since it has nothing to do with assuring the competence of those actually performing the functions of providing care. As we shall see below, however, the

---

[2] A non-profit hospital can "own" an outpatient clinic or emergency ward in which physicians on its payroll do things which look very much like medical practice. The Hudson's Bay Company, however, could not.

[3] The same prohibitions do not appear to apply in other countries, however. The long battle by U.S. physician associations against the "corporate practice of medicine" may at last be swinging against them, with the emergence in some states of what appear to be ambulatory medical practices owned by for-profit, non-medical corporations hiring salaried physicians.

economic dimension of licensure also has important implications for the cost and efficiency performance of private health practices.

TRANSACTIONS BETWEEN FIRM AND ENVIRONMENT: THE TIME HORIZONS OF DECISION

However it is defined, the firm in health care (or out of it) must interact with its economic environment in certain specific ways. It can be thought of as pursuing certain objectives, such as survival, professional self-expression, profits, growth, the interests of patients, or the "public interest" somehow defined, subject to constraints imposed by its environment. Its resulting behaviour and impact on that environment, expressed in terms of resources used up, goods and services produced, and patterns of income/wealth generated, can then be evaluated from a more general social standpoint. A significant part of health policy can be considered as attempting to mould the environment in which health care firms (including relevant government departments) function, so as to promote desirable behaviour and discourage undesirable.

"Cost explosions," for example, as a policy issue, can be interpreted as health care firms (public or private) either using up more inputs than necessary for what they produce, or producing too much of the wrong sort of output, or generating too large incomes for those who supply resources (principally skilled labour) to them. "Unmet needs," on the other hand, imply either that existing firms should expand or change their output patterns, or that new firms should be induced to enter the field, drawing in new inputs and expanding total output. One way to do the latter might be to train more professionals of a particular type—a specific set of skill bundles—but this most common response may be much more costly and less effective than alternative ways of increasing the output of the firms (practices, clinics, hospitals) where those skills are deployed, by adding other types of personnel and/or equipment.

For some purposes it is convenient to organize the various forms of interaction between firm and environment by time horizon, into short– middle– and long-run decisions, so long as one does not take these as water-tight categories. The firm's decisions and behaviour can then be classified according to the length of time taken to plan and execute a change, and the length of the subsequent period affected by the change. The long-run time horizon, for example, is a period long enough for all aspects of production to be modified. Long-run decisions include entry to or exit from an industry, or major expansions or contractions of capacity. Decisions by a person to enter or retire from a profession, to migrate across regions, to take specialty training, are long-run decisions, as are the establishment or closure of a hospital or professional school, a major expansion, or the launching or major modification of a public program. All such decisions have a significant investment aspect, long-term implications, and are costly to make or to reverse. In the short run, by contrast, are decisions on current levels of production and pricing. The private practitioner can adjust hours of work and appointment scheduling, modify treatment patterns, and (if not constrained by regulation or co-ordination) raise or lower prices, on very short notice. Hospitals, government departments, or larger private companies may take longer to decide, but in general any organization can speed up or slow down a production process much more quickly and cheaply than it can start one up *de novo*.

Thus questions as to how health care providers decide on current output patterns, choice of technique, or mix and volume of output, and how prices are set, fall into the short-run category, while issues of manpower availability and distribution, and hospital bed and facility capacity, are long-run, planning questions. In the middle ground we may classify changes such as adding or reducing auxiliary staff in a professional practice or changing standard operating procedures in a hospital. Technically, these changes could take place from day to day; in practice the costs of adjustment are great enough that adjustment is less frequent. But for a practitioner, taking a short course on a new technique is not the same as a change of speciality, nor is a hospital's replacing its radiology equipment in the same category as building a new wing, though obviously boundaries are fuzzy.

In the Canadian context, pricing decisions for hospitals and most medical practitioners have also become middle-run. Periodic collective fee negotiation and hospital budget determination (which sets prices implicitly, in conjunction with output levels) makes these adjustments costly (at least collectively) and possible only at defined intervals. Like staffing patterns, such prices are neither instantaneously variable nor set in concrete (or sheepskin) for years at a time.

THE "TEXTBOOK" FIRM: A SINGLE-EXIT MODEL

The archetypal firm whose behaviour is analysed in the economic theory of production makes these same sorts of decisions, though for simplicity it is often assumed to use only two inputs, continuously and costlessly variable "labour" (plus associated raw materials), and "capital" which takes time to acquire and to dispose of. Short-run decisions involve choice of labour input for given capital, long-run decisions involve adjustment of capital stock, and there is no middle ground.

More importantly, however, the theoretical firm in private competitive markets is so constrained as to have no degrees of freedom for independent discretionary behaviour; its responses to changes in its environment thus become perfectly predictable. These constraints are imposed by its objectives, its technology, and its market environment, although at root the first two considerations derive their binding force from the third. It is precisely because health care firms do not, in general, operate in a competitive market environment that a number of different dimensions of their behaviour become discretionary and of interest for policy analysis. Some of the same types of issues arise in the study of non-health care firms in imperfectly competitive markets.

Most obviously, a profit-maximizing firm must always seek to minimize its costs of production for any given level of output. Existing technology, expressed in the production function, will dictate the minimum quantities of resources which can be used to produce any particular level and pattern of output. Once the firm makes its output decision, there may be one, several, or a large number of combinations of different inputs which can be used to produce that output. But the firm will never choose a combination involving pure waste of inputs—it will always be on the production function. Furthermore, the price it pays for each input will be determinate, either beyond its control if it is a small buyer in a large market, or else an observable function of the amount it chooses to buy (defined as the input supply function) if the firm is such a large participant in the input market that its decisions alone affect price. In either case, however, the minimum cost input combination corresponding to each output level is determinate, and *must* be chosen by the profit-maximizing firm.

But prices in output markets are also either given to the firm (perfect competition) or determined by its decisions as to how much to produce and sell. In the latter case, the firm with monopoly power is assumed to face an externally determined demand curve; it can choose how much to sell, or at what price, but not both. Once one is set, so is the other, and so are all input decisions. Furthermore, the profit-maximization objective determines which price/output combination will be chosen. Analytic structures of this sort are known as ''single-exit models''; the firm's field of choice is narrowed down to a single variable, which in turn has a single optimal value. And the firm's objectives require it to choose that value.

The firm's middle– and long-run decisions are determined in the same way. As more choices of technique, capacity, or field of activity become available with the lengthening of the planning horizon, the relationship between output chosen and cost of production changes, and the profit-maximizing output shifts.[4] Moves into more profitable geographic or

---

[4] It may also become less predictable, and the firm's behaviour will then depend on its forecasting capabilities and its attitudes toward risk, but that raises additional complications which are immaterial here.

product markets become possible. In general, the scale of the firm's response, in terms of change of quantity or mix of output, to any change in its environment will be increased as the time horizon and the range of potentially variable inputs increases. (Long-run supply functions are more elastic.) But the basic structure of optimization under constraint remains. The firm's short– and long-run behaviour will respond to shifts in the external environment—in product demand, input availability, taxes or subsidies, technological knowledge—in a determinate and rather simplistic way. Its internal decision processes are unknown, or at least ignored in the economic theory of production—the firm is a "black box," a transformation function. In any case such internal decision processes are uninteresting, since their outcome is externally determined.

HEALTH CARE FIRMS: A CHOICE OF OBJECTIVES

The health care firm is quite another matter. The organization and institutional environment of most such firms is deliberately structured so as to relieve them in whole or in part from competitive pressures, on the presumption that the resulting resource allocation in health care will be more effective, from a broader social perspective.[5] Accordingly, such firms are free to, and do, pursue a wide range of other objectives, additional to or in place of profit-seeking.[6]

Not-for-profit (NFP) firms include hospitals (other than proprietary), voluntary societies, government departments—all organizations which lack a "residual claimant" with legal title to any surplus of revenue over expenditure generated by operations.[7] The objectives that guide the behaviour of such organizations are various, complex, and rather obscure;

---

[5] The argument for this presumption was developed in chapter 4; it will be recalled that, if it is rejected, the social justification for all of licensure and self-government, regulation, and protection of non-profit organizations disappears.

[6] Economists frequently treat the assumed profit-maximization objective as if it were a datum, presumably rooted in psychology, imposed by the nature of man and the universe. In fact, it rests in turn on market structure conditions of free entry and competition which require such behaviour as a condition of survival. There is no obvious reason why a private monopolist (protected from capital market takeover) should maximize profit. Human beings as individuals or in groups have numerous objectives besides money, and to assume such behaviour universally is simply naive (and wrong) amateur psychology.

[7] Not-for-profit is preferable to non-profit, as such firms may quite frequently earn a surplus of revenue over expense (as U.S. voluntary hospitals usually do). And of course "ownership" of such surpluses is clearly vested in the organization (or in the case of a government department, the Crown). But no participant is entitled to appropriate the surplus for other purposes; as might a shareholder or the owner of a practice. And the generation of persistent surpluses indicates for a not-for-profit firm either too high prices (revenues) or too low expenditures.

as discussed in chapter 8, there is no satisfactory unified theory of the not-for-profit sector. But profit per se has neither a priori appeal nor empirical support as an objective, though it might be a means to other ends such as future growth or administrative discretion.[8] Whatever else the organization is trying to do, it is not in the final analysis trying to make a profit, much less to earn maximum possible profits.

Professionally owned and directed practices and clinics, and perhaps some proprietary hospitals, nursing homes, or pharmacies, can best be described as not-only-for-profit (NOFP). Any surplus (or deficit) from operations forms part of the income of the firm owner(s), who also either is, or appoints and directs, the management. Accordingly one would expect the firm's behaviour to respond, to some degree at least, to opportunities for profit. But the self-employed practitioner is also a supplier of skilled labour and (sometimes) physical capital to the firm; payments to these inputs must be deducted, along with other expenses, from firm revenue before arriving at (positive or negative) profit.[9] Thus the proportion of total income accruing to owners of not-only-for-profit health care firms which is actually "profit" in the economic sense may be quite small compared with return to labour and human or non-human capital, and its generation must compete with other objectives of the owner/management. The firm is run in part for profit, but not exclusively for that purpose, hence NOFP.

Moreover, the process of training and socialization, the regulation of practice conduct by professional bodies, and public expectations all tend to discourage pure profit-seeking behaviour and to encourage the substitution or addition of objectives based on professional self-image or perceptions of patient interests. Indeed as emphasized in chapter 4, the social, as opposed to private professional, justification for the significant economic privileges conferred by licensure and self-government is the *quid*

---

[8] In the U.S., however, it appears that voluntary "not-for-profit" hospitals which have borrowed heavily in private markets to finance capital expansion may find themselves forced to behave like for-profit hospitals, at least in the short run, to earn a surplus to finance debt servicing (Wilson *et al.* 1982). More generally, an NOFP firm may strive at least to break even on operations, if that is a condition of survival and the continued pursuit of the organization's (non-profit) objectives.

[9] In principle one should deduct from the gross revenues or receipts of the practice/firm the opportunity costs of all inputs used in order to arrive at true economic profit. In the case of arm's-length transactions, amounts actually paid correspond to opportunity cost, at least from the firm's perspective. But non-arm's-length transactions may overstate true costs. The cost of office rental or of practice management services may be overstated for tax reasons if these are purchased from firms controlled by the practitioner; the above-market profits of such firms are thus indirectly a form of practice income, and will show up as consumption by, or increase in the assets of, the practice owner. Such overstatements should, in principle, be added back to net income before subtracting the opportunity cost of the practitioner's own services to compute true profit.

pro quo of professional acceptance of a responsibility to undertake the agency role and to make patient interests dominant over, or at least competitive with, private economic interests. If one assumes profit-maximizing behaviour by professionals, one has explicitly denied the agency role, and thus undercut the rationale for self-government, which then becomes solely an economic "conspiracy" against the public. Insofar as particular health care firms do act as profit-maximizers, the logical concomitant of deregulation and a return to competitive private markets becomes increasingly appealing.

Such deregulatory policy becomes particularly significant at the boundaries of the NOFP field. The agency role of physicians, particularly with respect to highly sophisticated interventions or physically or mentally dependent patients, is central to the utilization process. But for others (paediatricians providing well-baby care?) the informational asymmetry may be much less pronounced. In dentistry, the agency role becomes even more attenuated, while in community pharmacy it is difficult to discover at all. Informational problems may remain, but it is not at all clear that agency and self-government are an appropriate response. And while a small, owner-managed community pharmacy may claim, perhaps genuinely, to have objectives other than "the bottom line," and an interest in promoting the health of its customers, large firms or chains such as Boots or Shoppers Drug Mart seem clearly in the strictly for-profit (FP) category. Their responsibility to their shareholders is to earn the maximum possible profit (subject to considerations of risk) from operations; all other activities are means to that end.

In general, for-profit firms supply commodities—drugs or medical equipment and devices—rather than services, and sell to hospitals, medical practices, or pharmacies rather than directly to patients. (Non-prescription drugs being the most obvious counter-example.) Private laboratories, however, sell diagnostic services, and appear in several provinces to be in the process of migrating from the NOFP to the FP sector, if not already there. Hospital laboratories in Canada are in the NFP sector. American private laboratories are now squarely in the corporate FP sector (Bailey 1977, 1979), and even NFP American hospitals treat their labs as profit centres. The maintenance of an administrative and regulatory structure based on the assumption of NOFP objectives characteristic of a professional practice seems inappropriate and unjustifiable, either for FP firms or for FP divisions of NFP firms, but the area appears still to be very much in flux.

OPENING UP THE "BLACK BOX": PERFORMANCE CRITERIA FOR HEALTH CARE FIRMS

The significance of this range of objectives, and of corresponding forms of firm organization, is that it opens up the relationship between resource inputs and goods-and-services outputs in health care. The firm can no longer be treated as a "black box" converting inputs into outputs in a deterministic manner. The theoretical for-profit firm in a competitive market is both led by the self-interest of its owners and forced, for competitive survival, to seek least-cost modes of production. Thus technically efficient behaviour follows from the assumed market structure. But health care firms in the NFP and NOFP sectors are under no such market constraints. Accordingly serious empirical and policy questions are raised concerning the efficiency with which hospitals or professional practices use the resources which they mobilize, or the extent to which they do or do not choose minimum cost combinations of resources. In both sectors there is considerable evidence of systematic biases away from least-cost production and of inefficient resource use.

In addition to being technically efficient, the hypothetical private firm in competitive markets is allocatively efficient. Such firms collectively produce the "right" amounts of different commodities, relative to buyers' preferences (as measured by their willingness to pay) and to the opportunity costs of the required resources. They will expand their outputs as long as there is a buyer willing to pay a price equal to or greater than the cost of producing the additional output. The output level reached in equilibrium is that at which market price equals marginal cost; no buyer willing to pay the going price, or more, is unsupplied, and no more can be produced at or below current costs. At this point one more unit of output would be valued by buyers at less than its resource cost (the value of other production opportunities represented by those resources) while reduction in output by one unit would require some user to give up something which she valued more than (or no less than) the freed-up resources.[10]

In the health care field, however, buyers' willingness-to-pay is considered to be too ill-informed (chapter 4) and sensitive to relative income levels (chapter 3) to serve as a guide to social priorities, even if it were not "distorted" by insurance (chapter 2). Firms in the NFP and NOFP

---

[10] The firm in monopolized markets, or with some degree of market power, will of course restrain output before this point is reached, leading to allocative inefficiency. Buyers would value additional output from the monopolized industry/firm at more than its resource cost, but profit-maximization by the firm is inconsistent with supplying this additional output. Hence the standard economists' condemnation of monopoly power as leading to inefficient resource use. In general, however, the profit-maximizing monopolist will be *technically* efficient, producing the chosen output at least cost. Relieved of competitive pressures, the monopolist need not be a profit maximizer either, but that issue has received less theoretical attention.

In health care, by contrast, market power of suppliers seems to co-exist with concerns about *oversupply*, not just in the willingness-to-pay sense (Figure 2-2) but relative to "need."

sectors are permitted, indeed encouraged, to substitute their own preferences and priorities for the dictates of the marketplace. In effect, producers' sovereignty is substituted for consumers' sovereignty. The presumption is that given the specific characteristics of health care, producers' sovereignty in the form of discretionary power over use patterns will lead to a pattern of resource allocation which is closer to what informed consumers would have wanted, for themselves and others, than would emerge in private competitive markets in which firms respond to buyers' willingness to pay.

And of course, firms do not merely respond. Advertising, and marketing in general, are normal activities of for-profit firms. Given the peculiar characteristics of health care, such marketing to inherently uninformed and vulnerable buyers can lead even further from what informed consumers would have chosen. The quack and the snake oil salesman are simply owners of for-profit firms following the rules of the competitive marketplace. But that does not invalidate the usual social judgement as to the consequences of their activities, which reflects the fact that these rules are inappropriate in some parts, at least, of the health care field. Hence the significance attached by providers, and the public generally, to restraining profit-seeking as well as encouraging the pursuit of professional and patient-focussed objectives.

But producers' sovereignty, though it may better approximate a social optimum, is not in general optimal. The freeing of health care firms to follow objectives other than profit does not ensure that they will become perfect agents, in terms of either information or motivation. Hence the issue arises of the clinical, as well as the technical and the allocative, efficiency of health care firms. Whether they are pursuing professional objectives or perceived patient interests, is the behaviour of such firms clinically effective? Or do they use resources in ways which have very little, or no, positive impact on health.[11]

Going beyond treatment patterns, to the making of location, expansion, specialization, programming, or research and innovation decisions, if health care firms do not respond wholly, or at all, to profit considerations, to what *do* they respond? And are their responses consistent with what

---

[11] The distinction between clinical and allocative inefficiency is a bit tricky, though each is well defined in its own realm of discourse. Provision of a clinically efficacious procedure, which improved health status, but whose value to (fully informed) patients and involved others was less than its true resource cost, would be allocatively inefficient. Similarly, an ineffective clinical intervention for which patients were prepared to pay the marginal resource cost, in the full knowledge that it was ineffective, would be allocatively efficient. But if, in the absence of any examples of fully informed consumers, we assume that they would want only efficacious care, then the two concepts converge.

informed consumers might reasonably be expected to want, on their own or others' behalf? If not, how can the external environment of such firms be modified to bring their decisions and behaviour closer to meeting the community interest? Subsidies for practice in remote areas and certificate-of-need restraints on expansion of American hospitals are examples from this wide class of "environmental" policies. For the hypothetical private for-profit firm, the very rigid constraints imposed by the market pre-determine the answers to all such questions. The simplest and most effective way to modify the behaviour of such a firm, if that is desired, is to change one or more of the prices which it faces in either input or output markets. But health care firms have diverse and multiple objectives and operate in a social environment whose expectations of the health care industry are much more complex and subtle than simply that it should meet the effective (dollar-backed) demand, whatever its source, at lowest cost. The policy issues are accordingly much more diverse. And interesting.

FUZZY BOUNDARIES: WHERE DO FIRMS END?

The next three chapters will discuss in more detail the behaviour of each of the different classes of health care firms distinguished by their apparent objectives. Before proceeding, however, it should be noted that, particularly in the NFP sector but to a lesser extent in the NOFP as well, there are significant questions as to where the boundaries of the firms themselves should be located (Evans 1981). The archetypal firm as a conceptual construct, transforming inputs into outputs, can also be thought of as the locus of certain kinds of decisions, over output, price, capacity, technology, etc., even if in certain market conditions its decisions may be determined by external forces. In the NFP sector, many of the decisions which themselves constitute firm activity are made external to the organization. The treatment decisions of hospitals, short run (dealing with individual patients) or middle run (standard procedures), are made primarily by the medical staff, individually or collectively. A salaried physician is clearly part of the hospital "firm," but a private practitioner is part of an independent firm. One could think of the hospital "selling" or at least supplying, intermediate goods and services to physicians; this is expressed in the saying that hospitals do not have patients, they have doctors. The physician regards the patient as "my" patient, expressing an exclusive economic as well as professional relationship. Yet the physician does not deal at arm's length with the hospital as an independent firm; the medical staff is an integral part of management. And patients or insurers deal directly with hospitals in reimbursement; they do not go through the physician.

Under the Canadian hospital insurance system, provincial governments negotiate hospital operating budgets annually, and also separately provide (or refuse) support for capacity expansion. They thus influence or take over the long-run managerial functions of the firm. Indeed, the province may have the power to take over and operate the hospital directly, "at pleasure" of the Lieutenant-Governor-in-Council, under a public trustee. And provincial governments have specific legislative responsibility and authority for ensuring the development of a "balanced and integrated" system of hospitals in the interests of the provincial population. Thus hospitals must share both long– and short-run "rights of management" with external organizations who are not at arm's length, in a pattern of "incomplete vertical integration." The decision-making spheres of such firms are not mutually exclusive, but interpenetrate each other.

The location of decision-making authority within professional practices is by contrast well-defined. But here too the referral network, the relationship with hospitals, and the co-ordination of different specialties (physicians and non-physicians) blurs the analytic boundaries. A solo practice, or a legal partnership of professionals, is each a single firm. But an association of solo practices, all located in a building owned jointly by their principals, with shared diagnostic services and active inter-practice referrals, is in a fuzzy middle ground between one firm and many. This blurring of firm boundaries must be constantly kept in mind. The analysis of scale economies or competitive behaviour in ambulatory medical practice, for example, or the attempt to elucidate the objectives underlying hospital behaviour, can go seriously astray if too narrow or rigid a view is taken of the relevant set of decision-makers.

CHAPTER 7

PROFESSIONAL PRACTICES:
THE NOT-ONLY-FOR-PROFIT FIRMS

THE SCALE OF THE NOFP SECTOR IN CANADA:
EXPENDITURES AND EMPLOYMENT

In the previous chapter we suggested that it would prove helpful for analytic purposes to categorize health care firms according to the objectives which they appear to pursue. Some health care firms, like most firms in the general economy, are organized for the purpose of earning as large a profit as possible for their owners, *e.g.*, the for-profit (FP) firms which dominate the drug and equipment industries. Others, like most hospitals, have no participants, whether managers or owners, with personal legal title to profits; whatever other objectives they pursue they are not organized and managed with profit as an objective (NFP). Intermediate are not-only-for-profit (NOFP) firms, in which a legal claimant to profits is well-defined, but profits represent only one among several competing objectives of the firm's ownership and management.

The NOFP sector in Canada is represented by a wide range of different types of firms owned and run by self-employed professional practitioners. Medical practices, however, account for by far the largest share of both employment and economic activity. The other large sub-sectors are dental practices and community pharmacies, although, as noted above, the latter shades into the corporate, for-profit sector. Both conceptual and statistical boundaries are difficult to draw with precision.

The scale of an industry may be variously described by its sales, its employment levels, or direct measures of its physical capacity. Sales data in the health context are usually referred to as expenditures; but of course each dollar of expenditure is simultaneously a dollar of revenue for the provider. Expenditures on medical and dental services were displayed in Table 1-1; in 1982 these items amounted to $4.4 billion and $1.7 billion respectively. They made up a fifth of all health spending, and nearly 2 percent of GNP. The NOFP sector also includes services provided by other professional practices, chiropractors, optometrists, and others, but these in 1982 totalled under half a billion, and their share has been declining slowly over time.

The treatment of drugs and appliances is more problematic. These accounted for $3.3 billion in sales in 1982, of which prescribed drugs were $1.5 billion. But even if one counted all the dispensing activities of pharmacies as part of the NOFP sector, that would represent only somewhat over half of prescribed drug sales. The rest, cost of goods sold, is the output of the (strictly FP) drug manufacturing sector. And of course many non-prescribed drugs (total sales $1.4 billion) are sold else-where in the retail sector, while the "professional" content of their sale even by pharmacies is questionable to non-existent. On balance, then, the most generous addition to NOFP firm sales from the drug and appliance field would be about $0.8 billion, just over half prescription drug sales, with the true figure being perhaps much less.

Medical and dental practices not only make up the bulk of the NOFP sector, they also display the most variation through time. As Table 1-1 showed, physicians almost doubled their share of national income from 1951 to 1971, moving from 0.71 percent to 1.32 percent as their total sales rose from $153.0 million to $1250.4 million. But by 1976 they had dropped back sharply, to 1.10 percent, despite sales of $2103.2 million, and this share remained fairly constant through to 1981 (1.10 percent and $3741.0 million), rising to 1.24 percent on sales of $4414.3 million in 1982. Dentists, on the other hand, moved their share up sharply during the 1970s, after two decades of relative stability. In both 1946 and 1971 they accounted for 0.33 percent of GNP—recovering after a fall in the late 1940s—but by 1979 they had added nearly a third to their share, up to 0.42 percent, and in 1982 reached 0.47 percent. Between 1970 and 1982 dentist billings grew by a factor of 6—the second fastest increase of any health care component. ("Homes for Special Care" or care of the aged rose over nine times.) These swings in expenditure patterns do not show up in the smaller and/or more questionable components of the NOFP sector, whose shares of total national income have been relatively stable in the post-war period. Medical and dental practices appear to be where the action, as well as most of the money, is.

But the significance of such swings in expenditure/sales data depends on the reliability of the data themselves. And this, of course, varies according to the source. Data on billings by firms is most readily available and reliable under a universal public health insurance scheme; thus expenditure data improved in quality and coverage during the 1960s as the public plans developed. The existence of extra-billing (billing both patient and insurer) and opting-out, as well as various forms of uninsured services, renders this source still incomplete. Taxation statistics from self-employed practitioners form another source of gross and net income data, but they suffer from their own biases. Moreover published data are for net practitioner incomes only, not gross practice receipts, except for special tabulations prepared periodically by Health and Welfare Canada.[1]

---

[1] A comprehensive discussion of the physician income data is provided by Wolfson *et al.* (1980).

Expenditure/sales data also reflect changes in relative prices and incomes as well as shifts in actual scale of economic activity. Much of the increase in expenditures on physician services from 1951 to 1971, for example, was a result of increases in the relative price of their services, increases in both fees charged and collections ratios. Industry employment data, on the other hand, provide an indication of the actual resources, at least of human time and skills, used up in the sector. They are at best only a first approximation to real output levels, however, since those depend also on changes in productivity per person employed.

Table 7-1 presents data showing the growth through time in the stock of physicians, dentists, and pharmacists, relative to the total labour force. Almost a third of licensed physicians are employed in other than fee-for-service practice, which places them outside the NOFP sector. Most are employed in NFP firms, hospitals or other institutions. Dentists, by contrast, are almost entirely in fee-for-service practice; of 11095 licensed dentists in 1980, 9877 were reported by Health and Welfare Canada (see Data Sources Appendix) as self-employed practitioners, and some of the remainder would be salaried in private practice. Pharmacists likewise are predominantly in (salaried or self-employed) community pharmacy; about 10 percent would be working in hospitals or other NFP institutional settings, and a small proportion in FP drug manufacture or distribution.

Other than these three groups, self-employed private practitioners whose practices might be included in the NOFP sector are rich in variety but small in overall numbers. As of 1981 there were 74065 licensed physicians, dentists, and pharmacists; by contrast, other health professionals who would often be in self-employed practice were: chiropractors, 2412; optometrists, 2070 (opticians, 2726); osteopaths, 48; podiatrists, 259; veterinarians, 4236 (Canada, Health and Welfare Canada 1983*b*). Table 7-1 thus covers almost all the NOFP sector.

Employment in the NOFP sector excludes professional personnel in academic, government, or administrative roles. But it includes employees in professional practices other than licensed professionals themselves. Table 7-2 shows Census data for 1961 and 1971 on employment in selected professional practices. Unfortunately, the Census data do not distinguish licensed professionals (owners or employees) in professional practices from other types of personnel, so that one cannot directly determine the extent of other employment. An idea of its significance can, however, be derived from the reported sex data. These can be used to calculate a minimum (lower bound) estimate of the numbers of people, other than licensed professionals, working in professional practices. This minimum estimate assumes that all female professionals work in private practice, and that no male non-professionals do—more realistic assumptions would raise the estimate of non-professional employees.

In 1971, the Census reported 9325 females working in dental practices, but only 310 licensed female dentists. At least 9015 females, other than

TABLE 7-1

Professional Manpower in the NOFP Sector, 1946–1981, Relative to the Overall Labour Force ('000)

	Active Civilian Physicians	Physicians in Fee-For-Service Practice	Licensed Dentists	Licensed Pharmacists	Labour Force (000)
1946	12831	6343	4649	6000	4829
	(0.266)	(0.131)	(0.096)	(0.124)	
1951	14325	8790	5019	6400	5223
	(0.274)	(0.168)	(0.096)	(0.122)	
1956	17871	11868	5549	7856	5782
	(0.309)	(0.205)	(0.096)	(0.136)	
1961	21290	14588	5986	9022	6521
	(0.326)	(0.224)	(0.092)	(0.138)	
1966	26528	15361	6399	9863	7420
	(0.358)	(0.027)	(0.086)	(0.133)	
1971	32942	20742	7453	11330	8631
	(0.382)	(0.240)	(0.086)	(0.131)	
1976	40130	27395	9401	14687	10206
	(0.393)	(0.268)	(0.092)	(0.144)	
1977	41398	26586	10058	15328	10498
	(0.394)	(0.253)	(0.096)	(0.146)	
1978	42238	26819	10451	15709	10882
	(0.388)	(0.246)	(0.096)	(0.144)	
1979	43192	27419	10763	16052	11207
	(0.385)	(0.245)	(0.096)	(0.143)	
1980	44275	28739	11095	16588	11522
	(0.384)	(0.249)	(0.096)	(0.144)	
1981	45542	29633	11484	17039	11830
	(0.385)	(0.250)	(0.097)	(0.144)	

SOURCES: See Data Sources Appendix.

Bracketed figures are percentages of labour force. "Physicians in Fee-For-Service Practice" is measured by taxable returns of self-employed practitioners.

dentists, must therefore have been working in dental practices. The 1971 Census also reported 2890 female physicians, and 2170 female pharmacists, implying at least 22695 female non-physician employees in medical practice, and 21530 female non-pharmacists in drug stores. Since not all female professionals will be in private practice, and some males in such practices will be employees who are not members of the profession controlling the practice, one can estimate that there was at least one non-physician employee for each physician in private practice in 1971, and at least three other employees for each dentist. Indeed, males working in drug stores (14735) substantially exceeds reported licensed male pharmacists (7240) so that even if *all* licensed pharmacists were in community practice, there would be three additional employees for each pharmacist.

TABLE 7-2

Canadian Labour Force Working in Professional Practices, Census Data, 1961 and 1971

	1961		1971	
Offices of Physicians and Surgeons:				
Total	25902		43285	
Male		14006		17690
Female		11896		25585
Offices of Dentists:				
Total	9385		15445	
Male		5143		6120
Female		4242		9325
Offices of Paramedical Practitioners:				
Total			7830	
Male				3070
Female				4755
Drug Stores:				
Total	26933		38455	
Male		14171		14735
Female		12762		23700

SOURCE: See Data Sources Appendix.

Census data from 1961 for physicians' and dentists' practices permit a similar computation, showing at least 4007 female non-dentist employees and 10441 female non-physician. These minimal estimates of practice auxiliaries make up 42.7 percent and 40.3 percent of total practice employment; the corresponding 1971 percentages are 58.4 percent and 52.4 percent. This indicates a significant increase in non-professional employment in these professional practices over the decade of the 1960s, and the 1981 Census data will be of considerable interest to see if the trend continues.

Linking Tables 7-1 and 7-2, moreover, permits one to compare the professional employment patterns. The increase in numbers of physicians as a proportion of the labour force is quite striking; from 1946 to 1971 this proportion rose by 50 percent, though it has been relatively stable since. A substantial increase in share took place from 1961 to 1971, 17.2 percent, but employees of physician practices rose even faster. There were 67.1 percent more people reported as working in medical practices in 1971 than in 1961, while licensed physicians increased 54.7 percent, and physicians in fee-for-service practice rose only 47.5 percent. These comparisons underline the incompleteness of professional manpower data alone as descriptors of the economic significance of the NOFP sector, or of its growth.

Dental practice data make a similar point. Table 7-1 shows that the proportion of the Canadian labour force made up of dentists was identical in 1946 and 1980, having dipped about 10 percent by 1971 and recovered by 1980. Table 1-1 showed that the share of national income accounted for by dental expenditures/sales was similarly more or less constant from 1946 to 1971, but the rise since 1971 greatly exceeded the roughly 10 percent increase in proportion of dentists in the labour force. Similarly, the fall in the share of medical expenditures in national income since 1971 has occurred without parallel labour force shifts. Between 1961 and 1971, however, numbers of employees in dental practices rose 64.6 percent, while numbers of licensed dentists rose only 24.5 percent, so resource input to the sector was expanding much faster than professional manpower data would suggest. Once again, better understanding of the growth of the NOFP sector in the 1970s must wait on 1981 Census data—no other source reports practice manpower.[2]

Employment in the various NOFP sectors is an indicator of the opportunity or resource costs, the human time and skills, used up in those activities. Expenditure data, on the other hand, are the product of output and price levels. Output can be expanded through productivity improvement and technological change even while employment is constant. But some discussions of productivity in professional practices follow the tendency of the data sources to neglect information on salaried employees of professionals, with the result that increases in productivity are measured per professional only. If such increases result from more use of other personnel per peak professional, the result may or may not be an increase in productivity from a social perspective. If output per professional can be doubled by adding one auxiliary employee, then (unless such employees are as expensive as professionals) productivity is clearly increased. But if five auxiliaries are needed (in the practice or elsewhere, such as in a hospital) for such doubling, then overall, "total factor productivity" will have fallen. Yet if the output generates revenue in the practice, and the employees can be placed on someone else's payroll, they may still be added.

In Table 7-3 we present indices of "real" volumes of physicians' and of dentists' services; that is, expenditure data adjusted for estimates of fee change. These are then used to derive indices of "real" service use per capita and output per professional—active civilian physicians and licensed dentists, respectively. These are *not* indices of output per full-time equivalent private practitioner, which one would prefer, but will deviate only insofar as the proportion of professionals in full-time private

---

[2] The Census data are, of course, far from perfect. In particular, they are not full-time equivalents, a weakness which may be even more severe for practice employees than for practitioners themselves.

TABLE 7-3

Indices of Quantity of Physicians' and Dentists' Services, Adjusted for Price Change, and of Relative Prices, 1946–1982

	Physicians' Services			Dentists' Services			Relative Fees (Over CPI)	
	Total	Per Capita	Per Physician	Total	Per Capita	Per Dentist	Medical	Dental
1946	23.5	41.3	60.4	37.5*	60.2*	58.6*	64.8	63.5*
1951	27.4	42.3	63.0	40.4	62.2	60.0	67.7	61.4
1956	39.1	52.5	72.0	54.5	73.1	73.2	71.7	70.1
1961	50.8	60.1	78.5	64.3	76.0	80.1	81.5	77.7
1966	71.9	77.6	89.4	77.6	83.6	90.4	80.6	87.4
1971	100.0	100.0	100.0	100.0	100.0	100.0	100.0	100.0
1976	138.1	129.4	113.4	142.7	133.7	113.1	81.8	105.7
1977	139.9	129.6	111.3	157.4	145.8	116.6	82.1	105.0
1978	145.1	132.8	113.2	168.4	154.6	120.1	80.0	103.8
1979	151.0	136.4	115.2	177.2	159.1	122.7	78.9	104.8
1980	159.4	142.7	118.6	187.0	167.5	125.6	78.3	105.0
1981	162.4	143.8	117.5	193.9	171.6	125.8	77.8	103.6
1982	169.5	149.2	117.8	197.3	173.7	123.8	79.4	104.3

Annualized Rates of Change (%)

1946–56	5.22	2.43	1.77	5.49*	2.81*	3.23*	1.02	1.42*
1956–66	6.28	3.98	2.19	3.60	1.35	2.13	1.18	2.23
1966–76	6.74	5.25	2.41	6.28	4.81	2.27	0.15	1.92
1976–82	3.47	2.40	0.64	5.55	4.46	1.52	−0.50	−0.22

SOURCES: See Data Sources Appendix.

*Dental fees are from 1949, not 1946.

practice has changed over time. The dental fee index used in these calculations is simply the Consumer Price Index dental care component; the medical care fee is derived by linking earlier CPI data with later medical care fee schedule data and adjusting for estimated rates of collection (Barer and Evans 1983). Since 1971 it has followed the national fee indices prepared by Health and Welfare Canada, thus failing to capture the effects of changes in extra-billing patterns. Table 7-3 also displays movements through time in medical and dental fees relative to the overall Consumer Price Index.

From these data we can see the steady growth in output, or at least fee-adjusted billings, per professional, at about 2 to 2.5 percent per year over most of the post-war period. Only for dentistry in the 1949-51 period, medicine post-1976, and dentistry since 1980 do we see any break in this pattern. This growth is presumably a result both of increases in other inputs per professional—capital equipment and auxiliary personnel—and of "true" productivity increase or greater output per some index of inputs weighted by their cost.[3] The increases in other inputs may in turn be within the practice—an increase in hired auxiliaries per dentist, for example—or outside it. The expansion of the hospital system in the 1950s and 1960s clearly increased the levels of output which physicians could generate and bill for. And the sudden drop in rates of increase of output per physician in the late 1970s may be, in part, a result of the restraints on hospital expansion and the consequent reduction in hospital equipment and personnel available per physician.

The prices of medical and dental services, relative to the general price level, both moved substantially in the post-war period. Both escalated rapidly and steadily up to 1971. Estimated medical fees (adjusted for changed collections ratios) rose at an average of 1.75 percent faster than the general price level over the whole thirty-five year period 1946-71, to end 53.4 percent higher in real terms, while dental fees rose even faster, 2.09 percent per year from 1949 to 1971, for a total gain of 57.5 percent.

But after 1971, the pattern changes. Medical fees, presumably under the influence of the public insurance plans, fell sharply from 1971 to 1976, back to their relative level of 1961. They have continued to move down, though much more slowly, in the 1976-81 period. Dental fees slowed their rate of increase, but continued to escalate about 1 percent per year faster than the general price level during the early 1970s. Since then, they have run very slightly behind the CPI.

Utilization levels per capita for medical and dental care have also shown substantial movement, though with somewhat different timing. Per capita dental billings adjusted for fee schedule change moved up steadily in the 1946-66 period, about 1.95 percent per year. But in the latter half of the 1960s they speeded up sharply, and rose even faster in the late 1970s. Medical care use, on the other hand, speeded up earlier. It more or less paralleled dental care use increases in the first post-war decade, ran well ahead after 1956 and up to 1971, grew slightly more slowly 1971-76, and in the late 1970s and early 1980s ran well behind. The combination of continued restraints on physician numbers and billing patterns, compared with dental markets which are controlled only by the profession itself, can be expected to lead to continuing divergence in these trends. In referring to these differences as "productivity," however, we must keep in mind the problematic nature of the linkages between reported billings and care supplied, and between health care and health status.

---

[3] Whether the increase in billings corresponds to improvements in health status, or even the extent to which it represents increased servicing as opposed to re-labelling of existing services, is a difficult and important question. Here, we sidestep it.

In any case, a focus on licensed self-employed personnel alone seriously understates both the level of employment and the growth of output, or at least fee-adjusted billings, in the NOFP sector. Moreover, a significant amount of medical, and some dental, service production takes place outside owner-managed practices, in hospitals, public clinics, or other government agencies. The medical services industry and the collection of NOFP firms in medical care are not coterminous; we isolate NOFP firms in order to give a coherent description of their economic behaviour.

ECONOMISTS AND THE NOFP FIRM: THE BLIND MEN AND THE ELEPHANT

Economic analysis of NOFP firms can be traced through three successive phases, each emphasizing different aspects of such firms, or different characteristics distinguishing them from ''normal'' or text-book firms in private markets (Evans 1980). A broader discussion of the policy issues is provided by the papers in Slayton and Trebilcock (1978). Analysts have focussed in turn on the monopoly or cartel nature of self-regulation, on the self-employed, ''labour-managed'' nature of the firm itself, and on the direct influence of the firm over the demand for its own services implied by the professional relationship.[4] Each stage implies different assumptions about the NOFP firm's objectives and constraints, predictions about its behaviour, and recommendations as to appropriate policy.

PROFESSIONS AS MONOPOLIES: SUPPLY RESTRICTIONS

The monopoly or cartel approach has several variants, but all emphasize the role of licensure in restricting entry to particular professions. It is implicitly assumed that this in turn automatically restricts access to, and output offered in, particular service markets, although in practice that need not follow. The bitter jurisdictional disputes between dentists and denturists or dental mechanics, physicians and chiropractors, and outside health care, lawyers and notaries, chartered and certified general accountants, and engineers and architects, demonstrate that the definition of a profession does not uniquely determine the boundaries of its domain of exclusive practice rights. The ''senior'' profession in each of the above disputes, *i.e.*, the one claiming the broadest domain, has generally asserted the prerogative of setting its own boundaries. Much economic

---

[4] Of course the process of intellectual evolution does not correspond to a strict temporal sequence; one can still find analyses addressing the monopoly aspect in the context of assumed exogenous demand and profit-maximizing behaviour.

analysis has implicitly, and rather surprisingly, accepted and supported this political program by taking the scope of professional practice to be whatever the profession declares it to be.

In order to restrict the supply of services which professionals participate in producing, professional licensure must both restrict access to the profession itself and maintain the boundaries around the collection of activities which are defined as ''the practice of X.'' The law may or may not forbid unlicensed persons actually to *perform* such activities, but it clearly forbids firms other than those owned/controlled by licensed persons to *supply* such services to patient/consumers. Depending on the technology, however, restriction of supply may also require regulation of the structure and conduct of professionally-owned firms themselves. If the nature of the production process is such that one or a few licensed professionals may dramatically expand the output of their firms by hiring large numbers of non-licensed personnel, and delegating functions, then control of service output may require direct restrictions on production itself. Conduct regulation may specify maximum ratios of other personnel per licensed professional in each firm, or may specifically prohibit non-licensed personnel from performing certain functions. Similar constraints may be achieved through collective standards for defence in malpractice suits, or negotiated restrictions on insurance reimbursement.

In this framework, the essence of the professional firm is assumed to be supply restriction—''professional birth control.'' The market demand for professional services is assumed to be represented by a normal, exogenous demand curve; consumers choose utilization levels of professional services in response to market prices, and their own tastes and incomes. Total output/sales of professional services would then be inversely related to their prices, and all the agency issues of chapter 4 above are assumed away. Similarly, the individual firm faces an externally set demand for its services; the role of the professional in advising patients on utilization is assumed to be either non-existent or completely non-discretionary.

The nature of this externally set demand, however, varies, depending on the market structure assumed for the professional industry. At one extreme, firms might be assumed to be perfectly competitive price-takers, able to sell as much or as little as they choose at a given market price, but unable to affect that price. The restriction on entry would then ensure that this competitive market price was high enough to generate ''supra-normal'' profits or professional incomes, *i.e.*, incomes exceeding those available in non-professional occupations requiring similar training, skills, and effort. In a ''normal'' market, the existence of such supra-normal profits is an incentive to draw additional suppliers into the market, as well as a signal as to social, or at least buyers', priorities. But entry restriction blocks this process.

Behind the protective wall, however, the professional services market need not be perfectly competitive. More plausibly, locational factors and patients' perceptions of practitioner or firm characteristics create distinctions among firms so that each has some discretion over price setting. In such a "monopolistically competitive" environment, the volume of services each firm can sell varies inversely with its own price. For any given own-price, volume varies directly with the prices charged by others and inversely with the numbers of such competitors. By assumption, however, the firm cannot affect its own sales, except through the price it charges.

A variant on this approach, of some practical interest in medical care, is that in which the firm is assumed to be able to discriminate in price-setting, charging different prices to different patients, and perhaps even charging the same patient different unit prices for different amounts of care. In this environment the notion of "a" price for care becomes rather hazy; charges are set to yield whatever the traffic will bear, but the professional/firm's ability to discriminate in pricing will depend critically on the degree of competition it faces from other firms.

Finally, the most extreme form of cartel behaviour involves not only restrictions on entry and possibly scale of firm, but complete collusion, so that the entire group of firms acts like a single monopoly in its price and output-setting behaviour. Such a cartel, to be fully effective, would have to allocate output among its members (presumably by setting a structure of differential prices) and arrange for profit-sharing. A more limited form would merely involve agreement on a single pricing structure (a schedule of minimum fees) with some mutual understanding about appropriate patterns of price discrimination.

PROFESSIONAL EARNINGS: REWARDS OF MONOPOLY?

This simplest concept of a profession as a "conspiracy against the public" to enhance its members' incomes by staking out and enforcing exclusive rights to a market, and limiting competition among its members by regulation or collusion, clearly captures some important features of the industry. We do observe that average incomes in the self-regulating professions, and particularly the senior health professions, medicine and dentistry, are consistently at the top of the occupational lists. Table 7-4 shows average net incomes by year over the past thirty-five years for physicians, dentists, and other "representative" licensed professionals, relative to the average weekly wage, and indicates that while large swings have occurred over time, the top position of the health professions has

TABLE 7-4

Earnings of Selected Self-Employed Professionals, Relative to Average Weekly Wages and Salaries, 1946–1981

	Physicians (NHW Est.)*	Physicians	Dentists	Lawyers	Accountants	Architects Engineers	Average Weekly Wage × 50
1946	—	7466 (4.60)	5289 (3.26)	6529 (4.02)	—	5984 (3.68)	1624
1951	—	9975 (3.99)	6287 (2.51)	10214 (4.08)	8171 (3.27)	9628 (3.85)	2502
1956	—	13053 (4.05)	9230 (2.86)	12617 (3.92)	9940 (3.09)	13640 (4.23)	3222
1961	—	17006 (4.35)	12337 (3.15)	15718 (4.02)	11627 (2.97)	14692 (3.76)	3912
1966	—	24993 (5.19)	17212 (3.57)	21045 (4.37)	13946 (2.90)	21200 (4.40)	4817
1971	—	39555 (5.75)	25828 (3.75)	27862 (4.05)	18631 (2.71)	21648 (3.15)	6882
1976	51800 (4.54)	49310 (4.32)	43336 (3.80)	44858 (3.93)	36616 (3.21)	40626 (3.56)	11402
1980	72100 (4.54)	63411 (4.00)	56977 (3.59)	49481 (3.12)	43799 (2.76)	41052 (2.59)	15869
1981p	84000 (4.74)	68604 (3.87)	62497 (3.52)	56798 (3.20)	42113 (2.37)	43804 (2.47)	17736

SOURCE: See Data Sources Appendix.

NOTE: Bracketed figures are incomes relative to Average Weekly Wage × 50.

*Unpublished data from Health and Welfare Canada show a growing discrepancy between physicians' incomes reported in taxation statistics, and provincial insurance plan payments. These estimates have been prepared internally by HWC, and exclude Quebec.

not been challenged.[5] Indeed, Table 7-4 suggests that the income position of the leading non-health professionals has eroded somewhat, through time, while physicians rode a roller-coaster up to extraordinary (relative) heights in 1971, followed by a sharp readjustment toward earlier levels.

---

[5] The data, of course, *have* been challenged. In the course of physician fee negotiations, a great deal of nonsense has been talked about what physicians do or do not earn, involving confusion of full– and part-time practitioners, and some extraordinary manipulations of fringe benefit concepts. Wolfson *et al.* (1980) attempt to sort out the issues involved. It should be kept in mind that the data in Table 7-4, drawn from National Health and Welfare releases as of February 1983, are net incomes of *all* taxable self-employed practitioners, after expenses but before tax. They thus include part-timers, exclude salaried personnel, and exclude any expenses for tax purposes which re-emerge as income through other channels (as well as, of course, any undeclared income).

The extent of this adjustment, however, is difficult to determine in light of the significant discrepancies between incomes reported in tax data and those estimated by Health and Welfare Canada. The 1982 HWC estimate for average Canadian physician net incomes is $97,000, or 4.97 times the annualized average weekly wage.

Dentists, however, have shown a steady relative advance (discounting the rather questionable 1946 figure) and have narrowed the gap between themselves and physicians since 1971. Indeed, allowing for workload differences and possible tax advantages, dentists may now be as well or better paid, on a per hour basis at least. But the most recent HWC estimates show physicians pulling away again.

Of course, occupations with long training periods and long hours require higher average earnings to compensate. But most studies of earnings in the health professions indicate over-compensation.[6] Moreover, we find unsatisfied demand for entry to the medical and dental professions in particular, in the form of queues of applicants for limited numbers of training places, and apparently qualified candidates being turned away.[7] And it is widely observed that professional associations *do* restrict the economic behaviour of their members, discouraging price competition, forbidding advertising, and placing specific restrictions on practice organization, in all the ways the "monopoly" model would predict.

Moreover, the tradition of sliding-scale billing, or tailoring charges to the patient's resources, either directly or through varying efforts at collection, is readily reinterpreted as price discrimination or charging what the traffic will bear. The provider who attempts to ensure that no one will be denied service through inability to pay may also be maintaining a high level of "sales" by setting fees just below each patient's "reservation price," the level at which the patient would forego care (or go elsewhere) (Kessel 1958).

In the case of physicians' services, of course, the existence of public insurance plans negotiating uniform province-wide reimbursement schedules is the major (in some provinces the only) factor determining fee levels. But it has been the declared policy of several provincial medical associations to encourage their members to bill patients directly above this level. And while upholding in principle the freedom of the practitioner to set her own fees,[8] medical associations in extra-billing provinces continue to issue fee guides to co-ordinate billing behaviour and to discourage

---

[6] There is a line of argument to the effect that the effort and other costs of entry adjust to dissipate any monopoly gains. But the required informational/expectational assumptions are very specific, asymmetric, and quite implausible.

[7] Of course the question of what constitutes appropriate qualification is eminently debatable.

[8] Indeed, a direct attempt to regulate fee-setting behaviour by a medical association or College might be a criminal offence under federal anti-combines law.

competitive pricing. This sort of co-ordination and guidance can be re-markably effective; internal surveys of the British Columbia College of Dental Surgeons (which doubles as the British Columbia Dental Association, combining the public statutory and the private trade association functions) indicate that over 80 percent of its members follow the (purely voluntary) provincial fee guide unilaterally promulgated by the College).

The effectiveness of such co-ordination, however, depends on the se-curity of a professional group's control over its exclusive domain. Thus the existence of self-governing professions with overlapping claims of competence represents a constant threat of the outbreak of competitive behaviour which cannot be controlled within the professional framework. Friction and bitterness is common on such interprofessional boundaries. The general response of senior professions (physicians, dentists, lawyers, chartered accountants) to "professional insurgency" seems to alternate between denying the legitimacy of competitive professions or the com-petence of their members, and trying to draw current members into the "professional team," while suppressing new entry to the competitive profession—exactly as the profession-as-monopoly model would predict (Evans and Stanbury 1981).

The implications of the simple "monopoly model" for economic anal-ysis and public policy are rather straightforward. Professional organiza-tions lead to underprovision of professionalized services—prices are "too high," quantities are "too low." The opportunity cost of the marginal resources (not) used in producing professional services, their value in alternative activities, is below the value which users would have placed on the professional services foregone. The result is both an allocative distortion—society's productive resources are not being devoted to the production of things people value most—and a transfer of wealth (as a result of the elevated prices) from service users (or tax and/or premium payers, if the service is collectively funded) to professionals. The appro-priate policy response is to lower entry barriers and expand supply by more of the same or of competing types of professionals. This will lead, on the assumptions of the monopoly model, to more output and a com-petitive bidding down of prices so that the additional output can be sold. The recent analysis of professional incomes by Muzondo and Pazderka (1979) follows this approach.

If insurance is widespread (dentistry) or universal (medicine), things become a bit more complex; the monopoly presupposes a substantial degree of consumer/patient price responsiveness. In its pure form, how-ever, it encounters no difficulty from insurance. Competition among sup-pliers could take the form of cash rebates to their customers. If, on the other hand, prices are effectively fixed, more entry will drive down work loads and incomes until "supra-normal" profits are eliminated; whether this represents excess capacity will depend on where the fixed price is set. Advocates of a competitive market and of the curbing or dissolution of professional "monopoly" powers usually recommend policies to reduce insurance coverage as well, and minimization or elimination of public insurance.[9]

INADEQUACIES OF THE MONOPOLY MODEL

The "professional monopoly" viewpoint, however, is incomplete or misleading in several respects. Most obviously, it assumes that professional associations control entry directly, which is of course untrue (at least in Canada and for the health professions). Provincial governments, acting through universities and other post-secondary institutions, ultimately determine the numbers of training places available. Professional associations may attempt to influence such decisions, but as the decision in the late 1970s to expand the University of British Columbia medical school showed, they may fail. On the other hand, in most provinces most of the time (Quebec being an apparent exception) professional associations have exercised very powerful influence over their own governing legislation, and are able to make regulations under it subject only to scrutiny of varying effect by the Lieutenant-Governor-in-Council. The control over conduct appears more effective than that over professional numbers.

At a more fundamental level, by assuming both the existence and the policy relevance of an independent consumer demand curve, and by assuming away the agency role of the professional, the monopoly model in effect ignores the basic social (as opposed to private or conspiratorial) justification for the *existence* of self-regulating professions. If consumer/patient/clients are assumed to make their own decisions about how much care to use, responding to out-of-pocket prices and consulting their own incomes and "tastes" but not responding to the advice (as opposed to prices) of professionals, and further, if by the assumption of consumer sovereignty, we accept such decisions (however well or badly informed) as the choices which *ought* to govern production and distribution, then it is not surprising that the result is a policy recommendation to dismantle the professions, or at least to reduce significantly their control over the economic conduct of their members.

In this framework, the quantity and mix of services which consumer/patients choose to take off the market is always the "right" one for them, at the current level and pattern of prices which they face. Underuse, or inappropriate use, is defined only in terms of a faulty price structure—

---

[9] Some analysts advocate roll-back and privatization of insurance *without* removal of the professional "monopoly," which seems, at the very least, intellectually inconsistent.

"too high" as a result of restricted entry and/or collusive behaviour, just as in chapter 2 it was "too low" as a result of insurance. The issues of effectiveness (or harm) and the relation between care and health status or other ultimate objectives are simply ignored. The customer is always right, or else is, on average, closer to right than anyone else can be on her behalf.

In a number of currently "professionalized" markets, these full (or at least best available) information and consumer sovereignty assumptions, and their associated policy implications, do seem to be defensible. But in health care, particularly in its more complex and life/limb threatening aspects, they are highly dubious, if not silly. In any case, intellectual consistency requires either that consumers *are* sufficiently informed to, and do, make their own decisions, or that they are not. If they are, and do, then the exogenous demand curve is a valid tool of analysis, but the agency role of the professional is superfluous. If they do not, then the professional has a role as analysed in chapter 4 (which may nevertheless be well or badly performed), but the exogenous demand curve cannot serve either as a description of utilization behaviour (in response *inter alia* to prices) or as a standard for what levels or mixes *ought* to be. One cannot logically have it both ways. (Not that that prevents many analysts from doing so.)

The monopoly model also adopts the conventional assumption that the professional "firm" is a profit-maximizing entity, responding either to fixed input and output prices or to input and output supply and demand schedules. Once past the entry barriers, and except for specific regulations (and perhaps unofficial provincial constraints and threats), the professional firm attempts to minimize its costs and maximize its profits like any other private business. This assumption, in turn, makes the firm's short-run output decisions determinate, matching marginal revenue to marginal cost across each class of output. In the middle and longer run, decisions over use of capital and other labour inputs, choice of specialty, and location and migration decisions are all governed by the same profit-maximizing objective. The firm will always choose the minimum cost (subject to regulatory constraint) way of producing whatever its consumer/patients wish to buy (as represented by the assumed exogenous demand curve) and will go into whatever line or location of production which consumer willingness to pay dictates. Thus the model provides simple answers to a wide class of policy questions. Technical efficiency is, by assumption, always assured, and problems of location and specialization, if they exist, are easily dealt with through manipulation of prices or subsidies. Whatever behaviour is desired, which the market does not automatically yield, can be achieved by the creation of profit opportunities.[10]

---

[10] Some might argue that whatever the market does not yield, should not be desired; but that is an ideological input to economic analysis, not a conclusion from it.

Again, the model has some practical relevance. It seems clear, for example, that problems of undersupply of services in remote regions *can* be mitigated by "flooding the market" with providers or by fee differentials or subsidies such that incomes are higher in less than in more desirable regions. People do respond to income incentives. But it is a substantial step from there to the assumption that the professional firm "maximizes profits." The unrealism of that assumption emerges at both empirical and theoretical levels.

SYSTEMATIC DEPARTURES FROM COST-MINIMIZATION: THE (NON) USE OF AUXILIARIES

The empirical evidence bearing on profit maximization, which in turn implies (but is not implied by) cost minimization, is of several forms. The most extensively studied area relates to cost-minimization, in particular to the use of auxiliary personnel in medical, dental, and pharmaceutical practice. The comparison of group with solo (and, where permitted, chain or corporate) practice, and the question of the optimal scale and organization of practices, also open the issue of what motivates practitioners and the practices they control. Similarly, concerns over the distribution of practice capacity (usually expressed in terms of distribution of practitioners) across regions or specialties arise from the observation that factors other than income/profit possibilities strongly influence such career choices.

For at least twenty years, there has been a growing interest in the possibility of using "intermediate-level health practitioners," less neutrally described as paraprofessionals, or ancillaries, to perform a number of the functions currently performed by physicians, dentists, or pharmacists. An extensive literature, based in part on experimental and field experience, has developed which demonstrates the technical feasibility of such substitution over a wide range of functions, while maintaining quality standards equal to or better than those achieved by the "peak professionals."[11] And the problem of diagnosis of abnormality, of identifying those problems which have gone beyond the skills of the intermediate-level practitioner, turns out in practice not to be a difficulty. Diagnosing the existence of abnormality, of the unusual or complex problem, is of a lower order of difficulty from determining the nature of, and appropriate response to, the complexity itself.

The monopoly model predicts, of course, that established professions will attempt to suppress the entry of new types of professional "firms" into the service marketplace. The denturist/dental mechanic, the optometrist, the chiropractor, and the clinical psychologist are all selling

---

[11] As examples only: Reinhardt 1973, 1975; Rafferty 1974; Spitzer 1978; Evans and Williamson 1978; Record 1981; Denton *et al.* 1982.

services which compete directly with some of those offered by physicians or dentists, while self-employed dental hygienists, midwives, nurse practitioners, or dental nurses[12] would dramatically widen the range of contested territory. The pressure by other types of therapists, acupuncturists, for example, represents the same threat—more firms of diverse types sharing a market already overcrowded with physicians, dentists, and pharmacists, and practitioners with diverse professional backgrounds and cultures such that economic co-ordination would be more difficult. It is not therefore suprising that the entry and/or spread of such competitors has been bitterly contested, either by attacks on their professional legitimacy and competence or, where possible, by direct regulation, without any serious attempt at justification (as opposed to bald assertion) in terms of patient protection. The relatively slow growth, compared with their potential, in numbers and capacity of professional firms run by/employing substitutes for physicians contrasts sharply with the rapid expansion of occupations, particularly in hospitals, which are complementary to physicians in the sense of increasing their ability to serve (and bill for) patients.

What the monopoly model does not predict, however, is the failure of firms run by peak professionals to take up the opportunity to *hire* such personnel. Practitioner time is the principal cost of production of the NOFP firm. The professional owner(s) may hire other professionals as well as other employees, in which case the compensation of the hired professional shows up directly as a cost of production. But the self-employed individual must also be credited with an implicit wage. Profit in the economic (as opposed to accounting) sense is the net revenue (positive or negative) remaining after such deduction. Accordingly, the substitution of less costly auxiliary time for expensive own-time will lower the professional firm's cost of production and raise its profits. A truly profit-maximizing professional sector would still resist with all weapons available the entry of new independent firms as competitors, but existing firms would be willing to hire any and all auxiliaries so long as the resulting additions to total billings (marginal revenue product per employee) exceeded the increases in wage and overhead costs (marginal outlay per employee) including the implicit costs of supervision. Yet the evidence is extensive that this does not happen.

One possible explanation is external constraint. Under the Canadian Medicare program, for example, practitioners are not permitted to bill for services provided by employees, but only for their own services. Parts of a task may be delegated to assistants, but not the task as a whole.

---

[12] A dental auxiliary with about twenty months post-secondary training, who can interpret X-rays and "drill and fill" teeth requiring plastic restorations, to quality standards at least as high as those of a general dentist.

Clearly this discourages the use of more highly qualified assistants, such as nurse practitioners or midwives, who are specifically trained to perform entire services. And the measured productivity gains from task sharing are much less than those from task delegation.

If Medicare regulations were the explanation, however, the problem of underuse of auxiliaries would be confined to Canadian physicians. Yet most of the studies identifying underuse are American, and the problem appears at least as serious in dentistry (on both sides of the border), where no universal plan applies. The phenomenon is far too general to be explained by the payment rules of a particular insurance program.

Self-regulation also imposes constraints; dentists, for example, may not legally employ dental nurses even if they wish to. And physicians who go beyond their colleagues' norms in task delegation may be much more vulnerable to malpractice charges, regardless of whether any unfortunate outcome was in fact linked to delegation. Such collective restraint of the individual can be interpreted in the cartel form of the monopoly model—practitioners collectively recognize that if as individuals they begin to expand capacity and output, the resulting expansion in total supply will drive down price, while the new auxiliaries add to costs.

But collective constraints, while clearly significant in preventing the deployment of certain types of personnel, are also an incomplete explanation. Underuse is not restricted to regulatory blockage of specific occupations such as midwife or dental nurse; even legally permitted forms of auxiliaries are utilized well short of the cost-minimizing, profit-maximizing level by individual NOFP firms.

ADDITIONAL, OR ALTERNATIVE, OBJECTIVES FOR THE FIRM: BEHAVIOURAL AND POLICY IMPLICATIONS

The available explanations seem to be twofold, and both require us to modify and extend the simple monopoly model.[13] One is that practitioner/owners have "tastes" for particular practice styles: they enjoy doing things themselves, for example, and dislike directing and administering teams of other people (Reinhardt 1972). And the umbrella of protection against competition, created by restrictions on entry and collective self-regulation of economic conduct, enables practitioners to indulge these tastes without giving up an unacceptable amount of income. The objectives of the firm must then be extended to include not only "profit" but

---

[13] An "explanation" sometimes offered by professional associations, that patient/consumers will not accept services from intermediate-level personnel, has been shown to be without foundation whenever it has been tested.

attainment of the practitioner's preferred practice style. The practitioner's utility or level of welfare depends on both. The NOFP firm is now a utility-maximizer; profit being only one contributor to the practitioner's well-being.

The second explanation points in the same direction. The root weakness of the profit-maximizing assumption is that it neglects the identity between the practitioner as practice owner and residual claimant to net revenues, and the practitioner as supplier of labour and skills to the practice (Evans and Williamson 1978; Evans 1980). The major component of cost to the practice, the practitioner's implicit wage, is also the major component of the practitioner's earnings. A "cost-reducing" substitution of auxiliary for professional labour input will in fact lower the practitioner's income; profits rise but implicit wage falls, unless the total practice output can be expanded to maintain the level of employment of practitioner time. Accordingly, we find auxiliaries more extensively employed where professional/population ratios are low, and practitioners feel "over-worked" (a situation which is inexplicable for a profit-maximizing firm, at least in equilibrium—it just raises prices). Conversely, as professional practitioner to population ratios rise, collective hostility to intermediate-level practitioners increases, and their employment falls.

The bias of professional practices towards overuse of the "high-priced help," and underuse of less expensive auxiliaries, is thus explicable if we shift our focus from the profits of the firm to a more plausible objective, the net income of the firm's owner(s). But net income maximization alone is an implausible objective; formally, such an objective predicts twenty-four-hour work-days, 365 (or 366) days per year. Instead, we postulate maximization of a more general set of objectives which include both net income and leisure time, as well as elements of practice style—hence the NOFP designation. The firm's behaviour will only respond to profit opportunities which pay off in terms of some combination of net income and reduced or more professionally satisfying work load, subject also to the practitioner's preferences for particular working environments or practice styles.

This extended view of the NOFP firm retains the assumption that service demand is exogenous and price dependent, that firms individually and collectively are constrained by a demand relationship which uniquely (and inversely) links the volume of services they can sell with the price the consumer/patient/client must pay for them. It is thus, like the monopoly model, unable to explain the existence of self-regulation as other than a conspiracy against the public interest to constrain supply and elevate price. What it does do, however, is to open more dimensions of firm behaviour in a way which seems more closely to approximate reality. It requires us to re-interpret the "costs" of self-regulation and professional organization.

In the monopoly model, these "costs" were simply allocative distortions, too low total output from the NOFP sector and too high relative prices. Society as a whole would be better off, according to this model, if more resources were diverted from other sectors into expanding the NOFP sector. In addition to the allocative distortion, wealth is transferred to firm or resource owners in the NOFP sector in the form of higher prices and incomes, and away from those who pay for such services.[14]

The extended view of NOFP firms' objectives, however, shifts attention away from allocative distortions and towards the issue of the technical efficiency with which such firms use resources. By unnecessarily using the time and skills of the most costly practitioners, and failing to use equally effective, less costly substitutes, NOFP firms appear systematically to waste resources. And this form of waste is on a large scale. Estimates by various authors for several of the NOFP sectors in Canada and the United States suggest that reductions of as much as 40 percent of total expenditures on dental services, pharmaceutical dispensing, and ophthalmic goods could be achieved through rationalization of production and use of less expensive personnel, without loss of quality (Benham 1972; Benham and Benham 1975; Evans and Williamson 1978). Similar savings estimates for medical services are harder to develop, but in Canada are very conservatively put in the neighbourhood of 10-15 percent for all medical care and 16-24 percent for ambulatory care (Denton *et al.* 1982). For ambulatory primary care in the United States they run into billions of dollars (Record 1981). The most extreme estimated costs of allocative distortions, under the assumption that production of services is technically efficient, are by contrast almost certainly less than 10 percent, and quite likely below 5 percent.[15] And the simple monopoly model's policy "solution" to allocative distortions—increase the supply of professionals—is likely to exacerbate the more serious technical inefficiencies.

EVIDENCE FROM GROUP PRACTICES: TECHNICAL EFFICIENCY

The issue of the technical efficiency of the NOFP sector goes beyond the use of auxiliaries as substitutes for peak professionals. The discussion

---

[14] Wealth-transfer effects may or may not be viewed as a "cost," depending on one's distributional objectives.

[15] Assume, for example, that monopoly power in an industry has advanced prices by 50 percent, so that removal of the distortion would drop prices by a third. Further assume unit elasticity of demand, so that the price decrease would increase quantity sold by 50 percent (total sales remain constant). The allocative burden as a percent of total expenditure would be $(^{1}/_{3})P(^{1}/_{2})Q(^{1}/_{2}) \div PQ = 8.3$ percent. For the health care field as a whole, unit elasticity and 50 percent price enhancement are extreme assumptions.

of group versus solo practice, which has gone on for at least fifty years, has as one of its themes the issue of economies of scale and technical efficiency of production. It has been argued by proponents that group practices are able to make better use of "lumpy" forms of capital equipment or of auxiliaries for whom a solo practitioner could not provide full-time employment, and generally to gain from efficiencies in the scheduling and co-ordination of personnel and tasks in serving patients with multiple problems and needs. As evidence, one might observe higher rates of service output and of net income per practitioner in group than in solo practice. Yet if the profit-maximizing, cost-minimizing model of firm behaviour were correct, such discussion would be beside the point. Firms would adopt whatever structure they found to be cost-minimizing, and the persistence of both types of firms would indicate that each had a market niche, somehow defined. Promotion of one style or another rests on an implicit assumption that practitioner-owners of firms are either uninformed about opportunities for cost-minimization (implausible, in a world of rational profit-maximizers) or have tastes and perceptions about styles of practice which influence their behaviour but which could be modified. The latter view, of professionals with perceptions and tastes for particular practice styles which strongly influence practice mode independently of income opportunities, seems both a priori, and on the evidence, the more plausible.

But the focus of the group practice debate has shifted significantly over the last three decades. The earlier arguments for grouping per se, that taking a number of fee-for-service solo practitioners and combining them in a fee-for-service group would somehow increase efficiency, have largely been abandoned. The apparent income and output advantages of professionals in such groups have been shown to be largely a result of differences in product line rather than choice of production technique (Bailey 1970*a*, 1970*b*). The technology of particular medical specialties, such as diagnostic radiology and pathology, lends itself to large groupings with high auxiliary and equipment use per professional. But to compare such groups with solo or small group general or family practitioners, and to assume that large groups of primary care specialists would display the same behaviour as radiologists, is clearly illegitimate. Moreover, when primary care practitioners *do* form large groups, apparent increases in output per practitioner may result, not from greater efficiency in primary care, but from the establishment in-house of diagnostic services which were previously referred out. From a system-wide perspective, solo practitioners with a well-functioning referral network may be just as efficient as a formal group. Those functions which do display significant scale economies become specialized services available to several practitioners.

Significant advantages in efficiency have been consistently (though not universally) demonstrated for groups which not only assemble a number of practitioners but which are reimbursed on a capitation rather than a fee-for-service basis (Enthoven 1980; Luft 1981). Variously labelled as Community Health Centres or Health Services Organizations (HSOs) in Canada, Prepaid Group Practices, Closed-Panel Practices, or Health Maintenance Organizations (HMOs) in the United States, all such groups provide a combination of both professional and risk-bearing services. They serve a defined population group of enrollees, and their revenues are a fixed dollar amount per enrollee per time period. Enrollees are then provided with all "needed" services, as judged by the group's practitioners, either from the group itself or from external referrals at the group's expense. In the United States, an enrollee who self-refers for services outside the group pays their cost out of pocket; in Canada, the Medicare program relieves the patient of any personal liability. Depending on provincial arrangements, however, the cost of such services may be charged back to the group's budget.

Such organizations have achieved improvements in efficiency in two main ways. First, they have made significantly greater use of intermediate-level practitioners as substitutes for physicians than has the private practice, fee-for-service system. This observation tends to support the utility– rather than the revenue– or net income-maximizing model of the NOFP firm. It is of course true that a group which, when adding or replacing a professional, chooses a salaried nurse practitioner rather than a physician will, if revenues are unaffected, raise the surplus available for distribution among group members. But this is equally true for a fee-for-service group, if reimbursement agencies permit billing on behalf of auxiliaries. Differences in patterns of auxiliary use indicate that the shift in payment mode is associated with changes in management structure, such that practitioner preferences receive less weight. Or practitioners in such groups may be differentially self-selected and socialized. In any case, the evidence suggests that more efficient use of auxiliaries results from change in the reimbursement and management structure, the pattern of incentives and control, not from grouping and scale per se. Pure scale economics in medical practice, as opposed to more auxiliary substitution, do not seem to be pronounced.

PROVIDER INFLUENCE OVER USE: PREPAID GROUPS AND THE EXERCISE OF AGENCY

Secondly, and most important, the product mix of such prepaid groups differs substantially from fee-for-service practice. Numerous studies of different groups under different circumstances have shown reductions in hospital use of up to 40 percent for group enrollees, compared with similar patients in fee-for-service practices (Luft 1981). These results have accumulated over thirty years, and form one of the principal supports for present United States health policies of trying to contain health care costs by promoting the spread of HMOs. Similar findings in Canada have helped to keep alive an interest in alternatives to traditional self-employed fee-for-service medical practice, although the integration of such alternative forms of practice into a universal public insurance system is much more difficult (Vayda 1977; Luft *et al.* 1980; Stoddart and Seldon 1983).

For understanding the behaviour of NOFP firms and their practitioner-owners, the significance of such variations in output mix is twofold. First, it demonstrates the extent to which practitioners influence the demand for their own services, and thus supports the analysis of agency in chapter 4. The assumption that health care users display an exogenous "demand" for health care, using more when the prices they face are lower and conversely, requires that a difference in mix be associated with a difference in relative prices. If people enrolled in HMOs use less hospital care than patients of fee-for-service practitioners, then, according to that model, it must be because they face higher prices for hospital care, either absolutely or relative to ambulatory care. But significant differences in use are found in settings where patients are fully insured for either form of care. The obvious explanation, which is also that given by practitioners themselves, seems to be the correct one. Practitioners in capitation-based groups adopt, for economic and/or professional reasons, styles of practice which involve admitting patients to hospital less frequently and for shorter stays. The practitioners directly and powerfully influence the level of services which patients receive, independently of the prices which users do or do not pay.

ALTERNATIVES TO THE EXOGENOUS DEMAND CURVE: PROFESSIONAL ETHICS?

Such an inference may seem blindingly obvious, and is generally accepted by students of health care. But to a significant number of economists, principally but not entirely working in the United States, it has been unacceptable. Such intellectual resistance can be readily understood in terms of the fundamental role which the assumption of exogenous demand plays in "closing" the models above, and permitting the construction of consistent, if not necessarily accurate or enlightening, explanations of NOFP firm behaviour. Economists have a professional predilection for explaining individual or organizational behaviour as resulting from attempts to maximize or optimize with respect to some desired objective, subject to external constraints, and the external demand curve is a critical constraint. If practitioners can generate demand directly, why not do so indefinitely, and then raise prices to choke off that demand, thus achieving higher incomes at the same work load? What constrains utilization, if *not* the external demand curve?

An obvious answer is, professional ethics. Practitioners' concepts of "practice style" include views on how medicine, dentistry, etc., *ought* to be practiced, and a large part of their training is intended to inculcate such values. Providing services which they believe to be unnecessary, or even harmful, is clearly a source of professional dissatisfaction, as is imposing substantial economic burdens on their patients. The objectives of the NOFP firm must then be extended to include, not just practitioner net income, work load, and practice setting, but also the degree to which practice activity conforms to the professional, ethical principles of the individual practitioner (Evans 1972, 1974, 1976; Wolfson 1976; Reinhardt 1978; Wolfson and Tuohy 1980). Removing healthy organs, or drilling healthy teeth, has a negative impact on the practitioner's overall satisfaction, even if it is profitable and the patients, believing the organs/teeth were diseased, are satisfied. Professional ethics bound and constrain the demand-generation process.

But this approach is weakened by the second implication of hospital utilization differentials between capitation-based groups and fee-for-service practitioners. There is no observable difference in patient health or well-being between high-use and low-use groups. The inference is that the additional use is not "needed" in a technical, medical sense; such an inference obviously underlies all policies aimed at expanding the role of such groups. In terms of Figure 1-3, it appears that hospital use in aggregate has reached the flat of the health status curve, if not actually a downward sloped segment. The same inference can be drawn from observations of wide variations across regions in surgical rates, patterns of diagnostic testing, and hospital use within the self-employed fee-for-service system. Again, there is no evidence of impaired health status in low-use regions, and indeed in some cases there are grounds for believing that populations in high-use regions suffer as a result (Roos and Roos 1981). Thus if practitioners' ethics and preferences for practice style constrain them in influencing utilization, these preferences do not seem always to be linked to objective information on need. They may, of course, be linked to subjective assessments, and probably are. Most practitioners undoubtedly believe that the services they recommend and provide are genuinely needed in the sense of contributing to health status. Since the subjective views of different practitioners lead to such widely divergent (and expensive) results, however, the source of such views becomes a critical issue.

ARE ETHICS EXOGENOUS?

Hence the argument, which has considerable support from both expert opinion and research, that the appropriate response to problems of over-servicing and unnecessary use is better information and education for practitioners. The focus here is on overuse relative to objective criteria of need, not relative to willingness to pay; and in terms of modelling the NOFP firm the assumption is that the non-economic dimensions of the firm's objectives, the "professional" aspects of ethics and response to needs, are powerful enough motivators that better information can lead to better performance.

In contrast, a "structuralist" view focusses on the pattern of economic incentives implicit in fee-for-service practice. From this perspective, the educational approach involves a fallacy of composition. A convincing demonstration of the inefficacy of a procedure will eventually lead to its abandonment (although perhaps very slowly) as tonsillectomy indicates. (But circumcision?) But the overall level of activity will not be affected; NOFP firms will simply shift time and resources to other sectors. Since the objectives of the firm include economic as well as non-economic components, it will be prepared to trade off dollars against professional pride, or put another way, if income and work load shrink (say because physician-to-population ratios are rising), the practitioner will change the criteria which govern her recommendations to patients, and will generate more demand to keep the patient at the door and the wolf from it. The consistent response of utilization to numbers of practitioners, regardless of price levels, all over North America, is indicative of this trade-off in action. Moreover, standards of practice adapt over time in response to current practices, one's own and others. Thus a shift to recommending more servicing, which may initially be a response to economic factors, becomes over time the new standard.

THE ROLE OF FEES WHEN DEMAND IS ENDOGENOUS

In this process, price plays a role not so much in clearing markets, equating separately determined supplies and demands, but as an alternative instrument for trying to reach practitioner income objectives. The often-observed *positive* correlation of physician-to-population ratios with fee levels (though not incomes) is consistent with physicians reacting to the pressures of oversupply and falling incomes by pushing up prices as well as promoting utilization.

In the Canadian context, however, the fee schedule structure is critical. Many of the opportunities for increasing utilization without working longer hours have been removed. Practitioners are not paid for work done by auxiliaries or (except to a limited extent, by prior agreement, and varying by province) for privately provided diagnostic services. Further, the fee schedules provide limited opportunities for procedural reclassification. Thus, the very restrictive fee increases of the early and mid-1970s in Canada led to significant drops in practitioner real incomes, as shown in

TABLE 7-5

Selected Measures of Physicians' Services, Expenditures, and Use Annual Rates of Increase, 1971–72 to 1980–81

	1971–72 1974–75 %	1974–75 1979–80 %	1979–80 1980–81 %	1971–72 1980–81 %
Aggregate Fee Payments	10.1	11.7	15.9	11.6
Insured Population	1.4	1.1	1.3	1.2
Price	2.3	6.8	10.7	5.7
Utilization	7.6	4.6	4.7	5.6
Utilization Per Capita	6.2	3.5	3.4	4.4
Physician Supply	5.5	3.1	3.1	3.9
Output Per Physician	2.2	1.4	1.6	1.7
Consumer Price Index (All Items)	7.7	8.9	10.1	8.6

SOURCES: Canada, Health and Welfare Canada (1981, 1983a).

Table 7-4. They were offset to a limited degree by increased output per practitioner, but generating additional utilization imposed more time and energy costs on the practitioner. On the other hand, the expansion of practitioner numbers translated directly into increased utilization, as new NOFP firms built up "markets" for themselves. Table 7-5 displays price and utilization patterns during the 1970s, indicating the relatively steady 1–2 percent annual increase in billings per physician (adjusted for fee increases) over this period. Substantial increases in utilization are associated with increases in the physician supply. Since 1975, curtailment of physician immigration has reduced this growth somewhat, but physician-to-population ratios continue to climb.

The central significance of the organization and payment of professionals, and of physicians in particular, for utilization patterns is also illustrated by the experience of other countries. Sweden, for example, like Canada, experienced a dramatic increase in physician supply during the 1970s, 5.6 percent per year from 1970 to 1978. Yet the number of physician visits rose only 1.5 percent per year, and visits per physician fell 3.8 percent annually, or 27.2 percent over the period (Jönsson 1981). Sweden's physicians are salaried; when the population per physician drops, so apparently does the work load. Canada's fee-for-service physicians provide more services per patient. In the United States, an intermediate response seems to have occurred. Visit rates per capita do not appear to have responded to the increase in physician supply (which may reflect the fact that Americans pay a significant proportion of physician costs out of pocket), but the intensity of servicing per visit, billings per visit adjusted for fee changes (which the physician controls) has risen steadily.[16] In none of these settings does the independent decision-making of the patient appear to play a significant role.

We have moved a long way from the simple "monopoly model" of professional firms, gaining in richness and realism at the expense of complexity and increasing uncertainty of predictions. The monopoly model addressed only a single issue, the role of professional entry restrictions/conduct control in elevating service prices above, and depressing outputs below, their socially optimal levels. Profit-maximizing firms were assumed to ensure that production was fully efficient and that regional, specialty, or other types of sub-markets were all served equally adequately or inadequately, relative to consumer willingness to pay, while informed consumers ensured that whatever was produced and used was appropriate. The only policy issues in such a world concern who, if anyone, should impose restraints on entry and conduct, and on what criteria? Is any regulation necessary? If so what kind, and by whom? Expansion of entry and limitation of self-regulatory power are anticipated to lead to increased output and lower prices.

While identifying a part of the elephant, the monopoly model is unable to enlighten or even to express a number of aspects of the real world or of the concerns of health policy. Opening up the supply side of the model, by abandoning the profit-maximizing assumption, reveals serious concerns about the technical efficiency of professional service production and about the responsiveness of professional firms to the needs/demands of various sub-markets. From this broader perspective, it appears that professionalization generates unnecessarily high costs of production, and that these excess costs far outweigh those of the allocative distortions created by monopoly per se. Moreover, such excess costs appear to be *increased* by increases in the supply of professionals, so long as legal restraints permit only professionals to own/manage professional services

---

[16] From 1950 to 1979, expenditures on physicians' services in the United States rose on average 9.7% per year, while the Consumer Price Index Physicians' Services component rose 5.22%, and population rose 1.37% (United States, Department of Health and Human Services 1980, Tables 64 and 69; Gibson *et al*. 1983). Thus physicians' services per capita rose about 2.85% per year over this period, to finish about 125% higher, while visit rates per capita were relatively stable (Andersen and Anderson 1967; Aday and Andersen 1975; Aday *et al*. 1980; United States, *op cit*. 1980). The growth in services per visit proceeds relatively evenly over this whole period. Over the same period, physician supply per capita was increasing at an average rate of 1.06% per year, total increase 35.9%, while physician services prices (unadjusted for changes in collection rates) outstripped the general price level by 1.34% per year or 47.3% over the whole period. Fee-adjusted billings per physician, "productivity," rose 63.4% or 1.7% per year. The substantial increase in relative prices thus accompanied a dramatic increase in total output, and the trends show no sign of abating.

firms. More physicians/dentists trained leads to less use of auxiliaries, and higher costs of production.

In this environment, the appropriate response may be to open up the licensure process in one of two ways. If restrictions on practice ownership were removed, so that non-professionals, including public corporations, could own and manage practices (though not performing the activities and functions of professionals), then the economic disincentive to auxiliary use would disappear. Such a policy would operate in conjunction with licensure of more intermediate-level professionals themselves (midwives or dental nurses, *e.g.*) to lower the cost of providing professional services. Alternatively, one could adopt a policy of licensing more intermediate-level professionals to compete directly for parts of the professional market, as dental mechanics or optometrists now do.[17] The evidence is more than ample that such practitioners in either setting are capable of performing a significant range of additional functions. Professions do indeed function in part as monopolies, restricting supply and elevating price, but the simple response of training more peak professionals is likely to do more harm than good.

The influence of the preferences of professionals-as-persons on the behaviour of professional-practices-as-firms also opens the issue of service distribution and the adequacy of supply in sub-markets. Profit-maximizing firms go wherever effective demand is sufficient to cover costs. But people have preferences as to location and specialization, such that equal income opportunities may lead to very unequal distributions of service. In theory, a competitive market system would lead to the emergence of price differentials with lower prices and incomes for the same time and effort level in more desirable areas or specialties, to equalize net advantages. And as a rising tide lifts all the boats, expansion of supply should increase availability in both desirable and undesirable areas.

The latter effect does indeed seem to occur, but the differential prices, lower in desirable, overserviced areas, do not emerge. This is perhaps unsurprising, since much professional activity is devoted to ensuring that markets for such services are not price-competitive. The implication of extending the firm's objective beyond profit-maximization, however, is that redistribution of services across regions or specialties, if desired on whatever social grounds, may be sought through other mechanisms than the price-income link. Price differentials are not the only, or even necessarily the most effective, way to redistribute capacity or personnel. Changes in the education system, either recruitment or training processes, may be more successful and/or cheaper. Yet ironically, the possibility of a systematic test of the role of price differentials in allocating professionals

---

[17] One would also have to permit, and indeed encourage, open advertising and price competition if such a policy were to be effective.

across regions or specialties is greater in a system of uniform negotiated fee schedules, as in the Canadian provinces, than among independently price-setting practices. One can ensure that the desired differentials are in fact established.

Once we abandon the demand-side assumption that the utilization of professional services is determined by informed consumers responding to price signals, however, the world becomes a good deal more complex. Changes in organization which promise to increase efficiency and competition in service supply, by introducing for-profit corporate ownership, *e.g.*, may also degrade the performance of the agency function. Efficient overservicing is not an obvious gain. Bailey (1977, 1979) argues that this has occurred in the United States commercial laboratory industry, and similar developments may be underway in Canada. And the general presumption that "monopoly" leads to too little service at too high a price becomes misleading, irrelevant, or just plain wrong, if a public policy-induced oversupply of practitioners leads to both unnecessary servicing and inefficient production. Neither expanding professional through-put nor opening the industry to for-profit corporate enterprise is likely to improve the situation.

The model of the NOFP firm, from this more general perspective, suggests two distinct classes of policies (Evans 1980). One, a combination of research, education, and regulation, would seek to influence practitioner behaviour directly to improve the effectiveness of the services being provided. This would be combined with restrictions on the supply of new practitioners, plus removal of self-regulatory barriers to, and perhaps provision of direct incentives for, the use of more intermediate-level personnel. The second approach would involve attempting to redefine the nature of the services or products being provided, as the American HMOs do in offering packages of insurance plus "needed" services at a fixed price, rather than fees per service. For such redefined products, a combination of consumer information and/or regulation of product (as opposed to provider) characteristics may make a competitive market more effective. Both of these approaches will be dealt with in more detail below.

If the generalized model of the NOFP firm is realistic, however, any sort of policy response to the problems of appropriate servicing levels and efficiency in production will be made extremely difficult by the manpower policies of the past fifteen years. In the late 1950s and early 1960s, decisions were taken which substantially increased the supply of physicians in Canada. In part these were a response to population forecasts which turned out to be in error—the Hall Commission forecast 28.2 million Canadians in 1981, about four million too high—and in part they reflected some combination of perceptions of "unmet" need which public insurance would reveal, and of physician "shortages" indicated by rising (relative) prices and incomes. Increases in training places, plus immigration, led to an increase of about 50 percent in the physician-to-population ratio between 1962 and 1979, while output per physician was expanding as well (Barer and Evans 1983). This flood of new supply effectively foreclosed the opportunity to create and deploy less costly substitutes for physicians and led to the expansion of per capita utilization rates which has continued through the 1970s, as displayed in Figure 7.5.

In February 1975, immigration of physicians was cut back sharply in recognition of the problem of emerging oversupply. But present numbers of training places and attrition patterns, combined with current population forecasts, indicate a steady, though slower, rise in the physician-to-population ratio into the far future. On the other hand, the downtrend in death rates at the end of the 1970s and early 1980s could lead over the long run to both a larger and a significantly older population than that implied by population forecasts at the turn of the decade. Several studies (Boulet and Grenier 1978; Denton and Spencer 1983) have shown that if one assumes constant age-sex specific physician utilization rates, and calculates "needs" on the basis of population forecasts from the late 1970s, the aging of the population would not balance the growth of physician stock. But more recent data show relatively rapid increases in survival rates among the elderly, which may eventually justify current rates of production. In any case, one should not take for granted the appropriateness of current utilization patterns, and it remains true that such patterns could be provided by a very different mix of personnel.

Dentistry is experiencing similar dramatic increases in supply, an increase of 43 percent in active dentists per capita or over 3 percent per year, between 1969 and 1981 (Canada, Health and Welfare Canada 1980, 1983b). This increases the pressure on competitive auxiliary occupations and leads to efforts to promote prevention and cosmetics as ways of expanding servicing levels.[18] The environment of most NOFP firms in health care for the foreseeable future thus appears to be one of steadily expanding supply, and the implications for efficient resource allocation, given the present institutional framework, are not encouraging.

---

[18] This observation may appear inconsistent with data presented above, which show *increases* in numbers of auxiliaries per dentist in private practice. The concepts of complementarity and substitution in production provide the key. Classes of personnel which substitute for the skills of the dentist—the expanded function auxiliaries or dental nurses—which appeared in the early 1970s to be "the wave of the future" are now in the past; but complementary auxiliaries which add to the product line (hygienists) or expand the productivity and billing capacity of the dentist, are still popular. In the same way, physicians support the expansion of complementary hospital personnel who increase their billing opportunities, but resist competitive substitutes.

CHAPTER 8

HOSPITALS AND RELATED INSTITUTIONS: IF NOT-FOR-PROFIT THEN FOR WHAT?

THE SCALE AND GROWTH OF NFP INSTITUTIONS IN CANADA

The previous chapter traced out the way in which economists' analysis of professional practices, as special types of firms, has evolved over time. Earlier analyses attempted to treat practices as essentially similar to ordinary private, for-profit firms, differing only in their ability to limit (collectively) the rate of entry of new professionals/firms and to exercise some co-ordination of economic behaviour (particularly pricing). These profession-as-monopoly models explain some aspects of professional behaviour quite satisfactorily, but are clearly inadequate to capture its full diversity. More extended and sophisticated models of professional practices treat them as managed to seek a wider range of objectives, with broader sets of both constraints and strategies. The things that matter to professional practices, or rather to their owner/managers, include profits in the economic sense, but they also include other components of the professional's income, the style, nature and amount of work, and a professional interest in the well-being of the patient.

The process of balancing these multiple objectives, in the context of the economic freedom conferred by the legal status of the profession (particularly freedom to suppress potential competitors) generates a much wider range of questions about the relative efficiency and effectiveness of the outcomes. The greater realism and interest of such extended models, however, and the expanded range of issues they address, are gained at the expense of greater ambiguity in a priori predictive power, which must be supplemented by direct observation.

Throughout this evolution, however, models of NOFP firms have retained the conceptual framework of an owner/decisionmaker/residual claimant who directs the practice-firm's behaviour with some set of objectives in view. And those objectives include practice net revenues, whether expressed as profit or more realistically as practitioner net income. The owner (or owners) of the practice has the legal status of residual claimant to such net revenues: they belong to him/her; and this legal status is logically independent of the regulatory question of whether such residual claimant is a natural or a legal (corporate) person, or possesses a professional qualification.

While such firms are of central importance to the overall functioning of the Canadian health care system, their share in its economic activity (employment or sales) is substantially less than that of not-for-profit (NFP) firms. The leading example of these is the voluntary hospital, governed by a board of trustees on behalf of a voluntary society, municipality, or religious order who are the legal owners. But the category also includes government-run public health programs, co-operative-owned medical clinics, university programs providing health services or research, not-for-profit insurance plans, and in general any organization in which no individual can be identified as having a direct or indirect claim to net revenues.

In Canada, hospitals of all types (general and allied special, mental, and federal) made up 41.4 percent of total health care spending in 1982, compared with 21.8 percent for all professional services. Another 13.7 percent was spent in "homes for special care," split between the NFP and the for-profit sector. For-profit hospitals are virtually non-existent. Moreover, of the 12.2 percent expenditure on public health, research, prepayment, capital formation, and miscellaneous items, about three-quarters passes through the public sector and is thus controlled by NFP organizations.

The largest, most dynamic, and most extensively studied component of the NFP sector is, of course, hospitals. Table 8-1 displays the growth over time of the Canadian general and allied special (G. and A.S.) hospital sector ("allied special" includes chronic and convalescent), in terms of total spending, share of GNP, and share of total health spending. It includes, when available, other institutional spending and various components of all other health care net of institutions, professional services, and drugs and appliances (the "bureaucratized" sector). The latter, not wholly but largely NFP, has grown relatively slowly, while the hospital sector not only expanded dramatically in the general expansion of the 1950s and 1960s, but has been able to maintain some relative growth in the much more restrained climate of the 1970s. The G. & A.S. sector has had to absorb some of the workload of the provincial mental, and federal, hospitals, but it has also been able to shed some of the long-term maintenance of the elderly to the rapidly-growing "homes for special care" sector.

This continual growth in expenditure share has only to a limited extent been related to utilization patterns, at least as measured by admission and patient-day loads. As Table 8-2 indicates, the fast-growth period of general hospital bed capacity, relative to the population, was in the 1950s. Rates of hospital utilization continued to increase along with bed capacity during the 1960s, but they have been virtually stabilized by the restraints of the 1970s. The major sources of expenditure growth throughout the

TABLE 8-1

The Growth of the NFP Sector of the Canadian Health Care System, in $Mn and as Percentage of GNP (Bracketed Figures), 1946–1982

	G. & A.S. Hospitals	Other Hospitals	"Homes for Special Care"	Prepayment & Administration	Public Health	Capital Expenditures	Health Research
1946	150.7 (1.27)	—					
1951	326.4 (1.51)		—				
1956	380.8 (1.25)	149.0 (0.48)		—			
1961	722.1 (1.82)	227.0 (0.57)	—	52* (0.1)	81* (0.2)	176* (0.5)	9* (0.02)
1966	1319.0 (2.13)	349.7 (0.56)	—	83* (0.1)	110* (0.2)	221* (0.4)	31* (0.1)
1971	2585.5 (2.74)	567.2 (0.60)	516.0 (0.55)	123.4 (0.13)	214.7 (0.23)	420.2 (0.44)	78.3 (0.08)
1976	5778.4 (3.01)	793.1 (0.41)	1437.2 (0.75)	216.3 (0.11)	484.6 (0.25)	646.2 (0.34)	139.2 (0.07)
1977	6355.1 (3.02)	573.3 (0.28)	1743.3 (0.83)	256.5 (0.12)	544.5 (0.26)	668.3 (0.32)	168.3 (0.08)
1978	6929.3 (2.98)	554.2 (0.24)	2005.1 (0.86)	251.5 (0.11)	594.7 (0.26)	765.9 (0.33)	191.8 (0.08)
1979	7696.9 (2.91)	542.5 (0.21)	2293.4 (0.87)	273.8 (0.10)	697.1 (0.26)	822.7 (0.31)	206.2 (0.08)
1980	8920.4 (3.01)	564.4 (0.19)	2710.4 (0.91)	311.0 (0.10)	762.6 (0.26)	1219.8 (0.41)	243.4 (0.08)
1981	10364.8 (3.06)	359.6 (0.11)	3530.7 (1.04)	403.3 (0.12)	872.1 (0.26)	1332.4 (0.39)	290.2 (0.09)
1982	12045.4 (3.30)	424.6 (0.11)	4117.7 (1.15)	441.4 (0.12)	952.8 (0.27)	1585.4 (0.44)	327.1 (0.09)

SOURCES: See Data Sources Appendix.

*These data are for 1960 and 1965, not 1961 and 1966.

period are not population or utilization increases, but expenditure per admission or per patient-day.

Table 8-2 also shows that overall hospital capacity and use was relatively stable down to 1966, and has trended down since then, with dramatic reductions in mental and T.B. hospital use balancing the growth of the general hospital sector. Allied special hospitals, primarily long-term care, have shown the most consistent growth since 1961. But the most prominent growth pattern in the hospital sector has been the increase in costs per patient-day, adjusted for general inflation. Average annual increases in *per diems* of over seven percent, for thirty years, make up

TABLE 8-2

Hospital Bed Capacity and Utilization, Canada, 1946–1982/83

	Public General Hospitals				Public Allied Special Hospitals		All Hospitals	
	Beds per 1000 Pop'n	Patient-Days per 1000 Pop'n	Expenditure per patient-day $current	$1971	Beds per 1000 Pop'n	Patient-days per 1000 Pop'n	Beds per 1000 Pop'n	Patient-days per 1000 Pop'n
1946	3.87	1101.4	5.27	11.72	0.45	104.8	10.13	—
1951	4.19	1212.1	9.05	13.72	0.71	201.2	10.42	—
1956	4.67	1350.2	15.95	23.28	0.66	195.4	10.84	3202.3
1961	4.86	1434.4	24.34	32.47	0.65	205.1	10.58	3368.4
1966	5.27	1527.7	38.56	46.18	0.84	266.5	10.35	3261.4
1971	5.49	1595.9	66.61	66.61	0.92	300.8	9.78	3002.0
1975	5.66	1554.0	121.82	87.93	1.02	333.7	9.18	2675.7
1976	5.15	1435.0	140.13	94.13	1.55	500.9	7.19	2062.4
1977/78	5.25	1478.1	151.87	94.45	1.57	506.8	7.14	2075.1
1978/79	5.19	1472.9	166.26	94.90	1.57	515.9	7.10	2081.9
1979/80	5.11	1438.6	182.18	95.27	1.57	523.0	6.97	2079.2
1980/81	5.11	1474.8	208.89	99.20	—	513.5*	6.98	2039.4*
1981/82	—	1471.4	236.75	99.94	—	501.8*	—	2030.2*
1982/83	5.04	1464.2	276.67	105.40	1.51	493.4	6.82	2028.8
Annualized Rates of Growth:								
1946–61	1.53	1.78	10.74	7.03	2.48	4.58	0.29	—
1961–71	1.23	1.07	10.59	7.28	3.54	3.90	−0.78	−1.14
1971–75	0.77	−0.66	16.29	7.19	2.61	2.63	−1.57	−2.84
1976–82	−0.36	0.34	12.01	1.90	−0.43	−0.25*	−0.88	−0.27*

*These data are drawn from preliminary annual reports, which in earlier years are inconsistent with the subsequently published annual reports.

NOTE: Data from 1946 to 1975 are from Fraser (1983). Data from 1976 on are from Canada, Statistics Canada (1982, 1984). See also Data Sources Appendix. In the 1946-75 data, paediatric hospitals are included with "Public General," from 1976 on they are part of "Allied Special" as are maternity hospitals throughout. The "Allied Special" category is, however, predominantly long-term care. "All Hospitals" in 1976 and after excludes mental and tuberculosis hospitals. There appear to be additional inconsistencies between the two sources; pre– and post–1975 data are obviously not comparable. Expenditure per patient-day data are adjusted by the Consumer Price Index.

the lion's share of hospital, and indeed of health, cost increases over the post-war period. The second half of the 1970s represents a very significant break in this trend: virtually no increase from 1976 to 1979/80. Since then, costs per patient-day have averaged 3.43 percent per year growth, after adjustment for inflation, or about half the rate of the 1946 to 1976 period.

These increases reflect a combination of more intensive servicing per patient-day or per episode, and increasing costs of hospital "inputs."

The principal input to hospital care is, of course, human time and skills; thus the 1950s and early 1960s saw a substantial increase in hours worked per patient-day, from 9.2 in 1953, to 13.0 in 1965. Since the mid-1960s, paid hours per patient-day in G. & A.S. hospitals have fluctuated, from 13.3 in 1966, to 14.0 in 1968, back to 13.3 in 1971, up to 14.4 in 1975, and back to 13.9 in 1980/81.

At the same time, the incomes of hospital workers were rising substantially faster than those of the general population, a trend which continued through the 1970s. From 1960 to 1971, an index of hospital workers' wages (Barer and Evans 1983) rose at an average annual rate of 7.53 percent per year, compared with 5.58 percent for the industrial weekly wage, for a 2 percent per year relative gain. From 1971 to 1980, the same index rose 11.65 percent, and the average industrial wage rose 9.73 percent. In the late 1970s the relative gains of hospital workers were greatly slowed, to 9.08 percent per year from 1976 to 1980, compared with 8.62 percent for the average worker. Prices of non-labour inputs to hospital care, particularly food, fuel, and imported equipment (though not drugs), also rose faster than the general price level during the 1970s, but the main source of escalation is labour costs.

The patterns of increase in hospital costs in Canada find an interesting counterpoint in United States experience. The United States showed the same rapid increases in the 1950s and 1960s; between 1950 and 1970 hospital care moved from 1.35 percent of United States GNP to 2.79 percent. This compares with the Canadian percentages of 1.51 percent in 1951 and 2.74 percent in 1971. But by 1979 United States hospitals were up to 3.56 percent of GNP, compared with Canada's 2.87 percent, and the 1982 United States figure is 4.43 percent (Gibson *et al.* 1983). And, as in Canada, utilization changes have contributed little to these increases. In the 1970s, days of care per capita in short-stay hospitals were virtually static—from 1970 to 1978 community hospital beds per thousand people rose from 4.3 to 4.6, but occupancy fell from 77.3 percent to 73.2 percent (United States Department of Health and Human Services, 1980), implying an increase in patient-days per capita of only 1.3 percent over the period.

The chief difference seems to be the "intensity of servicing" factor. In the United States, it is estimated that after allowing for all increases in prices of hospital inputs, wages and other, increases in service intensity per day raised costs per day at an average annual rate of 4.5 percent from 1970 to 1978 (Freeland *et al.* 1979). A similar calculation for Canada, 1971-80, yields 1.7 percent (Barer and Evans 1983). On the other hand, the same United States source indicates substantially smaller relative wage gains for hospital workers. The indication, therefore, is that the cost impact of increasingly sophisticated technology in hospitals, ever more widely used, with more and more expensive people and machines, has been much less severe in Canada, and that this is the principal source of our cost advantage. On the other hand, the relative income status of hospital workers in Canada, compared to the rest of the population, has advanced more rapidly than in the United States.

Whereas the universal public health insurance program contains medical care costs through its impact on fee schedules—prices—and physician incomes, rather than outputs, it controls costs in hospitals by limiting the growth of service intensity, of quantities of services used. If this very broad generalization is correct, it immediately raises the issue of the potential cost in health benefits from such foregone servicing—the extent to which it is "needed" in the sense of chapter 1. If increased servicing levels per patient-day or stay would lead to improved outcomes, then the Canadian system may be underfunded. But if they do not, as is implicit, and sometimes explicit, in the widespread concern in the United States for controlling and containing hospital costs, then why do hospitals choose to provide them?

MODELLING HOSPITAL BEHAVIOUR: "ORGANIC" NFP FIRMS IN A HYPOTHETICAL MARKET ENVIRONMENT

Put another way, we can "explain" hospital cost trends, in an accounting sense, by identifying the various components of hospital expenditures—wages, prices, utilization, service intensity—and observing which appear to be the primary sources of increase. But this approach addresses only the "how" aspect of cost behaviour, not the "why." The more fundamental, but more difficult, explanation in terms of "why" requires us to explore the behaviour of individuals and organizations which underlies such trends. Whose decisions and acts, in response to what stimuli or constraints, are reflected in the aggregate data? If these questions can be answered, then one can begin to consider ways of influencing aggregate trends.

The most natural, indeed almost instinctive, approach to such questions by economists is to apply the theory of the firm developed in the private sector, treating the hospital (or the government bureau) as a single decision-making and transacting entity, creating what Jacobs (1974) calls "organic" models of the hospital. Hospitals *look* like firms. They have a well-defined physical plant and organizational/administrative structure, purchase productive inputs and convert them into services which are valued by customer/patients, and (depending on the reimbursement system) the "sales revenue" from such services makes up their budgets.

The role of physicians is a bit of a puzzle when this model is applied to North American hospital systems. Physicians admit patients, direct their treatment, and, through the medical staff, exercise important managerial powers, yet they are not paid by or (with some qualifications) responsible to the hospital administration. Are they customers or management? Organic models have tended to sweep this embarrassment under the rug, often with unfortunate results.

In these models, the hospital-as-firm is conceptualized as seeking some objective, or set of objectives, subject to constraints imposed by the external environment. The simplest version expresses the constraints in the usual demand curve form,[1] thus presupposing a reimbursement environment in which patients, or their insurers, pay the hospital on an arm's-length fee-for-service basis.[2] Patients are assumed to choose the type, amount, and source of hospital care they will utilize, responding *inter alia* to the price of such care in terms of out-of-pocket payments. Total care utilization then depends on the average level of hospital prices faced by users, while each individual hospital's output level also depends on its prices relative to the general average. Levels and patterns of utilization by patients with full insurance coverage are rather difficult to explain in this context; analyses applying such models usually include an implicit assumption that hospital insurance is of the private, for-profit variety, with significant patient cost-sharing. Again, the specific United States institutional environment underlies the "general" theoretical framework.

The only modification to the theory of the private firm in the simplest organic model is that hospitals are obviously not profit-maximizers. Some other objective must then be identified, to be maximized under the constraint of the demand curve. Total output is a natural alternative, on the grounds either that hospitals exist to serve the community, or that physicians (entering the model by the back door) value hospital services as "free" inputs to their own practices and also dominate hospital management. One might then postulate that hospitals try to produce as large a quantity of output as possible, subject to the constraints of the demand curve, the production function, and input supply functions.

Such a model has strong implications. Prices will be set as low as possible, to attract patients and increase output. If the hospital must break even financially it will price at average cost, but if it has access to external subsidies, it will price below cost and expand utilization to exhaust the subsidies. Cross-subsidization may occur—profits on some services covering losses on others—depending on the weights with which different types of services enter the overall hospital objective of "quantity" and on the price-responsiveness of demand for different services. In general,

---

[1] The production function and input markets also form part of the constraint set.

[2] The relevance of such analyses outside the United States (or in it!) is thus questionable, but they are useful in providing a bridge between the conventional economic theory of the firm, which presupposes arm's-length output markets, and subsequent attempts to provide a more realistic description of hospital behaviour.

price-insensitive services will be over-priced to subsidize the price-sensitive. But technological efficiency will be assured, since any excess costs due to inefficiency will have to be passed forward in higher prices and hence will lead to lower output.

Break-even operation assumes a static environment. More realistically, hospitals may try to earn surpluses in any one period in order to finance future growth. Since a surplus implies that prices could be lower, and the demand curve constraint implies that lower prices would draw more patients, any surplus represents failure to maximize output in that period. But the surplus can be used to expand or modernize facilities. These lead either to lower production costs for present output, or support anticipated future expansion, and may also induce an outward shift in the demand curve if capacity or "quality" are perceived by potential patients or their physicians as enhanced. Thus present output is traded for future, just as private firms invest by trading present profits for future.

The thrust of such analyses, however, is to divert attention away from the internal workings of hospitals. Whatever is done is assumed to be done efficiently, and the choice of what is to be done is determined externally by patients.[3] Thus, the focus of analysis comes to rest squarely on patients and, in particular, on the role of "excessive" insurance in encouraging "overuse" as discussed in chapter 2 (recall Figure 2-2). If input markets are competitive, hospital care production is technically efficient, and levels and patterns of use are patient determined, then (by prior assumption) nothing else *can* be wrong! Users of some variant of this model accordingly interpret the historical record of hospital cost escalation in terms of growth of hospital insurance stimulating patients to demand more care as out-of-pocket costs fell, thus moving the "demand curve" restraint outward, and enabling hospitals to expand supply.[4]

BRIDGING THE GAP FROM MODEL TO EXPERIENCE: THROW IN MORE ASSUMPTIONS

The apparently contrary observation that utilization increase has *not* been the primary source of expenditure growth in the last thirty years,

---

[3] The obvious weakness of this assumption may be shored up by assuming a "physician-patient pair" as the informed consuming unit. As noted in chapter 4, however, this dodge undercuts any independent theory of the provider; in this context it also assumes away the physician's role in hospital management.

[4] This opens the question as to why, if this interpretation is valid, insurance has become so over-extended, to which the reply is, "public provision plus tax subsidy to private provision." Presumably, in this framework, whatever level and form of insurance coverage, and associated hospital use, arose in an unsubsidized private insurance market would be optimal—Dr. Pangloss again. There is one remaining possible wrinkle, in that the long-run equilibrium scale of quantity-maximizing firms may differ from that of profit-maximizers, with cost implications if the long-run average cost curve is not flat in the relevant range. But in fact (chapter 9) it appears to be flat.

anywhere in North America, can be dealt with in two ways. First, one can postulate that despite the apparent existence of excess capacity in the hospital industry (occupancy rates in the United States typically average in the 70–75 percent range, in Canada about 80–85 percent), for various reasons the industry *is* in fact at full capacity well below 100 percent occupancy.[5] Thus increases in utilization stimulated by, for example, the introduction of a public hospital insurance program, either Canada's universal system in the late fifties or the United States limited form in the mid-sixties, cannot be immediately accommodated. In a United States-style system, prices would then rise to ration demand; in Canada, "direct rationing"—waiting lists, queuing, turning patients away—would according to this model be a necessary response.

The problem with this approach is that costs per patient-day rose rapidly after the introduction of public insurance in *both* countries, and in neither was the utilization response prominent. And the predicted associated phenomena did not appear, neither overt evidence of direct rationing in Canada in the sixties, nor a delayed surge of utilization in the United States in the late 1960s or 1970s. According to the model, the growth of insurance in a situation of capacity restraint should have led to an initial jump in United States hospital prices which would then fall back as capacity and utilization increased. The second stage has never occurred.

A second line of response, therefore, redefines output as it enters the hospital/firm's objectives. Patient-days, or admissions, per se are an implausible representation of the things which matter to hospital managements; "quality of care" is also important. The firm's objective function must reflect an interest in the dual aspects of care: quantity and quality. But quality of care requires resources, too. So an increase in costs per patient-day or per admission might be desired by hospital managements insofar as it corresponds to an increase in intensity of servicing, which *is defined as* increased quality (in this analysis), which is "good."

Furthermore, one may hypothesize that patients also value quality, so that they are willing to pay more for "higher quality" episodes or days of care. The demand curve constraint, defined over admissions or patient-days, thus moves outward to the right as service intensity increases, and there will be some optimal quality-quantity combination which responds to consumer willingness-to-pay and meets hospital management objectives. Increases in insurance coverage thus set off a two-stage increase in "quantity demanded." The demand curve for hospital care—utilization weighted by service intensity/"quality"—moves outward first as insurance coverage increases, lowering patients' out-of-pocket costs. In the

---

[5] Since many hospitals manage to function at occupancy rates of 95 percent plus, it is unclear why 75 percent or 80 percent represents a capacity constraint. A probabilistic definition of capacity based on ensuring that the probability of hitting 100 percent and turning patients away never exceeds some minimal level, neglects the fact that most hospitals have others nearby.

short run, prices of care increase, and the additional revenues are used to pay for more intensive servicing per day or care episode, which further expands consumer demand, which drives prices up further, and so on (Newhouse 1970; Feldstein 1971). Thus, the standard theoretical model of the consumer, determining utilization in response to price signals, can be reconciled with the observation that hospital cost increases are not associated with utilization increases as conventionally measured, either admissions or patient-days, and appear to be driven almost entirely by supply-side forces.

The concept of quality, in this framework, must play several different roles. In the hospital's objective function, "quality" is equated with service intensity. In terms of Donabedian's (1966) triad of structure, process, and outcome concepts of quality, this is a purely structuralist definition. More (input) is better. But as everyone who has thought about the quality of health care has emphasized, what matters to patients, and to society generally, is the quality of *outcomes*. Technological extravaganzas which leave the patient no better, or even worse, off are *not* quality in any meaningful sense, however satisfying they may be to the hospital where they occur or the personnel who carry them off. There is in fact no necessary relation between intensity of servicing and quality of care in the sense of improving health status, however plausible such intensity may be as a description of hospital objectives. Analyses which equate intensity of service—(price adjusted) input costs—with quality, and which then assume that such "quality" is of value to informed consumer/patients for its own sake, require one either to disregard the extensive clinical evidence that more is *not* in general better—more intervention does not always imply health improvement—or else to assume that patients derive direct utility from health care interventions independently of their health-enhancing effect—Münchausen's Syndrome again.[6]

The extended definition of output then brings the issue of cost inflation back to insurance coverage, sidestepping the apparently contradictory utilization data by redefining utilization. Patients are assumed to choose—demand—higher levels of intensity of service, in full knowledge of the effects. In this context, overuse and cost escalation are only problems insofar as knowledgeable consumers are demanding care which they would

---

[6] There is another alternative. One could accept the existence/validity of the clinical evidence on zero or negative health effects of "overservicing" (relative to need) yet assume that such overservicing either never occurs or more plausibly, occurs in some sense "optimally," *i.e.*, could not be reduced by any alternative institutional framework without excessive cost in some other dimension. In the complete absence of either supporting evidence, or the specification of any currently operational process yielding this result, such an assumption can be only a rather peculiar confession of faith—Pangloss, but not economics.

not want if they had to pay its full price, and the solution is to reduce insurance coverage. Any concept of ''need'' has, like the agency role of the physician, dropped out of the model.

A Canadian, or any resident of a country where hospitals are not financed through fee-for-service reimbursement by patients or their private insurers, might reasonably ask, if insurance leads to overuse, would it not be as effective to respond to the overuse by direct rationing rather than by reducing coverage? The answer is no, within this framework, for two reasons. First, consumer/patients are assumed to be the best judges of their own interests. Thus any level of overall expenditure and use achieved by direct rationing will be inferior to (or at least no better than) that achieved by price-rationing and consumer responses.[7] Moreover, and also by assumption, rationing techniques must themselves be costly. They must take the form of non-price barriers (*e.g.*, waiting times) which must rise to a point such that demand adapts itself to constrained supply. Such non-price barriers are a pure overhead cost to society, unlike price barriers which are also someone's income. Rising prices transfer wealth from buyer to seller; non-price barriers are deadweight losses. Since the agency relationship has been excluded by the perfect information assumption, there is no possibility in this model that rationing could take the form of professionals simply changing their criteria of what to advise, in which case the rationing per se could be largely costless. But, of course, in the real world that is precisely what happens.

Despite its manifold inadequacies, the analysis outlined above remains quite popular in the United States. This may be partly a result of its strong linkage with conventional economic theory; doctrinal familiarity is a value in and of itself independent of explanatory power. But it also serves important political objectives. The model presupposes a particular reimbursement environment, dominated by multiple, competitive private suppliers of insurance. And it recommends as a solution to cost escalation further reliance on the type of insurance, embodying group-specific deductible and coinsurance features, which private corporations have a comparative advantage in supplying. It has thus served to protect their market against the threat of universal public coverage which, whatever else it did, would greatly reduce the costs of insurance administration. These costs are the sales of private insurance companies (see chapter 2).

---

[7] There will obviously be distributional differences. Rich people will generally get more care in a price system; poor people in a directly rationed system. Thus advocates of reduced insurance coverage and a greater role for direct charges to patients are also required to accept the existing income/wealth distribution—which they appear prepared to do. They must also accept as equitable the pattern of distribution of burdens of ill-health, either pre– or post-insurance, a much more radical proposition which in most theoretical analysis is simply evaded or ignored. With good reason.

Moreover, the analysis also serves providers by diverting attention from the questions of the technical efficiency with which hospitals produce their services, or the appropriateness of the service mix. The former is assured because hospital managements are assumed to be trying to achieve the highest level of output, in terms of either quantity or quality of services, under the constraint of limited resource inputs. They will thus be under as strong incentives as any manager of a for-profit firm to use those resources efficiently in a technical sense, not to waste them in ways which do not contribute to output. The service mix which the hospital produces is also, by assumption, appropriate, since it is determined by whatever consumer/patients choose to use (the consumer sovereignty and informed consumer assumptions again).

It is literally unthinkable, in this analytic framework, that cost escalation or overuse could be the outcome of inappropriate behaviour by providers, either hospitals or physicians. Given the basic assumptions, it cannot happen, so need not be discussed. If there is an economic problem, or a misuse of resources, it is the fault of patients, wanting too much and shopping too carelessly, and behind them ''the government'' heedlessly providing or promoting excessive insurance coverage.

MAKING EXPLICIT THE PHYSICIAN'S ROLE: "CO-OPERATIVE" MODELS

The two most prominent weaknesses of this ''organic'' model of the hospital as a single firm, striving to maximize some combination of quantity and quality subject to an exogenous demand curve, are its neglect of the role, or even the existence, of physicians, and its assumption of an arm's-length relationship between hospitals and reimbursing agencies. The implausibility of the latter is most apparent in systems such as Canada's, where a single public reimbursing agency, now typically the provincial Ministry of Health, determines each hospital's annual operating budget as well as approving, and to a considerable extent funding, the hospital's capital expansion plans. Supposedly general economic theories of hospital behaviour, originating in the United States, tend to be seriously culture-bound. But the role of physicians, in determining who gets into hospital and what happens to them there, is of central significance in all jurisdictions. In this process physicians act on both sides of the demand-supply relationship, individually influencing the patient's desired utilization pattern, and then collectively, through the medical staff, influencing the hospital's response.

Alternative formal models of the hospital have therefore been constructed which make the physician's role explicit, and indeed bring her to centre stage. The hospital can be represented as a physician's co-operative, run by and for its physician staff members (Pauly and Redisch

1973). Such models retain the organic structure—the hospital is still managed with a specific end in view—but that end is now the net income of the physician staff members who form the effective management.[8]

In this model, physicians supply a comprehensive package commodity or service—treatment of or relief from, a state of illness. They are assumed to face the usual exogenous demand curve determining how much of this composite commodity can be sold at each price. In producing "care" they may use their own time and effort, the services of employees, or other inputs purchased directly by them. Or they may admit the patient to a hospital, where capital and labour services will be paid for through the hospital budget. But all hospital activity is directed by the physician.

The physician's net income is, in this model, the residual after hospital costs and practice expenses have been deducted from the amount patients are willing to pay for treatments. Accordingly it is in the physician's interest to ensure that hospital costs are minimized at every level of hospital activity. Not-for-profit hospital organization ensures that any surplus of payments by patients over input costs accrues to the physician. And the physician's interest in cost-minimization ensures that hospitals will neither waste resources in their production of hospital services (technical inefficiency) nor supply unnecessary hospital services, since unnecessary hospital use for any given patient condition reduces the net income left over for physicians from the treatment of that condition.

The total amount the patient is willing to pay for treatment of a given condition is thus assumed to be independent of the specific services received for it. This implicitly introduces once again the counterfactual assumption that patients are fully informed about how health care produces health, with all the usual consequences. In effect, the hospital has disappeared as an independent entity. The "physician's co-operative" model is a model, not of a hospital, but of a large physician-owned and managed clinic with overnight beds, and this clinic is assumed to be run to maximize profits, or utility as a function of income and leisure, for the physician-owners. The co-operative aspect introduces complications of the type found in the labour-managed firm literature (Evans and Williamson 1978, Chapter 6; Vanek 1977; Meade 1972, 1974). Physicians supply labour as well as owning the firm, and managerial decisions are

---

[8] While developed in the context of a North American hospital system, in which private medical practitioners treat their patients in, as well as out of, hospitals, the "physicians' co-operative" model appears to extend to systems with fully salaried hospital medical staffs. Insofar as physicians collectively "capture" the organization and manage it toward a set of objectives defined by themselves, the hospital becomes a co-op, although the definition of objectives is much more complex than simply practitioner net incomes. But of course practitioner net income is a wholly inadequate description of the objectives even of fee-for-service practitioners (see chapter 7).

made by a group whose size is itself a managerial decision. Under some assumptions, this can lead to inefficient "firm" sizes. But the issues of effective *hospital* operations, of technical efficiency, and of the appropriateness of utilization, are dismissed by the assumption of cost-minimizing behaviour under a demand curve constraint.

Overuse of hospitals *could* arise if hospital care were more extensively covered by insurance than physician care, in the sense that more costly forms of treatment in the hospital might then yield higher returns to physicians. But such overuse would be defined in the way depressingly familiar in economic models—as a response to price distortions created by insurance—rather than being related to medical need or its absence. The idea that overuse of hospitals results from asymmetric insurance coverage of inpatient and outpatient care is a very old one, and not just among economists. It has now been largely exploded by empirical findings that expanded insurance coverage of ambulatory care is as likely to *increase* hospital use, perhaps because it encourages more initial patient contacts with the health care system.

More generally, however, the usefulness of analytic models which define away the most significant policy problems in the hospital sector, the appropriateness of hospital use and the technical efficiency of production of hospital services, is distinctly limited. The further assumption in such models, that inputs and particularly labour inputs are purchased in competitive factor markets by cost-minimizing hospital firms, sidesteps the whole question of wage-determination in hospitals. As a result, the dramatic increases in hospital workers' relative wages over the past twenty-five years are dismissed, implicitly, as the result of external market shifts in supply which are unrelated to hospital behaviour.[9]

TRANSACTION MODELS: THE HOSPITAL AS A FRAMEWORK FOR NEGOTIATION

The very limited application of formal organic models to actual experience can be extended in an *ad hoc* manner by inserting additional variables in the managerial objective function. One might postulate that managers have a direct preference for "organizational slack"—inefficient production—because it economizes on managerial time and effort. Or they may derive prestige and gratification from high technology interventions ("conspicuous production"), or have a charitable interest in the incomes of their workers. In this way one can come to grips with some of the behavioural realities of the hospital sector, but the arbitrary nature

---

[9]   Except perhaps in the short run, if input supply functions are inelastic.

of the process casts doubts on the usefulness of the formal modelling exercise itself.

Accordingly, more recent efforts to describe and understand the economic behaviour of hospitals have moved away from formal organic models of the hospital as a single entity, seeking some well-defined objective(s) under constraint, and back toward an older tradition of the hospital as a setting where various groups with differing objectives interact with each other in a mixture of co-operation and competition. The characteristic "two lines of authority" in hospitals, administration and medical staff, and the problems created by conflicts between them (Smith 1958), can be represented as two separate firms-within-a-firm, in which the administration assembles inputs and produces services which are then supplied to physicians, who demand and direct such services on behalf of patients (Harris 1977). This transaction process will obviously be governed by the objectives and constraints of the two different internal "firms." But it is not a "market" in any conventional sense, nor can either set of transactors, administrators or physicians, be adequately characterized as profit or income maximizers, or as functioning at arm's-length from each other. Their relationship is a very complex, non-zero-sum game, not a sequence of self-contained spot contracts at explicit or implicit prices. Realistic description and analysis of such complex processes can lead to very useful generalizations about how hospitals are likely to behave, and to respond to changes in their external environments, but they may never be expressed in a formal analytic framework which is either realistic or useful.[10] In any case, it has not happened yet.

If this assessment is accurate, one may reasonably ask why economists have spent so much effort on attempts at formal modelling. The intent, hope, was to try to go beyond informed generalizations about a particular setting, and to construct a framework which would predict behavioural responses more universally, on the basis of relatively limited information. If the results have been unsatisfactory, the problem nevertheless remains. It cannot be too often emphasized, at least not in an economics text, that *any* statement or prediction about how an individual or organization will respond to a change (or even absence of change) in its environment necessarily implies some sort of model, some set of assumed cause and effect relationships, describing the entity whose behaviour is predicted. This is true in particular of all policy analysis—to formulate and predict the effects of a policy one must have, at least implicitly, models of the behaviour of the actors who will be affected thereby. The models may

---

[10] For an excellent analysis of the historical evolution of this situation in the U.S., see Starr (1982), Chapter 4.

be loose, probabilistic, perhaps inconsistent, but without them one cannot make policy at all. One can only make blind stabs of unpredictable effect.

HOSPITAL REIMBURSEMENT: TAKE THE MONEY AND . . .?

As an illustration, we move from the abstract field of hospital modelling to the intensely practical problem of hospital reimbursement. For years, hospital managements, reimbursers, and students of health care have criticized prevailing modes of hospital reimbursement in both Canada and the United States as failing to provide incentives for efficient management of hospitals, or worse, for providing perverse incentives. Yet efforts to develop and apply alternative systems embodying incentive patterns consistent with more general social objectives have consistently been unsuccessful.[11]

Such alternatives have sometimes been referred to as "incentive reimbursement" systems, but of course all forms of reimbursement create incentives insofar as they make an individual's or organization's access to resources conditional on some form of behaviour. Moreover the behavioural response to any such incentive pattern will depend on the objectives of the individual/organization, and on the constraints, resource or otherwise, which bind it. An economic model of an organization is simply an explicit representation of these objectives and constraints. Accordingly any criticism (or advocacy) of a particular reimbursement system must logically rest on some implicit or explicit model of the hospital. Explicit models tend to be oversimplified and unrealistic; implicit ones are more commonly internally inconsistent.

At present, hospitals in Canada are reimbursed on some version of a negotiated budget; a system referred to in the United States as "prospective reimbursement". The process varies in detail from province to province, but in general the budget is based on a forecast of the hospital's patient work load and associated programs, which then serves as a basis for determining manpower and other input requirements. Combined with

---

[11] The alert reader should note that in the process the implicit criteria for evaluation of hospital behaviour have shifted. The depiction of hospitals as simply firms with a rather peculiar set of objectives other than profit, but still constrained by an exogenous demand curve, carried with it the consumer sovereignty assumption that "appropriate" levels of output were to be judged in terms of their marginal production costs relative to consumer/patients' willingness to pay. The hospital reimbursement literature embodies implicit or explicit models of the hospital in order to predict the effects of different reimbursement systems or formulae; but most such analyses judge the effect of such systems in terms of technical "need" criteria and emphasize hospital or physician, not patient, behaviour. Over– or underservicing in this literature, which may be a response to inappropriate reimbursement incentives, is defined relative to health status and need, not to willingness to pay.

wage and price projections, these yield an estimate of the cost of total hospital operations during the year. A hospital which exceeds its budget may attempt to negotiate acceptance of this overrun for reimbursement; its success will depend on the general fiscal or political climate as well as the reimburser's perceptions of the reasons for the overrun. Unexpected and uncontrollable increases in work load, for example, might represent a justifiable overrun, though the allowed increase in budget would not in general be proportional to the load increase. Insofar as a significant proportion of a hospital's costs are believed to be fixed, invariant to work load, any budgetary adjustment would attempt to identify and reimburse only variable costs. Budgetary underruns are in general returned to the reimbursing agency. Some provinces permit the hospital to retain all or part of any surplus, but administrators tend to believe that such surpluses may be removed from next year's budget.

It is easy to see that almost any model of hospital objectives will, in this environment, lead to spending of all of the approved budget. Underruns will be a result of error. Overruns may or may not be encouraged, depending on the associated penalties; the hospital management will presumably have to predict the probability of an overrun's being accepted, and the cost to the institution or to management themselves if it is not. Negotiating effort will seek to maximize next year's budget, subject to the costs of negotiation itself.

Within the general pressure for "more," however, several different hospital responses are possible. The budgetary process per se encourages spending all one can get and getting all one can; it does not encourage efficient management of the resources available. Improved efficiency, as is frequently pointed out, will in the presence of given work-load targets lead to a loss of revenue. On the other hand, reimbursing agencies do try to keep in touch with actual hospital operations, so that egregiously inefficient management, if observed, might make future budget negotiations more difficult (or current overruns less acceptable). Indeed as noted above, quantity-maximizing models of hospital objectives, with or without "quality" (*i.e.*, service intensity) adjustment, predict that hospital management will still strive for maximum technical efficiency, minimum cost per service, in order to maximize output under the total expenditure constraint.[12] But they are silent as to the nature or effectiveness of the

---

[12] In an environment of universal insurance, however, the demand side of the utilization process in such models becomes a bit obscure. If the idea of an exogenous, price-dependent demand by independent decision-making consumers is preserved (for hospital care!?) presumably one must postulate permanent excess demand and some form of direct rationing. Otherwise, the hospital might run into a quantity constraint before the budget was exhausted. The few U.S. economists who glance sideways at Canada (as opposed to the much fewer who have actually studied it) do seem to take such consumer-driven excess demand for granted, apparently because their theoretical models require it to exist, not because it is observed.

hospital services which will be produced. If, of course, utilization were exogenously determined by "medical need," and such need were finite as in panel (a) of Figure 1-3, then conceivably hospital output would eventually reach this limit, and any additional budget would be either given back to the reimburser, eaten up in technical inefficiency or organizational slack, or passed through in workers' salaries. In fact, however, physicians' and hospitals' *perceptions* of need seem to follow more closely panel (b) of Figure 1-3,[13] and their direct influence over utilization enables them to keep it rising. Indeed, utilization increase, "unmet needs," is a standard and sometimes effective lever for negotiating budgetary increases. But it is difficult to separate the role of hospitals from that of physicians in this hospital utilization process.

Almost any behavioural model of a hospital, however, save one which postulated altruistic self-sacrificing administrators and Hippocratic physicians who had taken vows of poverty, will "predict" the obvious— upward pressure on budgets—in an environment of prospective budgetary reimbursement. The interesting questions are how reimbursing agencies acquire information and establish priorities to govern budget-setting. As noted in Tables 8-1 and 8-2, the per capita availability of hospital space and resources in Canada has remained relatively stable since 1971, with costs growing slightly faster than the overall economy. But the number of *physicians* has grown much more rapidly (Tables 1-2, 7-1). The average physician's access to hospital space has thus been significantly reduced. This in turn limits her billing capacity. If this dramatic expansion in physician supply had not occurred, pressure on hospital capacity might have been much reduced. We do not know to what extent hospitals *qua* hospitals, as distinct from the physicians who use them, can influence the use of their own services.[14]

PAYMENT BY UNIT OF SERVICE: LOWER UNIT COSTS, HIGHER TOTAL COSTS?

At the other end of the spectrum, one could reimburse hospitals as private insurers in the United States do, on the basis of a fixed price per unit for each type of services provided. Hospitals would set charges separately for each of the components of a care episode, a *per diem* for ward care (accommodation and meals) plus a specific price for each diagnostic or therapeutic intervention such as an operation, a lab test, a

---

[13] Or else panel (a) with N^* constantly shifting to the right as more resources become available, which comes to the same thing.

[14] U.S. experience with for-profit hospitals (Lewin *et al.* 1981; Pattison and Katz 1983) indicates that hospital ownership *does* affect patterns of medical practice, but this could be through medical staff selection.

CT scan, or an aspirin. In the United States setting, such charges often depart substantially from actual costs of production. Hospitals thus can, and do, cross-subsidize losses on some services with profits on others, while running an overall surplus on operations to finance new growth. The existence of such cross-subsidies indicates an absence of competitive market pressures. But a universal public insurance program could also, if it chose, reimburse hospitals on a fixed payment per unit of service basis, either individually itemized or as an inclusive cost *per diem.*

The usual argument against doing so is that it would encourage hospitals to expand output of services whose marginal cost, the cost of producing one more unit of output, is below the average charge or cost level at which reimbursement is usually set. (Variable reimbursement on a scale reflecting the dependence of cost on output would require enormous amounts of information.) A fixed payment *per diem* encourages hospitals to keep patients in longer so as to earn ''profits'' on late and less expensive days of stay; similarly, a fixed reimbursement per lab unit encourages additional testing at very low (so long as excess capacity is available) marginal cost. The ''profits'' thus earned can be used to finance expansion, or absorbed in other organizational objectives.

On the other hand, payment per service unit would presumably encourage efficiency in the narrow, technical sense of minimizing cost per unit of service, because the rate of reimbursement per test, procedure, or day of stay would be, or become, equalized across hospitals. Differences in the needs or severity of different hospitals' caseloads would be reflected in different patterns of service input per patient, but unless such services were inconsistently defined, such variation would not require different rates of reimbursement for the same service.[15]

In this system the ''span of control'' of efficient management is extended; over time more resources are assembled under their direction. High-cost hospitals, on the other hand, would have to cut back other programs to finance losses if their costs per unit of service exceeded the group rate of reimbursement. Eventually the whole group of hospitals would become more efficient, either because management was stimulated to improve, or because those whose performance remained sub-standard would see their institutions shrink in favour of growth by the more efficient. Hence the appeal of ''incentive'' reimbursement. It is analogous in its effects to profits in the private marketplace, which both reward the efficient directly, and provide them with additional resources at the expense of the inefficient.

---

[15] If each hospital could negotiate its own level of reimbursement for each individual service, of course, technical inefficiency (high cost production) in any one time period would contribute to future reimbursement levels. This would vitiate any efficiency incentives in the reimbursement process.

The underlying implicit model of the hospital is one which assumes an unlimited appetite for more resources with which to expand services, and a willingness to trade off the effort required to minimize costs per service unit in order to free up resources for program expansion. It differs from the quantity-maximizing model, however, in removing the assumed exogenous demand curve constraint on output. Rather the hospital, perhaps acting through the medical staff, is considered able to influence the intensity of servicing per episode of care provided, independent of the out-of-pocket charges, if any, to patients. The model also assumes atomistic, not collusive, behaviour by groups of hospitals. Individual hospitals are assumed to be motivated to seek out and use ways of lowering unit costs of services; this information could then be used by the reimbursing agency in setting future reimbursement levels for groups of hospitals. The long-term result would then be a relatively high degree of technical efficiency for the group as a whole in the production of particular services, but high and perhaps indefinitely expanding levels of servicing intensity per patient and associated cost increases.

The appropriateness of such a reimbursement program thus depends on the extent to which hospitals are, or are not, constrained in their determination of service intensity, and on the relative importance of service intensity and of technical inefficiency in contributing to expenditure growth.[16] Canadian reimbursing agencies, as well as government or non-profit (Blue-type) reimbursers in the United States, have generally tried to avoid such systems, presumably in the belief that service intensity is to a large extent under the control of the hospital or its medical staff, and/or that pure technical inefficiency is a less significant problem than (actual or potential) overservicing.

REIMBURSEMENT BY EPISODE OF CARE

A popular suggestion, dealing to some degree with the overservicing issue, has been a shift to ''case-based'' or episodic reimbursement. The hospital would be paid a fixed sum for each inpatient with a particular type of problem or complaint, the amount being based on the average cost across a group of similar hospitals of treating that patient according to current standards. The hospital would thus have an incentive, not only

---

[16] Of course one might take the view that increased servicing was a social desideratum, at least over some range. The curve in Figure 1-3 might be perceived as having a relatively steep positive slope. In the earlier years of public intervention in hospital financing, this does seem to have been a dominant notion; the problem was viewed as one of getting more resources into the hospital sector to increase servicing. It is not so viewed now (except, of course, by physicians' associations). The shift in perspective only makes sense in the context of our health care system having reaching a point on the Figure 1-3 curve which is flat, or almost so.

to hold down the costs of the specific services used in treatment, but to work with the patient's physician to determine *less* service intensive ways of achieving a satisfactory outcome. Again, hospitals which were able to innovate in treatment, say by the substitution of day care for inpatient surgery, would earn a substantial surplus on some surgical cases which could be used to expand other programs (either capital or operating costs). High-cost hospitals, either technically inefficient or prone to excessive servicing, would see their resource base shrinking and might eventually disappear or be taken over by the more efficient. The approach is very attractive as a stimulus to more innovative and less costly forms of care in hospitals, and could lead to a great deal more attention being paid to the efficacy and effectiveness of the services now being carried out. The lab test which adds little or nothing to the diagnosis, the unnecessarily prolonged patient stay, would in this system subtract from the hospital's free resources for other programs, in contrast to the service-unit-based form of reimbursement where they add resources (so long as reimbursement rate exceeds marginal cost). In the negotiated budget system, improved control over service intensity frees up resources within the budget period, but these will usually be recaptured by the reimbursing agency if not spent in that period, and may also be removed from future budgets.

Episode– or case-based systems of hospital reimbursement rest on an implicit model of hospital behaviour in which perceived needs or demands for care arise external to the hospital, being generated by economic or medico-technical forces, but patterns of service within the hospital are controlled or greatly influenced by the hospital itself, or its medical staff. Otherwise, there would be no point in focussing financial incentives on the hospital as an organization. Such systems are radically inconsistent with models of the hospital which view it as constrained by some exogenous demand curve that relates its volume of utilization uniquely to the out-of-pocket payments of its patients.[17]

It is thus rather ironic that it is in the United States, where economic analysts (with some outstanding exceptions) seem to have had the greatest difficulty moving beyond the concept of an exogenous demand for health care, that the most extensive experiment with case-based hospital reimbursement is underway.[18]

---

[17] One could, of course, have an exogenous, price-dependent demand for episodes of care (Stoddart and Barer 1981), but with the hospital controlling the service content of the episode. And it is generally accepted by all observers that in the U.S. it is the increase in servicing intensity, not in episodes of care per capita, which is driving hospital cost escalation.

[18] Since the designers and advocates of reimbursement policy rarely if ever make explicit their underlying analytic framework, and the articulators of formal analytic models rarely go beyond the academic journals to translate their work into public policy (other than those who advocate *no* public policy—the easy out), "la conversation des muets" is likely to continue.

The episode-based reimbursement system creates obvious and severe technical problems of classifying patients into reimbursement categories such that treatment protocols and costs are reasonably standardized *and* such that hospitals cannot manipulate the labelling system to increase revenue.[19] Procedural reclassification by physicians under fee-for-service reimbursement is a well-established phenomenon, and efforts to deal with it usually lead to fee schedules which are rather insensitive to differences among, for example, different types of office visits. Quality control problems may also become more severe, if one fears that hospitals will be encouraged to underservice patients, although the professional and public checks on that process probably outweigh any economic incentives. Definition of the episode is also a problem; for many chronic conditions discharge and readmission or transfer across hospitals may make it difficult to determine when one episode ends and another begins. And finally, the hospital is in effect encouraged to admit and process rapidly the simple, straight-forward and "cheap" cases, and to discourage admission of, or refer to others, patients whose age, complications, or other characteristics make a long or costly episode likely. The "cream-skimming" of which United States proprietary hospitals are often accused would be encouraged by episodic reimbursement. Yet these costly patients may have the greatest needs. The straight-forward surgical procedures, by contrast, which are frequently observed to vary dramatically in frequency across regions, and are often targetted as over-provided, would probably also be, at least at the margin, the most lucrative.

---

[19] This is the problem being addressed in the U.S. by the development of the system of Diagnosis-Related Groups (DRGs) which are being used as a basis for per case (episode) prospective hospital reimbursement under the U.S. federal Medicare program. This system defines a large number of categories of problems, on the basis of patient diagnosis, age, procedures undergone, and complications. Apart from the general difficulty of defining unambiguous sets of categories, the DRG system has two significant weaknesses.

First, within each DRG as presently defined it appears that the severity of patient problems, and associated costs, is highly variable. One can define a severity index, cutting across DRGs, which picks up much of this variation, but this index relies on a significant amount of subjective clinical judgement. Second, the DRG classification of a patient depends partly on the pattern of services received, enabling the hospital to influence its own level of reimbursement by its choice of interventions. (Use of a severity index in conjunction with DRGs has the same flaw; the process of index calculation is under the hospital's control, and much less well defined than patient age or diagnosis.)

On the other hand, the U.S. initiative marks an important step forward in reimbursement, which may also have some powerful positive effects, and in any case should generate a good deal of new information about both hospital behaviour and the range of therapeutic possibilities.

REIMBURSEMENT BY PERSON, NOT PATIENT, CARED FOR: CAPITATION

This in turn leads to suggestions that reimbursement be based, not on episode, but on capitation, on persons potentially under care. The hospital could be assigned a panel of persons, based on its geographic catchment area, or it could enter into agreements to serve with individuals or groups. It would receive a fixed sum per year for each person for whom it was responsible, suitably adjusted for age, sex, and other objectively determinable personal characteristics affecting probability of hospital use. The specifics would obviously vary, depending on the form of overall hospital funding system into which capitation reimbursement was being inserted. Referral hospitals would receive smaller amounts defined over a wider population. Such a system creates maximum incentives to control unnecessary hospital use, as well as to limit excessive servicing within hospitals and to discourage waste of resources in producing services. It also, however, implies substantial reorganization of medical practice to link physicians, as well as persons, with specific home base hospitals. In smaller communities this might be no great change, but in larger cities "choice" of hospital frequently follows from choice of physician. Under a capitation-based system the potential patient would be locked in, for a time at least, to a particular hospital (or group of hospitals) and would thus have to use a physician with privileges there.[20]

Suggestions for capitation reimbursement implicitly assume that the hospital's influence extends to the patient admission or case generation process, while retaining the assumption that hospital behaviour will be motivated by opportunities to earn surpluses, or free resources, on some activities which can then be used for other and unspecified hospital purposes. Thus it is anticipated that the overall number of episodes of hospital care, in addition to the pattern of servicing provided for each, might be reduced (with no deleterious effects on the health of the empanelled population) if the hospital reimbursement system embodied incentives to do so.

WIDER STILL AND WIDER . . . WHERE ARE THE BOUNDARIES OF THE HOSPITAL "FIRM"?

At this stage, however, the implicit model of the hospital is becoming stretched out of shape. It may be plausible to think of hospital managements—the administration—as having a predominant influence (not total)

---

[20] The intricacies of cross-institutional funding, and the location of payment responsibility when a patient uses services away from her "home" hospital, are critical to the actual functioning of such systems, but need not detain us here.

over the production and costs of particular services. Extending management to include the medical staff collectively, it may be plausible that they can influence servicing patterns. When we begin to look at the admission process, however, we have effectively shifted our focus from management-as-administration to management-as-physicians, and it is not clear that the word "hospital" still refers to the same organization, group of people, or objectives.

If the reimbursement mechanism is to be used as an instrument for influencing the case generation process, the appropriate targets for such incentives are the physicians admitting to particular hospitals. Capitation-reimbursed organizations providing health care, community health centres or health service organizations, or, in the United States, prepaid group practices or health maintenance organizations, typically combine both physician services and hospital care within a single organizational structure. In industrial organization terms, capitation reimbursement is associated with vertical integration of production. This pattern of integration then internalizes all the appropriate efficiency incentives, to provide appropriate and effective care, at minimum cost, to a defined group of people.[21] The hospital as such ceases to be a self-contained firm in the conventional economic sense and becomes a component of a larger entity.[22]

The analysis of alternative reimbursement systems, and the combination of positive and perverse incentives with respect to efficiency embodied in each, thus points up a difficulty in our thinking about hospitals. The peculiar relationship between hospitals and physicians, at least in North America, can only be described as a form of incomplete vertical integration (Evans 1981). If the hospital-as-firm is defined to *exclude* (non-salaried) physicians, then it is a peculiar firm in which a significant share of the crucial resource-allocation decisions—what to produce and how—are made by people or groups who are not part of the firm's line management. If on the other hand the firm is defined so as to *include* admitting physicians, then, except for vertically integrated group practices, the management and financial structure of this broader assemblage is totally incoherent. It may be misleading, therefore, to think of the hospital as a firm at all, at least in the traditional economic sense of a set of well-defined production activities and managerial decisions under the control of a single transactor. To understand how hospitals behave,

---

[21] Quality control, assurance that care is both adequate and appropriate, is not necessarily achieved by this reimbursement mechanism—or any other.

[22] It would, of course, be possible for a group of physicians to accept reimbursement on a capitation basis for medical and hospital services, and then contract with an arm's-length hospital to provide services as directed by themselves. In this case, of course, the hospital might be reimbursed on a negotiated unit-of-service basis, since the hospital separate from the physician group would have relatively little direct influence over use.

and how hospital utilization, patterns of care, and expenditures will react to different incentives, it may be as, or more, useful to study physician behaviour and objectives, as to try to model hospital behaviour directly.

The shift from organic to transaction models referred to above represents a move in this direction. Yet the transactions involved are not at arm's-length, nor price-mediated. "Rights of management," or authority over and responsibility for production decisions, are in a process of continuous negotiation.

In Canada the pattern of incomplete vertical integration is even more complex, because it must be extended to include provincial governments. These have responsibility, and power, to ensure the provision of hospital services throughout their jurisdictions. This includes both operating cost reimbursement, and separate capital funding for hospitals, giving governments a predominant influence in new investment and patterns of hospital capital formation. In the United States, by contrast, hospitals' operating cost reimbursements from public and private insurers include the costs of capital services; these depreciation and interest payments provide funding for capital replacement and expansion. They also make public planning of hospital systems virtually impossible, as planning consists of trying to guide or prevent a hospital's spending of "its own" money. In Canada, funds for capital investment are provided, not through operating cost reimbursement, but (primarily) through separate government grants. This gives the public planning process financial "teeth." But it also means that yet another set of managerial decisions internal to the conventional economic firm, those over capital formation, are in Canadian hospitals shared with or taken over by an agency external to the hospital. From a province-wide perspective, hospitals could be thought of as operating units in a provincial public utility responsible for providing hospital care, like the individual generating plants of the provincial Hydro authority.

Of course this perspective is incomplete; hospitals are obviously owned and in theory at least managed by their own boards of trustees. But in some provinces it is explicit that the Lieutenant-Governor-in-Council may *at pleasure* appoint a public trustee to replace the board and assume any or all board functions—or any other administrative functions. And even apart from such extreme forms of intervention, the predominant influence of provincial governments over the investment process, either within hospitals or through the construction of new hospitals, makes them, like physicians, part of hospital management.

Indeed a major problem with incentive reimbursement systems in the Canadian context is precisely that their major incentive, that of offering hospitals the opportunity to earn free surplus funds through improvements in operating efficiency, is implicitly an alternative way of guiding and funding organizational expansion, which would dilute the influence of the provincial government. Efficient hospitals, like efficient business firms, are enabled to expand and add more functions; the inefficient shrink. But suppose all the efficient managers turn out to be in regions of low growth or decline in population, and the inefficient in boom towns? Governments have a responsibility to match facilities to population needs, and no organizational framework exists for efficient hospitals to expand in areas of need. They grow where they are; an efficient hospital in Nelson, British Columbia could not use its surplus funds to buy out an inefficient one in Prince George.[23] Thus the fundamental concept of incentive reimbursement, of an arm's-length financial relationship which can be structured so that payments by one party induce desired forms of behaviour by another, cuts directly across the alternative framework of public authority and responsibility for the development of a hospital system. If government assumed direct ownership of hospitals, the firm structure would become clear; provinces would be running hospital public utilities on the Hydro model. In the same way, if hospitals placed all their physicians on salary, or physician groups established their own hospitals, or a private company or not-for-profit agency hired physicians and built hospitals, the resulting integrated firm would have well-defined managerial boundaries. But in the current situation, in which managerial responsibility is shared with groups outside the administrative structure, it may be inappropriate for most purposes to conceptualize a hospital as an economic firm. It may be a physical, legal, or organizational entity, but in economic terms it may be either part of a larger "firm," or a collection of smaller ones. The difficulty which economists have had in devising realistic and useful models of hospitals may reflect, not lack of sufficient ingenuity, but the nature of the industry itself.[24]

---

[23] Over the long run, some variant of multi-unit management may modify this situation, but the problem of ownership remains.

[24] The development of for-profit or investor-owned hospitals in the U.S. may re-establish the hospital or hospital chain as a clear-cut economic firm. As a number of observers have pointed out, the consequences for the managerial role of physicians in such a structure will be profound. They may well find that they must either join the organization of the hospital and serve its objectives (profit) or deal with it at arm's-length as an independent economic transactor. See chapter 10 for further discussion.

CHAPTER 9

HOSPITALS CONTINUED:
FROM THEORY TO MEASUREMENT

GENERALIZATIONS FROM EXPERIENCE: INDUCTION AS WELL AS DEDUCTION

Whatever the difficulties of conceptualizing hospitals as firms, it is clear that the same economic processes which go on in firms also occur in and around hospitals. Decisions are made as to what services to produce, and how, what inputs to use, and how much to pay for the inputs/ charge for the services. Negotiation of a budget for reimbursement purposes involves setting implicit prices for hospital outputs, just as wage negotiation determines input prices. And concerns over hospital costs reflect concerns about the quality of decision-making in all these areas. Are the "right" sorts of hospital outputs being produced, or are people being over-hospitalized, provided with unnecessary care? Are there too many surgical procedures, unnecessary diagnostic tests, overly prolonged hospital stays? And do hospitals use the least-cost mixes of labour and other inputs in producing their services? All these are the standard questions of economic performance outlined in chapter 6, except that in health care, the issues of appropriate quantities and mixes of servicing relate back to health care needs rather than to the conventional criterion of consumer willingness-to-pay.

A substantial literature has grown up attempting to measure directly various aspects of hospital industry performance, a literature which has been at best loosely linked to theoretical models of hospital behaviour. On the whole the empirical literature has been rather more successful than the theoretical, in that it has given rise to certain generalizations about behaviour, based on statistical regularities, which do seem to have advanced our understanding somewhat. Such generalizations are of course always consistent with some implicit analytic model of hospital objectives and constraints, but unfortunately there are usually a large number of such models consistent with any particular empirical regularity.

For example, one of the most widely accepted generalizations about hospital use is Roemer's Law, that "a built bed is a filled bed." Holding all else (illness levels, incomes, insurance coverage, etc.) constant, if more beds per capita are available in a region, more will be used. (Though as noted in chapter 4, they may not be *fully* used.) And this is not because "demand" somehow defined always exceeds capacity, but because the availability of capacity modifies physicians' and hospitals' perceptions of appropriate patterns of use. Such an observed regularity, however, is consistent with a wide range of different postulates about hospital objectives.

It might appear to rule out models in which an exogenous "demand curve" specifies hospital use as depending only on out-of-pocket prices paid by users, as well as their incomes and "tastes" for hospital use, since capacity should then increase use only if it led to price cuts in a world of incomplete insurance. Roemer's Law is strongly suggestive of an agency relationship in which physicians' recommendations to patients as to hospital admissions and lengths of stay are influenced by their perceptions of bed availability. One might extend this process to include actions by hospital managements to encourage or discourage throughput, by facilitating or obstructing early discharge, for example, or use of day care surgery.

But exogenous demand models can always be salvaged by postulating "implicit prices," unobserved variables, such that capacity lowers access costs to patients either directly or through its effects on physicians. One could argue that when bed capacity is increased, some "full price" of hospital use, of which out-of-pocket charges if any are only a part, is reduced, and hence patients choose to use more care. Unobserved variables are a powerful device to reconcile preconceived theory with awkward fact; the direct agency process by contrast has the advantage of being readily visible, even if not reported in aggregate statistics.

Empirical economic studies of hospital activities may be roughly grouped into three categories:

(i) hospital cost function studies;
(ii) specific hospital program studies;
(iii) hospital utilization studies.

Cost function studies look at the hospital in aggregate, and make comparisons of performance across groups of hospitals each defined as a single unit of observation. Specific program studies focus on a particular set of illnesses, or of activities within the hospital—"disease costing" falls in this category—and analyse alternative ways of providing care or carrying out particular activities inside or outside hospitals. Utilization studies focus on differences in hospital use by populations compared across regions, over time, or in different systems of hospital and medical care delivery. Each type of study bears on a different aspect of the "efficiency," in the most general sense, of the hospital industry, and each has implications for the characteristics that an adequate analytic model of a hospital should have.

(i) Hospital Cost Function Studies

These studies, largely carried out by economists. have their roots in the conventional theory of the for-profit firm. Given a stable technology, expressed in a production function linking amounts of inputs of productive resources—labour time and skills, raw materials, plant and equipment services—with the maximum amounts of the firm's product(s) which can be produced thereby, there will exist a cost function which defines the minimum attainable cost per unit for each quantity of output produced. The short-run cost function defines minimum unit cost for given fixed capital, plant, and equipment, and hence shows unit cost rising beyond designed capacity and becoming infinite beyond absolute maximum capacity. The long-run function, however, is defined over a time horizon such that all inputs are variable and no capacity constraints apply. If plants can be replicated without increasing costs of co-ordination, then the long-run cost curve, the graph of unit cost against output, may beyond some minimum output level be horizontal—constant returns to scale— and unit costs will not depend on the size of the organization. Or the curve may be U-shaped, displaying a range of economies of scale— falling unit costs as organizational size increases—followed by diseconomies of scale as the organization becomes managerially unwieldy and unit costs rise. In the short run, of course, a U-shape is normal, as unit costs are usually elevated if a plant is being run well below or well above its designed capacity.

Whatever the shape of the cost function imposed by existing technology, the profit-maximizing, cost-minimizing firm should be operating at or near the "frontier" which it defines. Unit costs below the cost function are, by definition, technically impossible; costs above it reflect failure to minimize costs. Thus it should be possible actually to observe the cost function for different industries by plotting unit costs against scale of operations for different firms in the same industry. One could then identify efficient firms, as well as optimal scales, and infer a number of things about market behaviour which would interest students of industrial organization.[1]

The application of this statistical technique to hospitals is obvious. One could plot costs per patient-day or per admission for a group of hospitals against number of patient-days, admissions, or beds, and fit a regression line, or curve, through the scatter of points. The shape of the curve would indicate the existence or absence of scale economies or diseconomies, while outliers—hospitals with *per diem* or per admission costs well above

---

[1]   There is a great deal more to the story than this, both statistically and economically, but we cannot pursue it here.

or below the line—would be those with unusually efficient or inefficient managements.[2]

Such a relationship could be both a planning tool, in that it would show the optimal scale for building new hospitals, and a guide for reimbursement of hospitals either by arm's-length insurers or direct budget negotiators. A provincial government could squeeze the budgets of the high-cost hospitals while studying and trying to generalize the secrets of managerial success in the low-cost. And a United States insurance company or public agency might set its reimbursement rates on the basis of regional or group averages, and under-reimburse costs or charges of "above-the-curve" hospitals.

Formally, one could identify a statistical relation of the form:

$$PD_i = a + bBED_i + cBED^2_i + e_i$$

where PD_i is the average *per diem* cost (in a particular time period) of the ith hospital in the group, BED_i is its rated bed capacity (as an index of its scale of operations), BED^2_i allows for non-linearity—costs may first fall and then rise as scale increases—and e_i is the "error" specific to the ith hospital. If it is positive, the hospital has a higher *per diem* than its size warrants, and if negative, a lower, for unspecified reasons independent of the measure of size used.

Alternatively one could write:

$$CC_i = a + bBED_i + cBED^2_i + e_i$$

letting CC_i be the average cost per treated case or episode of care in hospital i. (The a, b, and c parameters are specific to each relationship, and are not constant across different equations.) CC_i would usually in practice be costs per separation (discharge or death) as an approximation to a care episode. Earlier studies tended to focus on the more familiar *per diem*, but costs per episode or at least per separation are both theoretically more satisfactory as a representation of hospital outputs—days of care are an intermediate product used in the "production" of treatment—and also lend themselves more naturally to statistical techniques of product standardization.

Figure 9-1 displays this cost/capacity relationship, each data point representing a single hospital, and shows outliers with unusually high and low costs. The parameters a, b, and c are constant across all hospitals in the group, and are defined by the curve of best fit (minimizing the sum of the squared e_i) to the observed scatter of points. If the relationship

---

[2]   The alert reader will notice that the concept of the production function defines the cost curve as a frontier of minimum attainable unit costs; the measurement process fits a line of best fit through a scatter of points. Beware of hobgoblins!

FIGURE 9-1

Hospital Costs per Unit of Output as a Function of Scale of Operation: Alternative Cost Curves

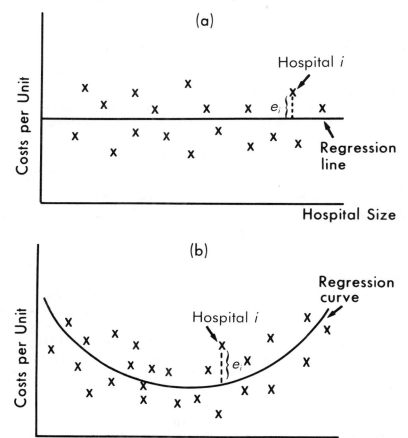

(a)

Hospital *i*

Costs per Unit

Regression line

Hospital Size

(b)

Regression curve

Hospital *i*

Costs per Unit

Hospital Size

Possible Measures of:

Hospital Size: Rated Bed Capacity, Total Patient Days

Output Units: Patient Days or Separations

is one of constant returns to scale, then b and c will be zero; size does not affect cost per day (Figure 9-1a). A U-shaped relation arises (Figure 9-1b) if b is negative and c positive.

One can also allow for short-run effects by extending the relationship to include, for example, occupancy rates. Two dimensions no longer suffice to graph the points, but one can "plot" each hospital *per diem*, bed stock, and occupancy rate mathematically, and fit a relationship:

$$PD_i = a + bBED_i + cBED^2_i + dOCC_i + fOCC^2_i + e_i$$

where now OCC_i is the occupancy rate of the *i*th hospital. If short-run variations in occupancy influence unit costs, then one might expect d to be negative, and f positive, indicating that for any given bed stock, costs per day fall as occupancy rises (fixed costs can be spread more widely), but at some point pressure on capacity reverses this relation. If *per diem* costs do depend on both long-run scale and short-run occupancy, then the e_i in the second relation should in general be smaller than the first. The variation across hospitals would be more completely "explained" by taking account of their differences in short-run utilization as well as in scale.

Indeed, the coefficients d and f, plus knowledge of the hospital's patient-day load, enable one to calculate the marginal costs, the amount by which total costs rise, when one more patient-day of care is provided, for each size of hospital. This can then be compared to the average *per diem*. The conventional wisdom is that "an empty bed costs almost as much as a full bed," *i.e.*, given that capacity exists, the marginal costs of increased utilization are low. This would be reflected in large d (and perhaps f) estimates. Reliable estimates of marginal costs would enable provincial reimbursement agencies to determine by how much a hospital's negotiated budget should be augmented if it suffers an unexpected increase in utilization. The lower the marginal cost, the less the cost implications of short-run variations in utilization. Small values of d and f would suggest that average unit costs do not vary much with occupancy; in this case costs rise more or less proportionately with patient load.

Unfortunately, the real world is somewhat more complex than this very brief outline suggests. (For a more complete discussion, see Barer 1981, 1982). Any attempt to draw conclusions about production technology from a simple plotting of unit cost against output rests, as one might expect, on an implicit model of hospital behaviour, and not a very plausible one. It assumes that hospitals do in fact attempt to minimize unit costs, which given their not-for-profit status is at least questionable. What is in fact measured is a statistical relation between cost and output which reflects a combination of technical constraints and behavioural regularities, and shows relative costliness within a group of hospitals. It is quite conceivable that all hospitals in any group lie above the technological minimum cost curve—if we knew where it was.

Furthermore, the measurement of costs per unit of output in terms of *per diems* or total costs per separation is badly misleading on several counts. First, if hospitals are firms, they are multiproduct firms producing some combination of inpatient care, outpatient services, education, research, and community services. Not all hospitals provide the full range, but many do, and few if any are confined to inpatient care alone. Secondly, inpatient care itself is very far from being a homogeneous process. The service intensity of a "patient-day," in terms of the diagnostic, therapeutic, and custodial services it embodies, varies widely over the range of different types and severities of problems cared for, as well as over the stages of the illness. It is obvious that some diagnoses require more intervention than others, that the severity of the "same" illness varies across patients, and that in general late days of stay for an illness episode are less costly than early. And finally, the outcome of treatment may vary with the quality of care provided, which may be connected (either positively or negatively!) with service intensity. A "treated case" of whatever type is not a measure of output uniform across hospitals if the probability of survival, or some other significant outcome dimension, varies substantially across hospitals.[3]

Quite apart from the problems of standardizing hospital cost data for differences in the nature of their patient load, the cost function as an instrument of management evaluation or reimbursement policy has the serious disadvantage that it assumes exogeneity of utilization. Patients appear on the hospital doorstep, are admitted, and after a time are discharged, by a process which except for absolute capacity constraints is beyond the hospital's influence. On these assumptions it is reasonable to evaluate hospitals by comparing the costs which they incur in responding to these externally generated needs or demands.

On the other hand, if hospital managements can by their administrative practices or by discussions with the medical staff influence lengths of stay, then they can influence costs per day and per separation as well. Pressures for "efficiency" focussed on *per diem* costs may encourage delays in discharge; "cheap" late days of stay serve to lower average costs. Costs per admission may be held down by admitting cases of low severity and referring high severity ones elsewhere, or by discharging and readmitting the same patient several times. Thus the simple cost comparisons may be reflecting either real differences in efficiency or just different ways of manipulating the denominators. The behavioural responses which in chapter 8 undermined the effectiveness of incentive reimbursement, may here invalidate statistical inferences.

This litany of problems has to some extent been dealt with in the course

---

[3] Cost comparisons among hospitals will also be distorted by differences in wage rates or other input prices faced by different hospitals. It is assumed here and elsewhere that such variations have been adjusted out, although this is by no means a trivial exercise.

of development of "hospital cost function" studies over about twenty years. In early studies, the multiproduct problem was dealt with by inserting additional variables into the right-hand side of the PD_i relationship above, *e.g.*, to reflect the presence or absence of a medical school affiliation or to measure the numbers of outpatient visits. The Canadian hospital statistical reporting system, however, permits one to identify in each hospital the direct costs of non-inpatient activities such as outpatient care or education. By removing these, plus an appropriate share of overhead costs, one can derive an estimate of the hospital's operating (not capital) costs for inpatient care, a measure which should be more closely related to inpatient utilization than is global expenditure.[4] Some variant of this estimate of inpatient costs has thus been used in most Canadian studies.

Variations across hospitals in the nature and severity of inpatient load have been dealt with in various ways, depending on the information available on patients. Early United States studies attempted to infer severity or complexity of illness from the intensity of servicing, and so measured surgical rates and diagnostic procedures per day or case. But this approach has the same circularity problems as the measurement of "quality" by servicing intensity described in chapter 8; a hospital which overtreats simple cases would be considered to have complex cases.

It is now generally accepted that characteristics of the patient must be used to standardize for patient load differences, since (except for misreporting) they are beyond the hospital's control. Age, sex, and diagnostic mix of patient load have been used in various transformations to try to adjust for interhospital differences. In these analyses, the separation records generated by the Canadian hospital insurance system have been extremely useful. While the specific record contents may vary across provinces, and extensive additional data are available from PAS or HMRI reports, at the very least each separation is identified by age, sex, residence, length of stay, discharge diagnoses, and operative procedure(s) if any. From these data one can develop profiles of the characteristics of each hospital's case load.

Some patient classification systems rely solely on patient age and diagnosis; others build in additional information on whether or not surgery occurred or on length of stay. In general such additional information makes systems of classification more sensitive to differences in severity within diagnostic groups, but at the cost of making a hospital's relative

---

[4] Students of the wool and mutton problem will know that "joint costs are joint," and will be dubious of accountants' allocation rules as used here. Given some ideal, very large sample with plenty of observational variance, one might prefer statistical techniques for cost allocation, but in practice the accounting approach seems to yield much better results. (Judged how? A priori plausibility . . .)

position, in terms of the difficulty of its case load, more sensitive to its own behaviour as well as the external needs to which it is responding. Whichever system is used, however, the adjustment process takes place in two stages. Patients are first classified into groups of differential difficulty, severity, or complexity (labels vary), and then some aggregation rule is used to construct one or several hospital-specific measures of the difficulty of the overall case load.[5]

Certain very specific results have arisen from these studies (Barer 1981, 1982). First, the initial interest in scale economies has been seen to have been misplaced. Early United States studies gave widely divergent results (Berki 1972; Lave and Lave 1979); Canadian studies consistently showed unit costs rising with scale, more or less indefinitely, unless adjustment is made for differences in case load characteristics between small and large hospitals. After such adjustment, scale effects become rather unimportant. The characteristics of patients treated, as represented by age, sex, and diagnosis, exert a much more significant influence on relative costs, explaining half to two-thirds of differences across hospitals in costs per separation. Inpatient costs in teaching hospitals appear to be significantly higher than in non-teaching, even after deduction of costs directly allocated to education. Short-run utilization variables—occupancy, length of stay, case flow rate (cases per bed per year)—usually have the anticipated effects; costs per day fall as utilization rises, indicating that hospitals are mostly on the falling (negatively sloped) segment of the short-run average cost curve. Cost per episode of course rises with length of stay, but not proportionately. Marginal costs per case or per day are significant—an empty bed is not as costly as a filled bed—but are perhaps in the neighbourhood of half of average costs.

Most striking of all, Canadian studies consistently show that a combination of scale, short-run utilization level, and patient characteristics variables "explain" a very large proportion of inter-hospital variation in costs per day or per case—usually in the range of 70–90 percent and in

---

[5] In Canada, such measures could be used to rank hospitals for budget negotiation purposes; in the U.S. it might appear that a global hospital measure or measures were unnecessary. If, for example, one could partition the hospital's case load into a number of mutually exclusive and collectively exhaustive categories, each believed more or less internally homogeneous with respect to its needs for treatment resources per case, then reimbursing agencies could pay each hospital the same amount, X_i, for each case in group or category i. But the relative amounts paid for different categories, the ratios X_i/X_j, would then be the aggregators yielding a single index for each hospital, which would, in fact, be its reimbursement level. And the information required to determine the X_i, X_j, X_k does not arise from the grouping process itself. The use of Diagnosis Related Groups (DRGs) in the U.S. is intended to categorize patients insured by their federal Medicare program, but the actual rates of reimbursement will be set on the basis of average actual experience for groups of "similar" hospitals.

some studies close to 95 percent. This finding indicates a very high degree of managerial uniformity, presumably induced by the centralized reimbursement system and associated oversight. It does not indicate either uniform efficiency or uniform inefficiency, of course, but only that most *variations* can be "explained by," or associated with, identifiable characteristics of the hospital's situation, not differences in management.

Thus far, such aggregate statistical studies of hospitals do not appear to have been much used as input to the hospital budget negotiation process in Canada, although Quebec has applied an extension of the technique, and Alberta has some experimental work underway. Apart from the complexity of the statistical techniques, and their unfamiliarity to hospitals and to provincial negotiators, there remain some problems with the analysis.

First, variations in severity within diagnostic categories have not been allowed for, except insofar as they correlate with age and sex. One hospital's cases of diagnosis D *may* typically be "sicker" than another's. Some progress has been made with patient care classification systems in hospitals, particularly for nurse staffing, but this has not been linked to aggregate cost functions. Some United States classification systems go beyond diagnosis to include procedures performed, or direct assignments of level of severity, but as noted they are then sensitive to the hospital's choice of treatment patterns, as well as to subjective judgements of severity.

Secondly, measures of cost per "case" are based on separations—discharges and deaths—which are assumed to represent episodes of care. But an episode may involve re-admissions or transfers, thus generating several separations. Present studies have not adjusted for this, so its impact is unknown.

Thirdly, comparisons are made of costs per unit of *output*, not *outcome*; almost nothing has been done to test for differences in outcomes across hospitals. These in turn would represent, if adjusted for difficulty of patient load and resource availability, the differences across hospitals in quality of care. Some results do exist which indicate that mortality outcomes, at least, do not correlate with intensity of input use, whether or not one adjusts for patient characteristics. These findings cast further doubt on the identification of service intensity with "quality." But even this limited information has not been integrated with aggregate cost function analysis (Lundman 1982).

Finally, as emphasized above, analyses at the hospital-wide level cannot deal with the issue of the appropriateness of hospital use itself. Insofar as they focus on comparisons of costs per episode, they can help to identify a combination of technical efficiency (or inefficiency) in the production of particular services, and (assuming equivalent outcomes across hospitals) more or less intensive use of resources for a given set of illness episodes. But such analyses could easily identify as highly efficient a hospital which was providing unnecessary services, admitting patients who did not need care. It is usually cheaper to look after healthy people than sick ones. The significance of such analyses depends on the extent to which one identifies general managerial efficiency or inefficiency in running inpatient services as an important policy issue in hospital care. Broader issues of over– or underuse, or of innovative techniques in substituting forms of non-institutional care, are beyond their scope.

(ii) Specific Hospital Program Studies

At a less aggregated level, a number of studies have examined the resources used and costs generated in caring for particular groups of patients in hospitals. These include comparisons across several hospitals caring for patients with the same problems, or of alternative modes of treatment in the same hospital—day care versus inpatient surgery, radiation versus surgery for cancer—or comparisons between hospital and non-hospital programs (home care, for example) for dealing with similar problems. The focus here shifts from the hospital to the patient or group of similar patients as the unit of analysis.

Such a study is a form of program analysis, which is discussed in more detail in chapter 11. There, however, the focus is on the methodology of such studies; in this chapter we are interested in particular results and in the implications they have for our understanding of hospital behaviour.

Studies of this type indicate that there exists substantial variation across hospitals in the process of treatment for, and costs of, similar problems. Variations shows up most readily in differences in lengths of stay; more detailed analysis shows differences in frequencies of diagnostic procedures or of surgical or other therapeutic interventions. Hospitals also differ significantly within or across regions in their use of substitutes for conventional inpatient care. Day care surgery, for example, represents a much larger proportion of total surgical load in some hospitals and provinces than in others (Evans and Robinson 1980). Care-by-parent wards for children are another, though much less widely used, form of care which has been shown to improve care quality, or at least patient/parent satisfaction, and lower costs of care (Evans and Robinson 1983). Yet implementation has been glacially slow, and highly localized.

Often the choice of program alternatives is between low and high technology interventions. A pair of widely quoted randomized trials of home care versus intensive coronary care units for survivors of a first heart attack (Mather *et al.* 1971; Hill *et al.* 1978) indicated no significant difference in outcome between the two forms of therapy—of radically different costs. A survey of literature on the efficacy of electronic foetal monitoring (Banta and Thacker 1979) indicated that this procedure might on balance be doing more harm than good. Its high false positive rate can lead to unnecessary interventions—Caesarian section to deliver babies "in distress" who in fact were not. This technology, widely adopted apparently without full evaluation, may be to a significant degree responsible for the current epidemic of Caesarian sections. Variations in patterns of laboratory diagnostic testing across regions and time have led to serious concerns, particularly among pathologists, as to the growing incidence of investigation without information, of costly testing with at best zero therapeutic payoff, in hospital as well as ambulatory care.

It would be neither useful nor possible to provide here a survey of the vast array of studies on specific hospital programs. What emerges from such studies, however, is a rejection of "cost-minimizing" models of hospital behaviour. Over and over, one finds differences in techniques across hospitals which have significant cost implications without apparent associated outcome differences. Yet these differences do not lead to any response by the high-cost hospital(s), at once or ever. Unlike private sector management, hospital management is not under any institutionalized pressure to seek out and adopt less costly ways of providing care.

As an example, but only an example, expert opinion in Canada holds strongly that tonsillectomy cannot safely be performed as a day surgical procedure.[6] Although its frequency of performance has dropped dramatically in the last decade, this procedure still accounts for a very large number of paediatric admissions. Yet in British Columbia, two hospitals were each reported as having performed about a hundred such operations per year, on surgical day care, over a period of more than a decade. The important point is not whether "expert opinion" was right or wrong in this case, but that other hospitals felt no necessity to observe the discrepancy and react to it. Apparently no effort was made to find out if the "deviant" hospitals were taking undue risks, or if the conventional approach imposed undue costs.[7]

At a less local level, the serious questions raised by the randomized trial of coronary care units or the analysis of electronic foetal monitoring do not appear to have had any impact on the utilization of these technologies. The finding that halving lengths of stay for heart attack victims who have no complications in the first four days of stay had no adverse effects on patients (McNeer *et al.* 1978) has not led to drastic cuts in this major component of hospital utilization. Early discharge programs for

---

[6] How often it should be performed, if at all, is a separate issue.

[7] British Columbia Ministry of Health, Reports on Day Care Surgery (Annual), 1968 through to 1980/81. In the last five years, "expert opinion" in the U.S. has shifted to the point that day care surgery for tonsillectomy is becoming more common, a development apparently ignored by Canadian practice.

obstetrical patients and newborns are just beginning, and struggling against apparent indifference among most physicians and hospital administrators. It is hard to see how such massive inertia in response to new technological information on ways to reduce costs while maintaining care outcomes can be reconciled with theoretical models of hospital behaviour which assume cost-minimizing behaviour a priori.

Indeed, the incentives in hospitals seem rather to be towards the adoption of more costly, more resource-intensive techniques, so long as the budgetary climate is sufficiently permissive. Far from cost-minimization, as implied by quantity-maximization under budget constraint, the process appears to be one of intensity-maximization. But the fact that much of the resulting intensity of resource use, of servicing, cannot be linked to patient outcomes, and in a number of cases can be shown *not* to be so linked, forbids us to refer to this process as "quality-maximization"—ineffective care is not quality.[8]

Apart from their implications for our understanding of hospital behaviour, specific program studies support several important generalizations. First, there appears to be a great deal of scope for lowering hospital costs, and improving the effectiveness and efficiency of the hospital "industry," in particular program areas. No one program innovation by itself will have a major impact—even if it were possible, say, to do all tonsillectomies on a day care basis, the influence on overall hospital use would be minimal. But across all forms of questionable utilization, the potential for reduced hospital use appears to be very large indeed. No one has yet attempted to assemble the literature on alternatives to conventional inpatient care, to see what the aggregate impact could be. A study which looked, diagnosis by diagnosis, at the savings in hospital use which have been demonstrated in some form of experimental or field trial, without deterioration of patient outcome, would almost certainly yield very large numbers indeed.[9]

Of course, hospital costs would not fall in direct proportion to utilization. A part of the savings would come from reductions in lengths of stay, and the late days of stay are those of lowest service intensity. One should not overemphasize this point, however, as it appears that the mere fact of being hospitalized is itself a risk factor for diagnostic intervention

---

[8] One might suggest that additional servicing can add to patient satisfaction even if it does not improve outcomes. But that depends on the service—more back rubs may do so, but more lab tests certainly do not. It seems a safe generalization that the more technical the service, the more likely it is to lower, not raise, patient satisfaction. TLC is not high tech.

[9] U.S. experience with HMOs represents an obvious first approximation, indicating potential savings of inpatient acute care use in the neighbourhood of 40 percent (Luft 1981).

(Hornbrook and Goldfarb 1981). Early discharge, or alternative forms of care such as surgical day care or care-by-parent for children, lead to less intensive diagnostic interventions, as well as less custodial care (Evans and Robinson 1980, 1983). And diagnostic intervention, given the inevitability of some false positives, leads on average to further care.

Reductions in hospital use lead to transfers in cost as well as reductions. People have to eat whether in hospital or out, for example, and part of the saving of hospital dietary costs by early discharge shows up in the patient's budget. Again, however, one must not overemphasize this point. Elaborate valuations of the time and effort of patients and their families at some hypothetical market wage rate can lead to rather peculiar cost imputations by simple failure to value the benefits of not being institutionalized. In general, people strongly prefer *not* to be in hospital, and enter or stay there only because they believe they "need" care.

It is important to emphasize the extensive evidence for potential improvements in hospital efficiency, because the impression is sometimes given, particularly in economic analyses, that hospital budgeting and health budgeting generally impose a grim trade-off between cost-control and death. If all diagnostic and therapeutic interventions in hospitals (or out of them) have some expected payoff in terms of health status, then we are on the curve in Figure 1-3b, and decisions on resource allocation in hospitals are indeed decisions as to who shall live and who shall die (or who shall live in what condition). How much shall we as a society give up to extend or improve the life of someone needing care? The point of the specific program studies is that we are *not* on the curve, but well below it.[10] The trade-off may be very real, and very grim, but system-wide we are not there yet. There is scope for either withdrawing resources from health care without reducing anyone's well-being, or for redeploying resources to achieve better results without having to spend more. Too much attention to the ultimate trade-off can distract our attention and our policies from these opportunities here and now.

But it is not in fact true that *no one's* well-being is reduced by changes. Patients may be better off, but providers are not. Day care surgery saves money by making ward nurses redundant. Lab tests which add nothing to diagnosis or therapy (*ex ante* or *ex post*) can add substantially to the provider's revenue, whether hospital or private lab. Since every dollar of expenditure is also a dollar of someone's income, there is a direct

---

[10] Note again the ambiguity of the definition of health care "outputs." We can think of a curve of the Figure 1-3 type relating, *e.g.*, resources devoted to laboratory testing and health status, in which case we are probably on or near the curve, but it appears to be flat (or even downward sloping) where we are. Or we can think of a curve defined over resources devoted to, *e.g.*, particular forms of inpatient care, in which case unnecessary testing is represented by a point below the curve.

interest in the hospital sector in resisting cost-reducing innovation. Fee-for-service medical practice makes the conflict of interest between patient (or insurer) and provider more explicit than does salaried care, but it is present in either case. Thus it is not surprising that the second point emerging from program studies is that innovations which add to costs (incomes) proliferate rapidly on the basis of relatively weak evidence of efficacy, while innovations which lower costs (incomes) make little headway and are held to much more rigorous standards of proof of efficacy. An intervention which can clearly be shown to be harmful to patients does, of course, die out quite quickly, but those whose effects are minimal, or for which the evidence is equivocal, seem to persist indefinitely.

The failure of hospital managements to seek out new information on efficient technique, or to respond to it when it is available, is partly a problem of incentives—not-for-profit organization and some form of cost reimbursement—and partly a reflection of the ambiguity of the definition of management at this level. How patients are to be cared for is traditionally the prerogative of the medical staff; the administration are responsible for the efficient assembly of the resources needed to provide that care. Thus the managerial failure implicit in ineffective or unnecessarily costly modes of care is in the first instance a failure of the medical staff, individually or collectively. But the information which might guide staff decisions is generally more readily available to administration. Thus the failure of medical staff to react to new knowledge is in part a failure of administration to assemble and present the information. In any case, the division of responsibilities in present hospital management structures appears to assign no one the responsibility for ensuring that the patterns of service which patients receive reflect the best available information on efficiency and effectiveness. And the cost implications of this failure seem much more important than the narrow questions of technical efficiency—of cost minimization per unit of service.

Indeed a third general point arises from the specific program studies, which is even more discouraging than the problem of information dissemination and uptake. In the present climate of economic restraint, which has lasted for a decade in Canada and is probably with us for the indefinite future, new programs are very frequently advocated on the basis of cost savings. CT scanning, for example, substitutes an ambulatory procedure for several different types of inpatient procedures, and thus might save enough in inpatient care to pay its costs. Home care or day hospitals for the elderly will save money by keeping people out of institutions. Day care surgery or shortened inpatient stays can significantly reduce utilization *by particular patients.*

It does not follow, however, that overall hospital costs will in fact fall, and indeed most specific program innovations seem to be associated with increased expenditures. Two different variants of Roemer's Law are at work.

First, innovations which free up capacity of any sort induce more utilization, just as does the construction of new capacity. Hospitals frequently point out that programs to shorten stay *increase* their costs. What they mean is that *per diem* costs rise as the "cheap" late days of stay are curtailed, *and* that new admissions flow in to maintain occupancy. If admission rates did not respond, *per diem* costs would still rise, but total costs would fall. Similarly, surgical day care lowers inpatient use for the class of procedures it serves, but other forms of inpatient use react to the newly available capacity (Evans *et al.* 1983). What started off as a cost-reducing substitution of one form of care for another becomes an add-on of more care and more costs. Indeed, some United States commentators on surgical day care specifically advocate its introduction only when inpatient use is at capacity, so that one can be sure it will yield add-on business (Robinson and Clarke 1980, chapter 11). Otherwise, the new service might lower inpatient use and hence lower the hospital's revenue base!

Secondly, new procedures which substitute for more expensive (and less effective or more uncomfortable or dangerous) old procedures, as CT scanning does for pneumoencephalography, rarely stop there. Again utilization rises to meet capacity; so the utilization and overall cost of the new technique will often substantially exceed that of the techniques it replaces. Automated laboratory testing has the same result—unit costs fall but total costs rise as volume expands. While the value of the new technique for some patients may be beyond question, at the margin it may be highly questionable. Or the new technique may simply be piggy-backed on the old—both are done "just in case."

New drug therapies show the same behaviour. Cimetidine, the H_2 receptor blocker, represented a major breakthrough in treatment of duodenal ulcer, and has been shown to improve outcomes and lower costs of care for DU cases who would otherwise have gone to surgery. Studies of its use in the field, however, show that it is being marketed and used for conditions for which its effectiveness has not been demonstrated, and is being used in conjunction with, not as a substitute for, other chemotherapy (Hall *et al.* 1981). Such widespread indiscriminate use suggests that the cost of the drug *as used* exceeds any savings of other forms of therapy it might yield; its very real effective use is surrounded by a very large penumbra of questionable and, in some cases, useless or harmful applications.

Nor is the "add-on" effect confined to technological interventions. Extended care for the elderly and chronically ill has long been promoted as a means of reducing pressure on acute care facilities by misplaced patients, with the suggestion that overall costs could be reduced if more appropriate care were available. About twenty years of experience, however, suggests that if new facilities are built, they will be used, *and* the acute care hospitals will remain full. More recently, chronically ill or elderly patients in acute care facilities have been referred to in some quarters as ''bed-blockers''—implicitly suggesting that if they could be housed somewhere (anywhere) else, new acute admissions would be generated to use the freed space.[11]

The extended versions of Roemer's Law, that available capacity of whatever sort induces increased utilization, are not the only sources of failure of the program substitution approach. The basic premise of substitution may in some cases simply be wrong—homemakers and/or day hospital services may not affect people's need for and use of acute care facilities, for example, or not enough to recoup their costs. The Roemer's Law effects, however, are of particular interest. In the first place, they underscore the inadequacy of attempts to interpret hospital utilization in terms of an exogenous demand curve constraint. Hospital models which postulate such a relationship as a crucial feature will be seriously misleading, as will policy recommendations derived from such a framework. If we are to understand, model, the behaviour of hospitals, we must take explicit account of the processes whereby they influence the utilization of their own services, independently of any prices paid by patients.[12] In this context, it is obvious that ''the hospital'' includes its medical staff.

But secondly, the influence of capacity on use implies that policy, by whatever means introduced, must to be successful be global not partial in its impact. If substitutes for inpatient care are introduced, then a corresponding component of inpatient capacity must simultaneously be withdrawn from service. A sequence of innovations successfully carried out piecemeal will not add up to a major change in efficiency unless there exists some global constraint, public or private, over the hospital system

---

[11] Indeed, the representative of one medical association has been quoted as saying that his members' earnings are suffering because of inadequate access to acute care facilities in which to ply their trades. ''Bed-blockers'' are part of this problem; despite ten years of expanding capacity in extended care there is still no reason to believe that further expansion by itself would cut acute care use.

[12] Of course this process does not operate without limit; like every other ''Law'' it is an approximation to reality in the relevant range of experience. A hospital system such as that in the U.S. which has adapted to serving significant numbers of people who are too poor to pay their own bills or to purchase private insurance, and whose costs are therefore reimbursed by government, will find itself in severe difficulty if those subsidies are withdrawn. The hospital may still be able to keep itself full, but the clientele simply cannot pay. The only financially viable response is to move ''up-market'' to serve those who can afford private coverage, or who pay their own bills; but this adjustment (currently underway) cannot be instantaneous, and there may be some bankruptcies along the way.

as a whole. Hence the impossibility of effective control in fragmented, multi-source funding systems, compared with either direct public regulation of capacity in a sole source funding system such as Canada's, or the private, closed-panel, prepaid group practices in the United States which own or contract with their own hospitals.

(iii) Population-Based Hospital Utilization Studies

The third class of studies focusses on population groups rather than hospitals or specific programs, and compares aspects of hospital utilization rather than costs, efficiency, or effectiveness. Their findings, however, also serve as a basis for inferences about hospital objectives, behaviour, and performance.

Cross-population comparisons may address total hospital utilization—patient-days and/or separations per thousand population—or subcategories such as surgical use, or utilization patterns for particular procedures such as appendectomy or cholecystectomy. The latter are distinguished from specific hospital program studies, however, in that they would compare, say, appendectomy rates in two or more defined populations rather than patterns of service use by appendectomy patients in two or more hospitals or other provider sites.

Populations may be compared across geographical regions—countries, large areas such as provinces or states within a country, or small areas such as counties or school districts within a province. Or they may be compared across different types of health care service organizations, as between enrollees of community health centres or prepaid group practices and users of private fee-for-service practitioner care. United States studies have also examined utilization differences between populations insured with private for-profit, private not-for-profit, and public insurance carriers.

Data assembly for such utilization studies has a number of standard problems. Definition of denominators, the population of interest, is fairly straightforward for geographic comparisons, though small-area boundaries often shift over time. But populations served by different systems of care are more ambiguous, particularly if people can as in Canada switch back and forth from, say, a community health centre to private practitioners, or can use both simultaneously without penalty. Defining utilization also poses problems, particuarly for small-area studies, if use data is assembled by institution, not by patient. People cross area borders to obtain care, and one cannot assume that care provided *in* a region corresponds to care received by residents *of* the region. For small areas in Canada, boundary crossing is systematic and significant, though in regionalized delivery systems like Sweden it may be less common. For larger regions, provinces or countries, this problem becomes less severe but is replaced by definitional problems. The specific definition of a day or episode of care may vary across national statistical systems, as may the borderlines between acute hospital care, various forms of extended or chronic care, and custodial care for the elderly or disabled. Furthermore, the representativeness of aggregate or average measures of population characteristics, demographic or socio-economic, becomes weaker as region size increases. The establishment of valid cross-population comparisons is thus not a trivial exercise.

Subject to these qualifications, a large number of comparative utilization studies have been carried out and certain strong and consistent patterns emerge.

First, there are substantial variations in hospital utilization across geographic regions at any level of aggregation. Marked variations across countries might not be surprising, as reflecting differences in population characteristics, both physiological and cultural, as well as significant differences in health care organization, delivery, and payment. But the extent of variation does not shrink as one moves to comparisons among large or small areas in individual countries. In Canada, for example, days of (public general) hospital care per capita in 1980-81 varied across the ten provinces from 25.6 percent above the national average (Saskatchewan), to 15.0 percent below (Newfoundland), and separations from +48.8 percent (Saskatchewan) to −22.1 percent (Quebec) (Canada, Statistics Canada 1982).

Surgical procedures have been most intensively studied, with comparisons between the United States and England and Wales showing utilization differences of 2:1. Canadian surgical rates exceed England by almost the same amount, while variations among the Canadian provinces for particular procedures are in the range of from 3:2 to 2:1, with some procedures as high as 3:1 (Vayda 1973; Vayda *et al.* 1975, 1976). Studies of high and low surgical regions in Manitoba show overall surgical rates about 50 percent higher in high-rate areas, while for particular procedures the ratio is from 2:1 to 3:1 (Roos and Roos 1981). In Ontario, for particular discretionary procedures, the rate per capita varied by 5:1 between the lowest and highest frequency countries (Stockwell and Vayda 1979).

Further information is, of course, necessary before one can draw inferences from such observations. It is possible that utilization differentials could correspond to different population "needs." These differentials, however, show up in age-sex adjusted data, which removes the principal correlate of hospital care "need" at the aggregate population level. And efforts to relate utilization differentials for particular procedures or diagnoses to other indicators of differential need have not in general been successful. Marked differences in length of stay for deliveries without mention of complications, for example, a well-defined procedure, hardly admit a "differential need" explanation.

Even if populations are essentially similar, or their relevant (to utilization) differences have been identified and standardized for, the observation of a differential, however large, does not in itself indicate whether one area overutilizes, or another underutilizes (or both). Additional information is necessary, usually by particular procedure or diagnosis, as to the consequences in terms of mortality or morbidity which should follow from under– or overuse. If high use regions represent appropriate use, in terms of meeting needs/contributing to health status, then since the discrepancies are so large, low use areas should reveal significant consequences of insufficient care.[13]

In general, however, efforts to observe differences in mortality or morbidity associated with differences in hospital use have turned up very little—except for the effects of differential use on surgical death rates. Case-fatality rates in surgery do not appear to vary with the level of utilization; apparently areas with a high rate of surgical use do not reach down to patients of lower average risk status. (Roos and Roos 1981). So deaths in surgery are proportional to the volume of surgery performed, consistent with findings that death rates fall in areas where hospitals or physicians go on strike.

It would appear that, in terms of Figure 1-3, levels of hospital utilization in Canada and probably in other countries as well are now out on the flat of the curve, beyond the point of payoff in terms of health status and perhaps even on the downward slope. And from the size of the interregional utilization differentials, we would seem to be a long way out on the flat. Substantial reductions in use would be possible in many regions without, apparently, risk to anyone's health.

If utilization differentials are not traceable to differences in population characteristics or needs and do not appear to lead to differences in population morbidity or mortality, one is led to consider explanations rooted in the delivery system itself. But simple-minded explanations in terms of physicians paid fee-for-service or hospitals mantaining their occupancy rates and revenue bases are also unsatisfactory, or at best incomplete.

There seems little question that the source of variation is in fact provider behaviour. Studies of the characteristic patterns of surgical utilization in small areas, by procedure, show stability over time but considerable

---

[13] We leave out of account here economic-theoretical explanations in terms of differences in unobserved consumer "tastes" for, *e.g.*, surgery, that might lead some populations to choose to consume more surgical operations just as they might prefer beef over mutton. Surgical procedures, like health care generally, are as noted in chapter 1 not direct arguments in the consumer's utility function—or at least not positive-weighted ones.

sensitivity to the interests, preferences, and beliefs of the local medical community (Wennberg and Gittelsohn 1982; Roos 1983). Entry or exit of particular physician's shifts the use pattern such that Wennberg and Gittelsohn refer to the physician's ''surgical signature'' or personal pattern of behaviour. Efforts to relate such variations to characteristics or beliefs of the underlying population have not succeeded. The key role of specific practitioners was clearly shown in Saskatchewan when hysterectomy rates fell by nearly half in one year in response to an announcement (made to physicians, *not* the public) that performance of this procedure was to be investigated (Dyck *et al.* 1977). Even greater changes were observed in tonsillectomy rates in parts of New England in response to changes in physician information (Wennberg and Gittelsohn 1982). At the more aggregated level, Roemer's Law seems to apply to surgeons as well as to hospital beds—where more are available more are used (Bunker 1970; Fuchs 1978).

But the relation is not a simple one. In university teaching centres, more beds and surgeons available do not appear to have the same impact, at least on common procedures, as in a non-academic environment. More generally, the effects of increased capacity, either physicians or hospital facilities, depend on the interests and preferences of the people involved and on institutional tradition and habit. There is no clear relationship, consistent across time and place, between capacity and *particular* forms of utilization.

Further evidence of the importance of the delivery system in influencing hospital use is given by the extensive information on prepaid group practices, community health centres, HMOs, HSOs, etc. in Canada and the U.S. Groups encompassing physicians and hospitals (owned or contracted) paid by capitation not fee-for-service, have been shown over and over again to generate rates of hospital utilization which are from 10 to 40 percent below those of populations served by fee-for-service physicians. The same questions of comparability of populations and adequacy of care have been raised in response to these findings, as to the regional comparisons. But population standardization and in some cases random assignment of people to a capitation-based practice and to fee-for-service alternatives have left these findings intact. How physicians are employed and paid strongly affects how much hospital care their patients use. And despite considerable efforts to identify inadequacies of care in such practices, the reductions in use do not appear to affect mortality or morbidity. On other measures of quality, such groups frequently score above the general system.

These observations, frequently repeated over the last thirty years, could be and have been interpreted in terms of the differential economic motivations in capitation versus fee-for-service reimbursement. Not only do capitation-paid groups not profit from more servicing, they may actually gain, in a variety of ways, from keeping their patients out of hospital. But as noted above, the simple economic determinism arguments are inadequate. Inter-country comparisons have shown relatively very high servicing rates by surgeons with little or no economic stake in performance. Lichtner and Pflanz (1971) studied the German experience with appendectomy, for example, finding it three to four times the rate in any other country, with correspondingly higher surgical mortality rates, but no evidence of a higher incidence of underlying conditions. But the surgeons were salaried, not paid for the procedure. Moreover, inter-area variation within Germany was also high. McPherson *et al.* (1982) report high levels of inter-area variation in surgical rates in countries with very different funding systems. And hospital utilization rates vary across regions for capitation-based practices just as they do for private fee-for-service care. Investigators of inter-regional variations in particular forms of surgery have had mixed results in trying to find a relation with physician availability or level of activity. An important factor may be simply the uncertainty of providers about the nature of "best practice," and the evolution of personal styles or habits of behaviour, resulting from training, early experience, peer behaviour, or personal skills and preferences. The existence of wide variations in use, unrelated to needs or outcomes, is extensively documented, but at present there is no fully satisfactory explanation as to why.

GENERALIZATIONS ABOUT WHOSE BEHAVIOUR?

Such findings are as much, or more, a description of medical practice as of the hospital "industry." As we move from the technical efficiency with which hospitals convert resources into specific services, to the pattern of services involved in the provision of an episode of hospital care, and finally to levels of hospital use in the population as a whole, it is clear that we move from the traditional domain of the hospital administrator to that of the physician. But the necessity of this shift, if we are to think at all sensibly about the evaluation or the effective organization of the hospital sector, should be readily apparent. Hospital management includes physicians, whatever their formal organizational arrangements, in that physicians' decisions are a critical determinant of what hospitals will or will not do, as well as how they will do it. In production theory terms, the decision as to how much of what types of output to produce is principally in the hands of the physician; the administrator's influence is not negligible, but is secondary. The "how" of production is the administrator's role. But management includes both.

On the whole, the various types of empirical studies of hospital behaviour and utilization have contributed more to our knowledge about resource-allocation processes and system performance in hospitals than have the attempts at formal modelling. They will support generalizations which are of relevance for policy formation and evaluation, even if they are not easily embedded in some consistent conceptual model of a hospital as a behaving transactor with clear-cut objectives and constraints. Indeed, they are clearly inconsistent with the simpler forms of such models. The specific program studies make it difficult to maintain that hospitals strive to minimize costs, at least for costs *per* any measure of output meaningful to the patient or the wider society. Minimizing the costs of production of an unnecessary test is not cost-minimization. Further, the study of hospital utilization patterns and their correlates is very difficult to reconcile with the exogenous patient demand for hospital care which plays a central constraining role in many formal models of hospitals.[14]

But the findings are also difficult to reconcile with the Medico-Technical model of physician and hospital behaviour, or of professsional behaviour generally, which assumes that there is a best way of doing everything and that the professional seeks it out on the patient's behalf. One is left with several alternative, but not mutually exclusive, hypotheses.

Physicians may recommend, and provide in hospitals, care which they know to be useless or harmful, or may deliberately choose inefficient modes of production. While this probably occurs from time to time, as in any area of human endeavour, it is difficult to believe that systematic malfeasance is sufficient to explain the discrepancies observed.

Secondly, providers may be doing what they think best, but be in error, and most importantly, have no particular incentive, and indeed postive disincentives, to seek out least cost modes of production or weed out ineffective hospital use. This seems the most plausible interpretation, leading to the question of what types of social mechanisms or organizational structures, informational or regulatory, might help to promote better (*i.e.*, more effective and efficient) performance.

Finally, one might interpret the diversity of professional behaviour as indicating that there is really no such thing as best practice or best technique, in which case it would be unsurprising that there were no consensus on it. The extreme form of this position is that medicine has nothing to do with health, so why expect hospital utilization patterns to be any more standardized than consumption of any other commodity or service? On this view, the design of curricula in professional schools would be rather difficult, to say nothing of the difficulty of justifying professional licensure and regulation. But even the advocates of such a view do not appear to take it seriously enough to follow it to its logical conclusions.

---

[14] Difficult, but not impossible. The reconciliation can be achieved with the aid of unobserved variables and circular reasoning, but the process is not particularly enlightening.

On balance, then, the most plausible interpretation of the available research seems to be that imperfections in the information available to, and incentives bearing on, the management of the hospital system—physicians and administrators—leads to problems of both ineffective and inefficient servicing which are quantitatively very significant. The seriousness of inefficiency in the narrower sense of resources used per procedure performed, cost per lab unit or therapeutic procedure, is less clear.

Possible institutional responses to this situation range along a continuum from efforts to stimulate efficiency through competition among hospitals in a deregulated private market-place, to a centralized public hospital service. Neither pole seems particularly attractive, or politically feasible, and certain intermediate possibilities will be considered in chapter 14, below.

CHAPTER 10

SERVING GOD AND MAMMON? HEALTH CARE FOR PROFIT

FOR-PROFIT HEALTH CARE IN CANADA: SMALL SCALE BUT WIDER SIGNIFICANCE

Amid "voluntary" not-for-profit institutions in the hospital sector, professional practices, government bureaux, and voluntary agencies, the strictly for-profit (FP) firm of conventional economic theory organized and operated solely to maximize the profits of its owners provides a very small proportion of health care services in Canada. For-profit organization persists primarily in the production and sale of specific commodities— drugs and supplies, medical equipment, eyeglasses, and prostheses. The for-profit insurance industry continues to provide some prepayment and administration services, in competition with not-for-profit carriers, for care expenditures outside the public programs. In some provinces, a significant proportion of nursing home care is provided by FP institutions, and (again only in some provinces) the non-hospital wing of the laboratory industry appears to be moving or to have moved into the FP sector. Overall, a reasonably generous estimate of the for-profit share of health care expenditures might be in the neighbourhood of 15 percent.[1]

But the importance of for-profit organization in health care delivery is greater than this small proportion might suggest, for three reasons. First, the sectoral division of health expenditures is on a final output, not a "value added" basis; it identifies only the firm or institution directly supplying the end user. But hospitals, for example, buy significant amounts of their inputs from the for-profit sector. About 30 percent of operating expense is non-labour cost, and though much of this is food, fuel, and

---

[1] In 1982, drugs and appliances expenditure was $3,275.3 million. From this, subtract half of prescription drug expense (a conservative estimate of dispensing charges) or $736.7 million. Then add one-third of prepayment and administration expense ($147.1 million) and 40 percent of nursing home expense ($1647.1 million) (thus assuming that the private sector financing proportions reported in Canada, Health and Welfare Canada (1979) are equivalent to the for-profit shares—a more dubious proposition for nursing homes) to yield $4332.8 million, or 14.4 percent of total expense. But some portion of prescription dispensing charges, as well as some portion of physicians' services expense (private labs) should be added back as well.

other inputs non-specific to health care, there remains a substantial share of hospital expense, probably between 10 and 20 percent, which goes to for-profit firms selling health-specific commodities—drugs, dressings, medical gases, equipment, and supplies. The same is true of capital investment. Facility construction may be carried out by for-profit general construction firms, but major equipment, diagnostic and therapeutic machinery, is purchased from for-profit firms or divisions of firms specialized to the health sector.

Professional practices likewise buy from the for-profit sector some share of the inputs they use in providing services, the significance of equipment and supplies being more obvious in some fields (ophthalmology, radiology, pathology, dentistry) than others (general practice or psychiatry). Moreover as pointed out above, some (rather difficult to determine) share of professional earnings in the NOFP sector is also profit, net earnings after deducting the cost of purchased or owner-supplied inputs to production.[2]

Secondly, the behaviour of for-profit firms influences the decisions made by other suppliers. The extraordinary marketing efforts made by for-profit drug companies to influence physician prescribing patterns and attitudes toward therapy generally have long been a subject for study and comment. (Torrance n.d. *i.e.* 1972). Medical equipment manufacturers have a similar interest in marketing technological change to physicians and hospitals, whose decisions determine their sales.

Public policy and program design also create or destroy profit opportunities. The willingness or otherwise of insurers to reimburse physicians, as opposed to hospitals, for particular procedures can dramatically affect equipment sales. In Canada, CT scanners are not sold to physicians, because they cannot be reimbursed for providing the service to patients. In the United States physician practices make up a large market for such equipment. Similarly, drug substitution or compulsory licensure laws can have a powerful influence on the distribution of industry sales and profits. The Canadian federal government's modification in 1969 of patent protection for prescription drugs, to require compulsory licensure by the

---

[2] In this context one must keep in mind the distinction between the accounting and economic conceptions of profit. An accountant will describe as profit the firm's net revenues after deduction of purchased production inputs (labour and materials), depreciation of capital equipment, and interest on borrowed capital. This form of profit includes a return to the equity invested by the firm's owner(s), and so should be positive for a healthy business. Economists attribute a "normal" return to that capital (normalized for risk), and define as profit, or supranormal profit, any surplus of net revenue after attribution to owner-supplied capital. In a well-functioning competitive market, supranormal profits in the economist's sense tend to zero. In self-employed practice, economic profit is defined as net revenue after deduction of a return to owner-supplied capital *and labour*, using some estimate of market wage in the next best opportunity.

patent holder of competitive domestic producers or importers of generic equivalents, clearly cut into the profits of the multinationals while opening up markets for small domestic firms and lowering prescription drug prices to the Canadian consumer. The multinational drug firms have lobbied against this provision ever since. And the economic interests of private sickness and accident insurers are obviously threatened by the development and spread of public health insurance programs—the overhead costs of insurance or the spread between premium incomes and benefits paid being the source of their incomes and profits (see chapter 2). Thus the marketing and lobbying efforts of private firms must inevitably be directed to influencing public policy as well as the behaviour of the NFP and NOFP sectors in order to protect and expand their own sales opportunities.

Finally, a number of proposals for policy change, and more-or-less radical restructuring of the health care delivery system, involve a more extensive role for for-profit institutions. Such proposals are more prominent in the United States, where the existing situation is perceived as being in much more need of radical reform. There, some advocate the complete deregulation of the industry and the opening of all aspects of supply to private for-profit providers. Apart from the fact that such a revolution would disregard all the peculiarities of health care as a commodity analysed in chapters 1–4, its political feasibility is probably zero in any developed society.[3] Nevertheless, the powerful theoretical incentives to cost control, and to process as well as product innovations, in competitive markets served by for-profit firms suggest that one give serious consideration to the conditions under which for-profit motivation might be consistent with the more efficient allocation of health care resources. There is considerable experience with for-profit organization in the drug and appliance field, and its role is expanding rapidly, in the United States at least, in hospital ownership and management as well as in diagnostic services (Gray 1983). Some general lessons should be available from this experience, as to the risks and benefits of trying to harness for-profit motivations to health care objectives.

BEYOND GOOD AND EVIL: THE ECONOMIC FUNCTION OF PROFITS

From the outset, however, it is important to emphasize that profit per se is associated with neither moral turpitude nor additional costs.[4] There

---

[3] One may therefore assume that the promotion of complete deregulation is a stalking-horse for other objectives, probably re-distributional.

[4] Nor with any unique moral or spiritual virtues either. If the predominant, or at least noisiest, ideology of the 1960s made profit a dirty word, that of the 1980s seems to regard any activity which generates profits in the private sector (and for which no one

is an in-grained hostility to profit-making organizations in health care, often of rather obscure motivation. Making profits from the misfortune of others sounds morally offensive. Yet the individuals who provide care in NFP or NOFP settings make their livings, and frequently very good ones, from that same source. And profit, in a well-functioning competitive market, is not an extra cost component which can be "saved" by non-profit organization. In equilibrium it is a return to invested capital which reflects the opportunity cost of that capital to society as a whole. Capital is not free; it is scarce and has alternative uses. And an organization, profit or non-profit, which does not account for the value of the capital services which it uses is undercounting its true costs of production. When markets are out of equilibrium, profits (or their absence) also serve as signals of changes in tastes, technology, or resource availability, and provide both information and incentives to redirect resources. They thus perform a critical social role in assuring the efficient use of scarce resources—in a well-functioning competitive market.

The real concern over for-profit motivation in health care, therefore, (other than that of NFP and NOFP providers who fear the competition as a threat to their own interests or incomes), reflects a judgement that the conditions for a well-functioning market do not exist, and perhaps cannot be created even approximately, in the provision of health care. If this is so, then not profit per se, but the actions of the profit-seeker, may have undesirable results. The problem of the "quack" is not that he makes money—"legitimate" practitioners in health care also make money, and often a great deal—but that in the process he does or recommends things to patients which are useless or dangerous, or which delay or preclude more effective treatment. Of course so may legitimate practitioners, but presumably not as often, or else their legitimacy and the licensure process itself would be unjustifiable.

To criticize for-profit motivation, therefore, one must argue both that poor quality practice—where "quality" is explicitly defined in terms of probable effect on patient health status, *not* on general feelings of well-being—would be more profitable than good quality, at least for some current or potential providers (or else no one would provide poor quality care), *and* that this profitability is a result of patient ignorance—informed patients would not buy poor quality (or else it is hard to justify interfering with their decisions). The argument for keeping FP firms out of particular market is presumably that they are more likely to try to take advantage of patients' ignorance.

---

has yet been convicted) as not only *definitionally* in the broader public interest, but also a source of particular satisfaction to the Most High. This requires a reinterpretation of ethical and religious tradition, and a definition of the Good which, while not previously unheard of, is distinctly unusual. If fully spelled out, it might not command universal assent.

The same behaviour which the defender of profit views as energetic pursuit of efficient production becomes dangerous dilution of quality of care, while the flexible response to a wide range of individual preferences is interpreted in the context of asymmetric information as the exploitation of a gullible and vulnerable public with useless or harmful products. The objection to for-profit organization is thus based on the same assumption of asymmetric information between patient and provider as is the case for professional licensure, or the rejection of the assumed independence of consumer demand from supplier behaviour in theoretical analyses of utilization.

Conversely, the advocates of for-profit organization who have thought the matter through[5] argue first that the regulatory response to informational asymmetry is not perfect—which is clearly true—and secondly that a for-profit delivery system can be established which would remain competitive and would over time develop processes of information transfer (such as brand and reputation effects) which would remedy or at least mitigate the effects of asymmetry. The remaining distortions would be at least no worse than under the current approach.

This second proposition, unfortunately, is a pure statement of faith, arising neither from economic theory, conventional or otherwise, nor from empirical experience. One can, however, explore the present behaviour and performance of for-profit firms in particular areas of the health care field, in an attempt to draw inferences about their strengths and weaknesses. From these, one may be able to judge which other sectors of health care delivery might meet conditions for successful introduction of for-profit organization, and what benefits or problems are likely to follow.

PHARMACEUTICALS: THE EXTENDED BOTTOM LINE

The pharmaceutical industry is the largest and most studied component of the for-profit sector in health care (*e.g.*, Silverman *et al.* 1981; Silverman and Lee 1974; Walker 1971; Klass 1975). Prescription and non-prescription drug sales to Canadian consumers amounted to $1473.4 million and $1357.7 million in 1982, although these include dispensing fees and retail margins respectively, so that cost of drugs sold might be perhaps half of these amounts. Hospital drug purchases (1982-83) are reported at $224.7 million. Nor are pharmaceutical firms' sales confined to drugs for human consumption.

Prescription drugs, which are of most interest to health care policy,

---

[5] As opposed to the zealots or the fuzzy-minded for whom profit is per se a social desideratum.

are sold in a market characterized by a dual form of "derived demand." The user wants, not the drug per se (which may have unpleasant or even dangerous side effects), but the improvement in health status which it is expected to yield. Demand for the drug is derived from demand for improvement in or maintenance of health. But the technical relation between drug use and patient health is not in general known by the patient, so the law interposes the physician's judgement in the form of the prescribing process. The physician's demand is then derived from the patient's demand. Hence the marketing effort of pharmaceutical firms is aimed at physicians, and rarely if at all at patients.[6]

The sequence of resource-allocation decisions in prescription drug use can be divided into several stages, each of which raises economic issues. For a given drug, the utilization sequence begins with a prescription, an order to dispense written by a physician or other individual licensed to do so.

The appropriateness of this prescription, its relationship to the patient's condition and its probability of improving health status, is central to the evaluation of the whole drug delivery system. Inappropriately prescribed drugs, like ineffective or harmful diagnostic or therapeutic interventions, represent wasted resources and potential damage to patients however efficiently their production and distribution may be organized. Equally important is patient compliance; if the patient fails to follow the prescription, whether or not she purchases the drug, then the production and distribution process becomes pointless.

Assuming that the drug is appropriately prescribed and the prescription is complied with, a series of issues then arise concerning the efficiency with which drugs are produced, distributed, and dispensed. This includes questions of pharmacy organization and regulation—issues of price competition, advertising, personnel use, and regulatory restrictions on pharmacy and pharmacist behaviour generally—bearing on the efficiency and effectiveness of the dispensing process itself. But it extends to questions of product selection and substitution, the supply of branded and unbranded versions of generically equivalent drugs, and the effects of marketing efforts and regulatory policies on the cost, reliability, and efficacy of the ingredients supplied in response to prescriptions.

Finally, lying behind the activities of prescription and supply is the process of research and development whereby new chemical compounds are developed, their therapeutic properties, side effects, and safety determined, and approval granted for their coming to market. The drug

---

[6] Some industry "image advertising" is directed to the general public, presumably in the hope of political and public policy benefit. And a certain amount of "ricochet" advertising has begun in the U.S. to encourage patients to request physicians to order particular tests which may lead to subsequent drug use. Non-prescription drug advertising is of course directed at the general public—patients or otherwise.

industry, even more than most, must be viewed in a dynamic context and its performance evaluated in terms of its ability to generate new products and extend the range of effective interventions, as well as to respond efficiently and effectively to needs for existing products.

PRESCRIBING APPROPRIATENESS: INFORMING OR MANIPULATING THE PHYSICIAN?

For-profit corporations[7] play a critical role at each stage of the drug utilization process, but the positive and negative aspects of that role have been matters of intense and sometimes bitter debate. At the prescribing stage, attention focusses on whether the enormous marketing efforts of pharmaceutical firms, aimed at influencing physicians' decisions to prescribe particular brands of particular drugs, contribute to or detract from the appropriateness of the result. On the one hand, given the complex and rapidly changing array of drugs available, it is obviously impossible for prescribers to fill the role of the perfectly informed professional agent. To some extent the marketing efforts of drug companies serve as an information system, a transmission belt to ensure that new product information is rapidly and widely disseminated among practitioners. If the resources were not spent for this purpose—detail men, direct mailings, journal advertising—either some other transmission mechanism would be necessary or the process of innovation would be slowed down.

On the other hand the value of any transmission system depends on the quality of the information it produces, and it is widely recognized that the present channels are biased. Drug companies are in business to sell drugs, not to run professional in-service education programs or to heal the sick. The latter are only particular means to the former end, which is in turn the source of profits, the famous "bottom line." If it were otherwise motivated, the firm would not be for-profit, but "an eleemosynary outfit." Accordingly information is biased toward claims of efficacy and away from reports of side effects. Public regulation, plus the possibility of legal liability, shift the balance somewhat in the other direction, but only somewhat. And the personal contact of detail man with practitioner is difficult to check for "truth in advertising."

Three sorts of questions arise in this debate: (i) how serious is the problem of prescribing appropriateness? (ii) if it is serious, to what extent

---

[7] It is important to distinguish the motivation or objectives of an organization from its actual beneficial ownership. A for-profit corporation may in fact be partly or wholly owned by government, such as Canada's Connaught Labs or now France's Rhône-Poulenc, yet organized on private firm lines and evaluated on its profitability, and thus little if at all distinguishable from a private firm. A public drug production or distribution service as an arm of a Ministry of Health could be expected to behave quite differently.

is it a result of the drive for sales underlying the behaviour of for-profit drug companies? (iii) if drug company promotion is a significant contributing factor, are there ''cures'' which are not worse than the disease?

Whether even the first question is answerable depends, of course, on the extent of efforts made to evaluate prescribing behaviour. One of the strongest arguments for a universal public pharmaceutical insurance plan is that it can generate the data base with which one can observe and evaluate current prescribing patterns and attempt to modify them. In the absence of such insurance data, one is left with research studies of particular drugs in particular settings.[8]

Data available from such universal public plans as exist, and from specific studies, consistently show that there are indeed significant problems of prescribing appropriateness, and of two types. The first type, which shows up most clearly in utilization data, is misuse of a particular drug independently of the patient's illness. Prescriptions in amounts well beyond maximum safe doses or for overly extended periods or in conjunction with dangerously interacting drugs, represent per se inappropriate prescribing. These seem to be traceable to particular physicians and to derive from imperfections in the process of professional training and continuing competence review rather than in the drug delivery system itself.[9]

The second form of prescribing inappropriateness, probably much more important in quantitative terms, is the mis-match between drug prescribed and patient's condition, which is much harder to detect from utilization data alone. A drug which has been clearly identified as safe and efficacious for a range of specific conditions may also be prescribed in circumstances well beyond its demonstrated usefulness. Cimetidine, which represents a major breakthrough in duodenal ulcer therapy, is an excellent example. While its efficacy, relative safety, and capacity to substitute for more expensive and dangerous forms of therapy have been demonstrated for patients who might otherwise go to surgery, studies of its use in actual

---

[8] It might be technically possible for private insurers or prescription drug suppliers to assemble similar data, and indeed extensive data on physician prescribing behaviour is assembled to support the marketing efforts of private firms. But it would be naive in the extreme to imagine that firms whose profits depend on drug sales, and on the goodwill of physicians, would or could take an interest in restraining unnecessary or inappropriate prescribing. Creating the *appearance* of such interest might from time to time help to hold off unfavourable public regulation, but that is quite another matter. ''For-profit'' means what it says.

[9] A comprehensive data system enables one to distinguish the inappropriate prescribing behaviour of a particular physician from so-called ''shopping'' patients who might accumulate hazardous quantities or combinations of drugs by contacting several different physicians. Apart from narcotics or other addictive drugs, the problem seems to be located, not surprisingly, at the prescribing level.

practice indicate that it is being prescribed (i) for conditions in which its efficacy has not been demonstrated (and is in some cases quite implausible), (ii) in conjunction with other therapies (antacid) for which it is a substitute and with whose effectiveness it is imcompatible, and (iii) in amounts and for lengths of time which go beyond its demonstrated effectiveness and raise unnecessary risks of side effects (Hall *et al.* 1981). But this pattern appears to be a common one for "popular" drugs, of which cimetidine is a leading example. Antibiotics, which may have been the greatest drug therapy advance of all, have been widely used against virus infections, for which they are ineffective, and merely pose risks to the patient and the wider society by encouraging immune responses in patients and in disease organisms. The "minor" tranquilizers, such as diazepam, are now under criticism for their addictive effects, as well as (unproven) suggestions of carcinogenic side effects. Concern over the "galloping consumption" of pharmaceuticals is widespread among students of health care delivery.

There are of course other pressures besides those from the pharmaceutical industry itself which may lie behind prescribing problems. The physician, particularly in a fee-for-service setting, may find the prescription a convenient way to end a visit, a tangible symbol that she has understood and is taking charge of the problem. And the patient, in a society which expects problems to have solutions, may see the prescription as that solution—the technological fix. In this context, however, it is important to note that studies of nurse practitioners suggest that they provide somewhat fewer prescriptions than physicians for (apparently) comparable problems, and that their patients are at least as satisfied as those of physicians (Spitzer 1978). Further, cross-system comparisons indicate that practitioners reimbursed by fee-for-service consistently write more prescriptions than do those receiving other forms of reimbursement.

But the primary pressure does seem to come from the for-profit industry, as indeed it would be very surprising if it did not. Firms in this industry incur very high research, testing, and approval costs for new drugs, after which costs of production are relatively small. Additional sales, therefore, translate into high gross profit margins, and so can and do support a very large selling expense. It would appear then that the social benefits of information transmission financed by the industry must be balanced against a significant share of the cost of unnecessary and inappropriate prescribing. The global amount of that cost would be difficult to estimate, since it would have to include not only the costs of the drugs themselves, but also of any additional therapy made necessary by the inappropriate prescription as well as any direct costs of additional illness to the patient.

Possible policy responses to this issue fall into two categories: limiting or modifying the marketing efforts of pharmaceutical firms, or trying to improve the quality of information available to prescribers.[10]

Drug advertising is already regulated as to the claims which can be made and the side effects which must be disclosed, but this merely sets challenges for the ingenuity of marketers in pursuing the basic goal of expanded sales. One could conceivably go further, either with direct limits on advertising budgets, or with limits on the deductibility of advertising expenses for tax purposes. Such global constraints might be more effective than attempts to modify advertising behaviour on a piece-meal basis. Even more effective might be the system of wholesale bulk purchase of generic drugs on tender by a purchasing agency, government or otherwise, as is used by Saskatchewan, the military, and a number of hospitals. By weakening or removing the physician's ability to specify brands of particular drugs, such purchasing on tender lowers the payoff to advertising any brand for which there are several generic substitutes, as such advertising may simply be promoting sales of a competitor's product.[11]

Improving the information available to prescribers might take the form of more extensive pharmacological training in medical school or of a public or publicly supported agency to assemble and disseminate drug information. The former approach has the problem that space in medical curricula is chronically tight and hotly competed for. In any case, the rate of change in pharmaceuticals is such that even better training would rapidly become obsolete. Attempts to provide continuing information may be more successful, although they would be in competition with corporations with finely honed marketing skills and enormous financial resources. Any attempt to increase the flow of drug information through non-commercial channels might require a corresponding limitation on commercial marketing if it were to be effective.

Medical journals are in an ambiguous position, playing as they do the dual role of reporters of scientific research and of the "trade press" in matters which interest physicians as businessmen. Since their budgets depend very heavily on pharmaceutical advertising, their very existence might be threatened by efforts to modify or reduce its scope.

An approach which does appear to have had considerable success in

---

[10] In principle one might also try to augment the information available to patients, but the practical prospects of this appear small. Better patient information might well improve compliance with the prescription once written, but reliance on patient information to improve the prescribing process itself is logically inconsistent. If patients are reasonably informed about a drug's effects, it should be available without prescription (again excepting addictive drugs).

[11] It is of course essential that competitive generic equivalents are available in the market; hence, the significance of Canada's compulsory licensure legislation in ensuring that market alternatives exist.

improving prescribing patterns is the expansion of the role of the pharmacist in advising physicians. The pharmacist in a hospital or community health centre setting can communicate directly with physicians, *before* the prescription is written, and introduce better information about the advantages and disadvantages of particular drugs in particular clinical situations. Attempts are underway in some provinces to extend this relationship to cover drug use by the institutionalized elderly, paying a particular pharmacist on a capitation basis for dispensing all the drugs used by an institutionalized group and encouraging her to consult with the relevant physician(s) over the nature of the on-going therapy.

This approach depends critically, however, on the existence of an institutional framework such that the pharmacist can participate in the prescribing process "upstream" of the actual writing of the prescription, as well as being reimbursed for advice independently of dispensing. The more common situation, in which the patient contacts a community pharmacist *after* the physician has selected the drug, makes effective intervention by the pharmacist difficult or impossible. In principle, the pharmacist might evaluate prescriptions at this point, checking for the appropriateness of the dose, for interactions among different drugs, and for anomalies in the patient's prescription history. Such potential monitoring is the subject of much discussion by pharmacists seeking to justify the existence of pharmacy as a self-regulating profession.

In practice, however, the setting of community pharmacy makes this virtually impossible. Pharmacists are paid by the prescription, so that (since they never see the prescriptions which should have been written but are not) the monitoring role if energetically carried out would lower prescription volume. It would also engender physician hostility, by pointing out errors in front of the patient. And it would, of course, require extra time and energy. It is not, therefore, surprising that the exigencies of small business operation, for profit, preclude a significant professional role, and that such evidence as there is suggests that despite professional exhortation, community pharmacists exercise little or no influence on the prescription process.

DRUG DISTRIBUTION: DISPENSING OR RETAILING?

Retailing of non-prescription drugs displays similar problems. It is argued, and with justification, that just because a drug is not on prescription does not mean that it is safe in any and all uses and amounts. Accordingly pharmacists have lobbied, in some jurisdictions with success, for public regulation to require that certain non-prescription drugs should be sold only under the pharmacist's supervision. This places the pharmacist in a quasi-prescriptive role—she can refuse to sell a drug which she feels to be inappropriate, or can give advice about its proper use. But it also prevents non-pharmacies—supermarkets, *e.g.*—from selling such drugs, and thus is obviously in the economic interest of pharmacists. Since retail mark-ups tend to be much higher in pharmacies than in their competitors, this restriction also raises costs to users. But reports suggest that in fact pharmacists exercise little or no active supervision—which would require time and effort and potentially reduce sales.[12] Thus quite apart from the serious issue of whether such supervision, if it occurred, would benefit users sufficiently to justify its extra cost, it appears that in practice "supervision" responds rather to the economic interests of pharmacies as for-profit firms than to the concerns of pharmacists as health care professionals (Gorecki 1981).

However prescriptions come to be written, drugs must be manufactured, distributed, and dispensed to meet them. The role of the for-profit corporation in manufacture does not appear to have been questioned, subject to the usual considerations of quality control which arise in any industry where quality failure may be undetectable by, but potentially harmful to, the end user. Discussions of the distribution system focus on two major issues, the efficiency of the dispensing process itself, and the competition between different brands (including generic) of the same chemical compound.

The economics of the dispensing process display many of the same problems as do NOFP professional practices generally, in or out of health care. The patterns seem to be characteristic of all firms owned/managed by self-regulating professionals. It has long been a source of amusement or concern that several years of university training are required to qualify one to count pills from a large bottle into a small one. But the manifest inefficiency of this underutilization of skilled manpower, Lieberman's (1978) "inconspicuous production," is no different in principle from a dentist instead of a dental nurse filling teeth, or a paediatrician providing well-baby care (or a lawyer drawing up transfers of residential property). Quantitatively, the waste of resources in pharmacy may even be less important—but it is more obvious.

---

[12] This is not to say that pharmacists may not respond to patients' requests for advice about particular non-prescription drugs, or in some cases supply informed diagnostic as well as "prescriptive" services. And a patient/consumer buying information along with a product may reasonably pay for that information through a higher product price. Thus the availability of non-prescription drugs in both pharmacies and supermarkets, at different prices, may be a perfectly reasonable market equilibrium. But it is quite another matter to use public regulatory power—direct or delegated—to *compel* customers to use the high-priced source. Such compulsion must be justified on the grounds that consumer protection requires active professional intervention to check *each* product choice, and this form of pharmacist supervision is clearly absent.

The dispensing industry also displays restrictions on firm structure and behaviour—no advertising of drug prices or dispensing fees, limits on non-pharmacist ownership, and specific restrictions on size, hours of operation, and other aspects of dispensary management which vary from jurisdiction to jurisdiction. The net effect is to hold up the costs of dispensing, which could with present technology be reduced by perhaps as much as 40 percent by optimal use of auxiliary personnel in a high-volume dispensary (Evans and Williamson 1978). These higher costs are passed forward to patients or public reimbursement agencies in the form of excessive prescription charge mark-ups over ingredient cost. Pharmacists receive not only a professional dispensing fee, but in many provinces a ''standard'' reimbursement for ingredients which significantly exceeds actual acquisition cost.

Despite professional restrictions, however, in British Columbia and Saskatchewan public drug reimbursement programs have had some success in controlling dispensing costs by a blend of public reimbursement and private competition among pharmacies (*The Vancouver Sun* 1983). British Columbia's Pharmacare reimburses actual acquisition cost plus a professional fee for its roughly one-third share of provincial prescription costs, and prohibits pharmacies from differential pricing of prescriptions. Saskatchewan purchases drugs on wholesale on tender and supplies pharmacies, letting them set (within a range) their own mark-ups, which patients must (above a base rate) pay out of pocket. In both provinces, prescription costs are apparently well below the rest of Canada, suggesting substantial scope for savings in other provinces. Even greater savings might follow from removal of regulatory restrictions on pharmacy pricing and auxiliary use.

And in pharmacy, unlike medicine or dentistry, the product volume and mix (prescriptions filled) is externally controlled. The possibility that more competition among for-profit suppliers would lead to more, and less appropriate, output does not arise.

Indeed the steady growth of corporate chain pharmacies suggests that the balance is tipping towards fully for-profit organization in dispensing, with the remaining regulatory structure serving to protect, not the professional role of the pharmacist, but the market of the pharmacy. Restrictions on price advertising and personnel use in particular prevent consumer/patients from receiving the benefits of price competition and efficiency, while an oversupply of pharmacists results in their becoming *de jure* or *de facto* corporate employees. In the end it may be that no one wins, economically, from the combination of the regulation characteristic of a self-regulatory profession, imposed on an industry of for-profit corporate firms. A very different form of regulatory environment may be necessary if we are not to have the worst of both worlds. The issue is of even broader significance, because it appears that (given current United States developments) dentistry, and perhaps eventually even medicine, could move in this direction.

More specific to pharmacy is the long debate over whose drug shall be used to fill the prescription. From the point of view of the large multinational drug firms, the most favourable market position is that in which a given chemical compound has extended patent protection and is marketed to physicians under a specific company brand name. Once the prescription is written for that brand, patient and pharmacist have no choice. No substitute is legally permitted. A potential competitor must then either invest in the discovery of an alternative compound of equivalent or related effect, or seek a licensing agreement with the patent-holder for the right to bring out an alternative brand of the same drug, on payment of royalty. But the competitor must also engage in the very expensive process of marketing the alternative drug to physicians. It is alleged that the large multinationals, who already have a large sales force in being, frequently cross-license drugs among themselves, but for a new entrant costs would be prohibitive. In this environment, prices of drugs can exceed production costs by hundreds or even thousands of percent, marketing expenses take up 20–30 percent of the sales dollar, and industry profit rates (on invested capital) are consistently well above manufacturing industry averages.[13]

This environment has been opened to more competition on a number of levels, whose effectiveness is inter-related (Gorecki 1981). Since 1969 Canadian patent law, as noted above, permits any firm to apply to the Commissioner of Patents for a licence to manufacture or import, and market (under another brand name), any drug patented in Canada, on payment of a royalty (usually 4 percent of sales) fixed by the Commissioner and payable to the patent holder. The number of competitive drugs and firms has significantly increased. At the dispensing level, legislation in several provinces permits the pharmacist in filling a prescription for a particular brand to substitute a generically equivalent alternative brand

---

[13] It is frequently argued by industry spokesmen that reported profit rates overstate ''true'' rates because the asset base of a drug company is understated. Costs of research and of marketing are expensed in the year incurred, whereas in fact they represent investment in intangible assets—knowledge and goodwill—which should be added to assets and depreciated over time. The argument is correct, as far as it goes, though its corollary, that expensing investments represents an extreme form of accelerated depreciation and therefore a subsidy from the taxpayer, is rarely emphasized. If research and marketing expense are ''really'' investment, then they should not be deductible from income for tax purposes, until they depreciate.

The issue then turns on choice of an appropriate depreciation schedule. If intangible assets *never* depreciated, the asset base could become indefinitely large and profit rates indefinitely small. But plausible adjustments still show pharmaceutical profits consistently above those of manufacturing generally (Temin 1979).

(at the same or lower price) unless the physician specifies no substitution. And at the prescribing level, the federal QUAD (Quality Assurance of Drugs) program seeks to assure physicians that generically equivalent drugs of different brands are in fact equivalent in quality, while Ontario's PARCOST manuals make available to the prescriber data on the relative costs of different brands of the same generic compound. In Saskatchewan the provincial government has simply taken over the wholesaling function, purchasing drugs in bulk on tender, and supplying the pharmacist (free) with the particular brand which is to be used to fill all prescriptions for that compound. At the same time a provincial formulary is established to determine which drugs are approved for purchase. British Columbia's Pharmacare program places pressures on pharmacies to bid down whole-sale drug costs.

Taken in total, these policies work to increase the price-sensitivity of the sales of particular brands of drugs. They may or may not have any effect on the demand for drugs in general, but the market share of each supplier of a drug should be more sensitive to the supplier's relative price. And indeed, the prices of prescription drugs (net of dispensing charges) in Canada do seem to have fallen, or at least risen less rapidly, during the 1970s, as a result of these policies (Fulda and Dickens 1979; Gorecki 1981). Gorecki concludes, however, that much of the saving has been appropriated by pharmacists, who have been able to widen the spread between actual ingredient acquisition costs and the "catalogue" prices which (along with professional dispensing fees) make up prescription charges. Stimulation of competition at the manufacturing level thus requires effective price competition in dispensing as well, if consumers are to benefit.

The possible sources of such savings are of particular interest. There is no evidence that increased competition and lowered price has led to a dilution of drug quality or efficacy or to adverse health effects. Given the for-profit orientation of pharmaceutical firms there is no reason to expect much scope for increased efficiency in drug manufacture and distribution. To some extent lowered prices will cut into the supranormal profits of drug firms, which strictly speaking represents, not a gain in efficiency of resource use, but a wealth transfer from firm shareholders to buyers of drugs. (Since most pharmaceutical sales in Canada are by foreign-owned firms, of course, this represents a real gain to Canadians.) But even a large reduction in profit rates would not represent a high proportion of net selling price; a 50 percent cut in profits, if profits are 20 percent of sales, represents only a 10 percent cut in selling price.

If competition drives prescription drug prices down toward marginal production and distribution costs, the principal source of savings will probably be marketing expenses. If drugs are bought generically on tender, there is little payoff to marketing effort directed at physicians; indeed all the procompetitive policies outlined above tend to lower the payoff to promoting particular brands through direct personal selling. This selling expense, representing 20–30 percent of product prices, is the major source of potential price reduction at the ingredient cost level. On the other hand, as noted above, selling expense may also serve to transmit information. If all of North America followed the Saskatchewan model, drug advertising would presumably be cut back sharply along with product prices. It is an interesting question whether the quality of prescriber information would rise or fall, but clearly some other institution(s) for information diffusion would have to be developed, which would require some resource investment.

RESEARCH AND DEVELOPMENT: DOES SHORT-RUN MONOPOLY BUY LONG-RUN PROGRESS AND COMPETITION?

More policy discussion has focussed on the issue of research costs, whose social role is perhaps less ambiguous than marketing activity. It is argued by pharmaceutical manufacturers that Canadian policy is "unfair" and if followed by other countries would lead to sub-optimal rates of investment in new drug research. The research required to discover a new drug, determine its safety and efficacy, and bring it to market is very costly and these costs must all be incurred before any sales revenue begins to flow. The selling price must exceed production and selling cost by enough to recover this investment over the expected life of the drug— *i.e.*, before it is made obsolete by new discoveries. Moreover research is a high-risk activity; the successful drugs must pay not only their own costs, but also those of the failures. The point of a patent system is to confer a monopoly of specified term on an innovating firm to enable it to recoup these costs. If, as in Canada, competitors can promptly copy the innovation on payment of a nominal royalty, innovation will cease to be profitable and will slow down or stop.

The underlying principle of the argument is valid. It raises an interesting philosophic question, however, in that Canada, as a small market, does not significantly affect the world payoff from, or effort devoted to, pharmaceutical research. Accordingly current Canadian policy enables us to "free ride" on research paid for by others. But why not? Free riding is perfectly rational. The pharmaceutical manufacturers' complaint is that it is immoral—an odd position for profit-maximizers to take![14]

---

[14] The question of whether or not the research is carried on *in Canada* is a complete red herring. It will be sited wherever the conductors think most profitable. To reverse present Canadian policy in return for more locally-conducted research would be to fund a rather specialized employment-creation program by an indirect tax on Canadian drug buyers, administered by the pharmaceutical companies, without even any guarantee that "tax" revenues would be limited to program expenditures. See also chapter 12, n. 17, below at p. 285.

The research expenditure share of the drug sales dollar appears to be substantially less than the marketing share, so a focus on research alone does miss the main point. Still, it is true that research costs have to be funded somehow. The issue is highly debatable, partly because economic theory dealing with intertemporal problems is rather weakly developed. There is presumably an optimal rate of innovation, since one can certainly imagine rates which are too large or too small. How much should a society invest, and through what institutional frameworks, to yield that optimal rate? It certainly cannot be shown that the rate generated by a collection of private firms, in highly imperfect competition with each other, meets more general social criteria of optimality, but the alternatives are not obvious either. In other areas of health care, research (or at least new knowledge) is treated as a public good and subsidized directly. But does the for-profit motivation lead to more efficient research? Its proponents say yes—the stimulus of profit and the test of the market encourage a high yield of useful (saleable) knowledge per dollar of research effort. Its detractors say no—the spur of profit in an imperfectly informed market leads to a heavy investment in molecule manipulation, "me-too" products to invent around others' patents, and highly promotable compounds of piggy-backed drugs of dubious efficacy.

Apart from the effect of marketing structures and short-run profitability on the rate of investment in innovation, the United States literature has also emphasized the influences of safety and efficacy testing. The more extensively new drugs must be tested, the more costly they are to develop and hence the less profitable for any given market conditions. Consequently, the greater the testing cost the lower the rate of innovation. Some analysts have claimed to observe a clear negative impact of more stringent United States testing regulations in the early 1960s on the rate of new drug innovation, and have even purported to show that the cost of this slowdown exceeds the estimated gain in terms of harmful side effects averted. The evaluation methodology in this area is rather soft, however, and these conclusions have been strongly attacked. Nevertheless, the trade-off clearly exists in principle. Again one is faced with the difficulty, and costs, of aligning private for-profit motivations with social objectives in an environment of highly imperfect user information.

The strengths and weaknesses of for-profit organization in the pharmaceutical field thus appear to be very much what theoretical considerations would predict. Competitive for-profit motivation leads to efficiency in production and distribution, in the sense of minimizing resource use and seeking out lowest-cost methods. It also encourages a proliferation of products, including genuinely new therapeutic agents, minor chemical variants on other chemical entities, and recombinations or different brands of previously existing drugs. But the severe imperfections of *physician*, much less patient, information about the effectiveness of different drugs leads to very heavy investment in brand promotion and serious questions about the efficacy of drug prescribing and utilization patterns. It may also result in serious market imperfections, failures of competition at least in the short run, which are remediable by public policy. The old question of whether imperfect competition at each point in time may lead to more effective long-run competition through rapid innovation arises in particularly clear form in this industry, but again the imperfections of prescriber or buyer information make it difficult to evaluate the social payoff to innovation in general. The most profitable innovation may or may not be the one with the greatest health payoff (as the case of diazepam suggests). The search for "healthy-people drugs" which everyone can take all the time (Robertson 1976), makes eminent commercial good sense, but has no (or negative) health payoff.

MEDICAL EQUIPMENT AND DEVICES; PROFITS AND PROLIFERATION OF TECHNOLOGY

The same issues arise in all other health sectors where for-profit organizations play a significant role—medical equipment and devices, diagnostic services, and in some jurisdictions, institutional care. Rapid innovation and attention to per-unit cost control must be balanced against concerns of excessive and inefficacious utilization and high marketing expense.

In the case of medical equipment, the proliferation of highly sophisticated monitoring and diagnostic devices is driven by private for-profit corporations which develop, manufacture, and market such equipment. The results have been a dramatic extension, and rapid dissemination, of technological capabilities in health care. Diagnostic imaging, the ability to observe in detail anatomical structures and physiological processes within the body, has made particularly dramatic strides, from radiography, to ultra-sound, to computerized axial tomography, to positron-emission tomography and nuclear magnetic resonance. Internal information is both better, and safer and cheaper to get. CT scanning, for example, which can be done as an outpatient procedure, substitutes for the uncomfortable and dangerous inpatient procedures of pneumoencephalography and (some of) angiography. And the speed of advance is quite clearly stimulated by the profit opportunities involved.

But, as in the case of prescription drugs, the genuine diagnostic or therapeutic breakthrough carries with it the problem of excessive and inappropriate use. The profit motive drives each indifferently. New equipment is tested for safety, not efficacy—that is presumably the responsibility of the physician. But the testing of efficacy is a sophisticated and often costly exercise for which practicing physicians are neither trained nor particularly motivated. And the costs of excessive or inappropriate use, as in the case of drugs, are not just economic, they include threats to health as well.

Electronic foetal monitoring provides a good example. Monitoring proliferated rapidly in the early 1970s as a way of lowering neonatal death rates by detecting foetal distress *in utero* and permitting early intervention by Caesarian section. It is now virtually a standard procedure in North American delivery rooms. Yet a later survey of research literature suggested that its payoff in terms of reduced deaths, as measured in randomized controlled trials, was much less than indicated by simply looking at time trends—the intervention was apparently being credited with improvements generated from other sources. And the high false positive rate of intervention appears to be a major factor in stimulating the epidemic of Caesarian sections in the late 1970s and early 1980s. On balance the intervention may well be doing more harm than good (Banta and Thacker 1979).

The same sort of questions arose earlier about specialized, highly equipped coronary care units, after randomized controlled trials indicated that survivors of a myocardial infarct might in fact be as well off sent home as sent to the high technology CCU or Intensive Care Unit. Indeed some practitioners have expressed concerns that the atmosphere of tension and of patient self-awareness in the CCU may *induce* some of the heart irregularities that the CCU is intended to control.

Such criticisms could be multiplied. Concern has been expressed that in the United States, CT scanning could be used on everyone with a headache. And the problem is *not* merely one of practitioners being unable to determine in advance who will and who will not benefit from intervention. It is possible to develop protocols for diagnostic and therapeutic interventions which will identify what types of patients and problems can expect to benefit, and in some cases it has been done. It is also, and most important, possible to communicate these probabilities to patients who may then make somewhat more informed choices about whether to undergo particular procedures.

But such pre-screening for efficacy makes no commercial sense for a for-profit firm, and accordingly the research studies casting doubt on the efficacy, at least in some applications, of high technology interventions are either contested or ignored. No serious attempt seems to have been made to confirm them and to apply the results. Providers of health care, hospitals and particularly physicians, share the economic interests of the for-profit firms in extending the reach of new technology without overly energetic investigation of its efficacy. In blunt terms, the epidemic of Caesarian sections in Canada has raised the average billings generated by each delivery and has thus helped to buffer the incomes of obstetricians during a period of rising MD/population ratios and stagnant or falling birth rates.[15] This is not to say that economic considerations *motivated* adoption of the technology—but they were consistent with it. Cardiac Care Units provide challenging and rewarding employment for nurses and other hospital personnel, as well as a high profile of technical sophistication in the "war against disease and death." More types of interventions imply more billing opportunities for fee-for-service practitioners and more growth opportunities for hospitals and their employees, in directions which are difficult to constrain through easily measurable but crude bed-population ratios.[16]

The interaction between for-profit firms and other NOFP or NFP providers may go further. Just as a new piece of equipment will be more marketable if it is economically rewarding for providers to buy and use, and will thus have allies against challenges to its efficacy, so a breakthrough which *reduces* billing opportunities for professionals or needs for hospital care is likely to meet much heavier resistance. Accordingly the rational for-profit firm should direct its research resources (which like any other are scarce and costly) toward innovations which increase, not reduce, the earning capacity of other providers—which increase health costs. This motivation may partly explain the peculiar situation that in "normal" economic activity technological advance is seen as, and is, a way to *lower* costs of production, while in health care it is usually identified as a source of cost *increase*. Market failure at the provider level thus feeds back into distorted (from the social perspective) incentives to for-profit firms supplying those providers.

THE SHIFT FROM PROFESSIONAL TO COMMERCIAL DIAGNOSTIC LABORATORIES

The clinical laboratory industry in the United States, which has since the mid-1960s been to a large extent taken over by for-profit firms,

---

[15] In 1961 there were 688 certified obstetrician/gynecologists in Canada, and 475,700 births, or 691 each. By 1981, there were 1391, and 371,346 births, or 267 each. Of course, this ratio takes no account of the role of GPs in obstetrical care, or the gynecological share of ob/gyn workload. But the increasing technological sophistication of the delivery process may have played a significant role in increasing obstetricians' "market share" of ob. work.

[16] Analysts of U.S. attempts to control hospital costs have generally concluded that certificate-of-need programs have controlled growth of new bed capacity, but not overall hospital investment, because hospitals have simply diverted their resources to equipment purchases and associated staff and supplies. Direct public controls over all hospital investment have been more successful, but at the political cost of accusations of failure to keep up with the latest technology. The key questions of whether the latest technologies are worth buying, and if so in what quantities, tend to be lost in the political debate—partly because, although critical, they are difficult to answer.

displays similar problems (Bailey 1979). Diagnostic testing services have traditionally been provided, in Canada and the United States, in hospital laboratories, private laboratories run as professional practices by pathologists, and special-purpose government laboratories. Physicians may also do some of their own diagnostic testing, depending on the test complexity and the rules of third-party reimbursement.

Such testing has generally been a very profitable activity, because the physician-owner of a laboratory is able to delegate a high proportion of the actual procedures and thus to extend her professional "reach" over a much higher volume of billings than if she were required physically to perform the functions involved. And the demand for tests originates almost entirely from physicians who do not themselves pay for them. Accordingly, growth of testing volume has been very rapid for many years, and, at least in the United States, mark-ups over cost are much higher than for, say, hospital ward services. (The mark-up on physician services in general is a bit difficult to identify statistically.)

There has also, however, long been a fringe group of "lay laboratories" in the United States owned and run by non-physicians (who may have other relevant professional qualifications), which has sought to share the testing market. Pathologist-run laboratories have tried to keep them out in the name of "quality." But with judicial decisions establishing that the reporting of a test result did not constitute the practice of medicine, the way was open for non-physician controlled, for-profit corporations to move into this field.

According to the standard economic models of firm behaviour in competitive markets, the results of this shift in ownership should have been generally beneficial to consumers. For-profit motivation should lead to the minimization of testing costs per unit, efficient production procedures, as well as to the development of new forms of tests which are useful to and convenient for practitioners. Physicians as (presumably) informed buyers should be able to choose the most convenient and effective testing procedures for their patients, and competition among firms should drive down testing prices to a level which yields a return on investment comparable to that in similar commercial services industries.

Issues of quality control remain, since a test result does not carry with it any way of validating its reliability. But quality control can be maintained by a public agency periodically submitting blind test samples, just as the products of food processors are periodically tested for foreign matter. One does not license canners of beans; one inspects the cans.

The actual outcome of for-profit organization in the clinical laboratory field, however, appears to be somewhat different. After studying the California experience, Bailey concludes that the change may well have reduced per unit testing costs, at least at the level of the testing firm. But these are partly a result of transferring some costs—specimen collection and handling—back to the physician. Such a transfer may or may not be optimal from the social point of view; it depends on the marginal opportunity cost of physician time, which may be low in a situation of physician oversupply. But it does mean that one must be careful in comparing for-profit and professional lab costs to ensure that the same bundle of services is being priced.

More important, the relationship of for-profit labs to practicing physicians involves a number of different financial arrangements, "compensating" the physician for her role in specimen handling and test interpretation, which serve to give her a substantial economic stake in the performance of tests. To the extent that for-profit labs are price competitive, they compete for the business of physicians, not patients, by offering a wider spread between the rate charged to patients or third parties, and the amount the physician pays the laboratory. Market failure in the physician/patient relationship thus again feeds back into the relation between physician and for-profit supplier, such that whatever benefits of efficiency and competition are generated, they do not appear to be passed through to patients. Bailey's interpretation here parallels Gorecki's conclusions above that Canadian pharmacists have absorbed the savings from competition among drug suppliers.

Of course there are various regulatory and professional ethical constraints on the nature of the physician-laboratory relationship—overt fee-splitting has long been an unethical practice. But as Bailey shows, the for-profit stimulus is strong enough to induce a variety of innovations in organizational form which serve to establish an economic link without violating ethical or legal prohibitions.

Economists are fond of pointing out, however, and quite correctly, that one must distinguish resource allocation and wealth transfer effects. If for-profit firms lower the resource costs of carrying out a given number of tests, then society collectively is better off, even if the benefits flow differentially to one particular group in society, physicians, rather than to patients. It does not follow, of course, that public policy should be indifferent as to issues of wealth distribution and therefore automatically accept or encourage the final result, but it is true that a saving is a saving, to whomsoever accruing.

The serious issues of efficient resource allocation arise, however, when one considers the effects of such arrangements on the overall volume of laboratory testing performed. If one adopts the framework of chapter 1, then the optimal investment of resources in laboratory testing has to be evaluated in terms of their marginal impact on health status.[17] This in

---

[17] An alternative, market evaluation of optimal testing in terms of patient willingness-to-pay could be formulated in theory, but the process of writing down its requirements in terms of locus of decision-making and availability of information is sufficient commentary on its plausibility.

turn is a combination of the payoff from a test, in terms of new diagnostic information in a given situation, and of the payoff to that information in terms of its effects on choice of effective therapy. A test may be inappropriate either because it could not reasonably be expected to yield additional information, or because the information it could yield would not affect treatment in such a way as to improve outcomes.

From this perspective a number of commentators, including pathologists, have expressed considerable concern about the extent to which laboratory testing activity currently outruns its usefulness, not only *ex post* (in the sense that in many cases nothing of value is learned) but also *ex ante* (in the sense that the test orderer knew, or with a little consideration could have known, in any case *should* have known, that it could not be of value). Various ways have been considered, and some tested, for trying to discourage test-ordering by clinicians (Schroeder *et al.* 1973; Martin *et al.* 1980; Hardwick *et al.* 1982).

In this context, the strong stimulus to ''more'' which is a consequence of for-profit motivation justifies serious concern. Unnecessary testing is pure waste of resources. But for-profit organization does not, cannot, recognize unnecessary testing as an intellectual concept. Sales are their own justification. Individual people in organizations may recognize and share concerns about appropriate use, but insofar as these concerns influence firm behaviour they represent a departure from profit-maximization and will, at least in a theoretical perfectly competitive market, be punished. Firms which fail to maximize profit disappear, or their managements are taken over. Bailey suggests that the professional orientation of the pathologist-run labs, in or out of hospitals, did serve as some limitation on the performance of unnecessary testing; this would be plausible since NOFP organization is intended to deal with the conflict between economic and patient or professional interests. FP organization is not.

FOR-PROFIT HOSPITALS AND RELATED INSTITUTIONS: THE UNITED STATES EXPERIENCE

The growth of FP organizations, the so-called ''investor-owneds,'' in the United States hospital and institutional services industry provides yet another example of the two-edged impact of FP organization. Optimistically, one might predict that FP hospitals would actively seek out ways of caring for patients which were less expensive than those employed in the NFP sector. The sorts of evidence alluded to in chapter 9 would suggest that there is significant scope for such economies. And indeed one does find examples in the United States of investor-owned freestanding surgical centres, offering care which would in many hospitals be provided on an inpatient basis, while some advocates of proprietary hospitals suggest that they achieve lower costs per inpatient day or episode of care.

In reply, it is often alleged that United States proprietaries "cream off" the less costly, less ill, and more fully insured patients. But the possibility of "cream-skimming," of selecting patients with higher ratios of (collected) charges to costs depends on anomalies, on cross-subsidization, in the charge or reimbursement structure of the NOFP sector. If hospital reimbursement represents a lower share of costs of "sicker" patients, this suggests that they are being subsidized by the less sick, or at least less service-using, and an FP hospital could bid away those more profitable patients. But in the absence of cross-subsidy, from one class to another, there is no incentive to skim.

More recently, however, comparisons of NOFP and FP hospitals have uncovered further interesting aspects of charge and cost behaviour (Lewin *et al.* 1981; Pattison and Katz 1983). Matched samples of each showed very little difference in patient population, at least as measured by age and insurance status. Also very similar were charges per patient-day for "hotel"—room and board—services. There were, however, marked differences in ancillary costs—specific diagnostic and therapeutic interventions—such that costs overall in the FP hospitals were significantly *higher*. These differences were a result both of higher mark-ups of charges over costs in FP hospitals, and of a higher rate of provision of ancillary services.

The higher mark-up is quite consistent with the standard theory of the firm selling in markets with different elasticities of demand. The patient or her physician can collect information on, and perhaps respond to, differences in "hotel" costs prior to entering hospital, and the service may be thought of as fairly standard. But once admitted, the patient has no recourse to alternative suppliers of drugs, tests, or therapy, and will accordingly be sensitive to price differences only insofar as those forms of utilization could be forecast before admission. (Assuming, of course, that such services are uninsured.)

The quantity differences, however, reflect the special features of health care. The FP supplier will be more likely to exploit the professional influence over utilization to stimulate greater sales at the same, or even higher, prices. And since bed use and length of stay are easily observed and compared, and have in the United States been subject to planning controls, ancillary services are the least noticeable and most profitable to stimulate.

Few other differences emerged; in particular administrative costs were *not* lower at the hospital level in FP hospitals. This suggests that the overhead costs of central office staff for FP chains do not offset local administration costs, and may be a form of marketing expense. There was some indication (Lewin *et al.* 1981) that the personnel mix in FP hospitals might include relatively fewer registered nurses, which could represent greater efficiency or lower quality depending on its effect on patient outcomes. Or it could indicate less ill patients—the study did not address these issues. Certainly there is no one-to-one relationship between quality of care and either numbers or qualifications of personnel, and efforts to represent the one by the other are generally recognized as circular reasoning, if not special pleading for the interests of particular personnel groups. Nevertheless, quality control is a serious concern in all health institutions, and these concerns become particularly severe in the FP environment. The extensive regulatory and evaluative systems which monitor hospital quality, as well as the high costs of adverse publicity, probably discourage quality dilution in acute-care hospitals, but very serious scandals have emerged in the American FP nursing home industry where patients are, in general, unable to protect themselves. And early experiences with FP health maintenance organizations, capitation-reim-bursed medical service plans, showed that the obvious profitability of signing up prospective patients and then providing inadequate, or no, services, had not escaped the notice of entrepreneurs with short time horizons.

CAN ONE MIX MOTIVATIONS, OR MUST FOR-PROFIT FIRMS BE ALL IN OR ALL OUT?

Experience with FP firms in a number of sectors of the health care industry thus all tends to reinforce the same conclusions. As theory and conventional wisdom predict, FP firms are very energetic and innovative in development of new products and services and, to a lesser extent, new ways of producing existing products. They bring a dynamism to the process of health care delivery which is often lacking in NFP or NOFP firms.

But FP firms do not, cannot by their very nature, respond both to profit objectives and to social concerns for the efficient provision of *effective* health care services. They do not serve two masters. Nor do they in any other sector of the economy. As Adam Smith pointed out, the butcher and the baker are led to serve us by our appeals not to their charity, but to their self-love. We speak to them not of our necessities, but of their advantages. It is the invisible hand of the competitive market which turns this selfishness to the general advantage.

But in health care the hand is not only invisible, but usually absent. Its functioning depends on rational informed consumers, making choices among numerous competitive suppliers and enjoying or suffering the consequences, direct and financial, of those choices. The problems of overutilization or inappropriate utilization arise because consumers are insufficiently informed to make their own choices. The process of choice is delegated to professionals, while the financial consequences are shifted to governments or private insurers, and through them to the wider community. But the professional agent's information is often incomplete as well, and her financial incentives are usually perverse—she benefits from overuse. In such an environment, to expect a for-profit seller to disseminate unbiased information is to misunderstand the whole dynamic of the private marketplace.

In thinking about the current role of FP organizations in health care, therefore, and their possible extension or restriction, the central question should be, In which sectors do the customers of FP organizations possess the combination of information and incentives such that they can collectively form a market which will constrain FP firms? Informed buyers, bearing the consequences of their decisions, do not buy useless or dangerous products, and if they (knowingly) choose what professionals regard as "low quality"—so what? Further, structural reorganization of some sectors could lead to a shift in product definition which would enable buyers to be better informed. This is the basic idea of the United States advocates of competitive HMOs, to redefine the product sold from specific services to a combination of insurance plus all "needed" services, bought for a fixed annual fee, such that consumers can make informed choices among these new composite commodities (Enthoven 1980).

An intriguing possibility in Canada for such product and buyer redefinition is raised by very recent initiatives in the for-profit contractual management of hospitals. In this context it is the management team, not the hospital itself, which is attempting to earn profits, by selling not hospital services, but managerial services. And the buyer, in the Canadian context, is the provincial reimbursement agency. This represents a crucial difference from earlier and more developed United States experience with for-profit contract management.

In the United States the client for managerial services is the hospital board, and its objectives are increased revenues, growth of operations, or in some cases sheer survival. "Successful" management has meant primarily elimination of deficits, and increases in occupancy and throughput. These have been achieved by better control of bad debts,[18] improved "marketing" of the hospital in the community, and expansion of high mark-up ancillary services. But of course all such activities, while they improve the financial position of the individual hospital, *add* to the costs of hospital care as experienced by the community as a whole. No provincial reimbursing agency in its right mind would pay a private team for aggravating its problems.

---

[18] This also implies more careful screening of patients on admission for insurance coverage or personal resources.

Thus the intriguing question is, Can one write contracts with such private managements which will reward improvements in efficiency rather than expansion in hospital revenues/costs? The answer *may* be yes, as there is some United States evidence that contract management has also had some constraining influence on hospital costs of production. But it is not their major influence. And such contracts will have to be written on a comprehensive capitation basis, so that managements are not rewarded for shifting high-cost patients to other hospitals, perhaps in other regions, or for spilling costs out into the medical care sector or elsewhere in public or private budgets. Moreover it is obvious that some form of external quality monitoring must be maintained.

If such contracts can be written, to reward for-profit managements for cost-containment rather than cost-shifting or quality-dilution (or as in the United States, cost-expansion!) then they may serve as a countervailing force with the appropriate incentives to confront providers of care within hospitals. As emphasized above, cost control *definitionally* requires income control of physicians or of hospital workers—lower hospital costs means fewer employed nurses, however it is done. At present, no individual or institution anywhere in the Canadian health care system (except of course government) has any personal incentive to limit costs. Private for-profit management *could*, if properly contracted, be a way of introducing such incentives. But the highly speculative nature of this approach must be emphasized, as the successes of such management in the United States have been with the very different problem of working *with* the hospital to *expand* costs.[19]

Other sectors of health care show even greater scope for potential redefinitions of product and buyer. Prepaid FP group practice in dentistry, for example, reimbursed by annual capitation payments and bidding competitively for the business of employee groups, shows promise of great improvements in efficiency and reductions in cost if it were not blocked by self-regulating professionals (Evans and Williamson 1978). Dispensing of drugs and sales of eyeglasses or other appliances can, in an appropriately structured market, be left to unregulated FP firms. Of course normal commercial regulations to ensure truth in advertising, periodic

---

[19] It is the institutional framework, not the personal characteristics or abilities of managers themselves, which is of interest in this discussion. There is no reason to believe that the *individual* managers working in present or potential FP environments are more skilled or energetic than present administrators of NFP institutions; indeed the combination of experience plus demonstrated survival capability in a very complex environment might point the other way. The key question is whether management teams, however composed, might exercise more cost control if provided with a different pattern of incentives and authority. If experiments should show some success, present NFP administration teams might well seek FP contracts.

product inspection, and anti-combines oversight to ensure maintenance of competition would be necessary as in any marketplace, but a special self-regulatory structure appears much more questionable. And FP organization may be essential to keep the competitive process going (Evans 1980).

But the largest share of health expenditure, acute care hospital and physicians' services and, increasingly, long-term care of the elderly, is provided to people for whom the postulate of rational informed choice is inappropriate, and it is likely to remain so under any conceivable organizational restructuring. Shifting the incentives to providers, as competitive HMOs do, has some promise, but even there the possibilities of adverse selection and quality dilution make it questionable if FP operation of such organizations is workable. And the ''first-mover'' advantages of a firm which has established the first phase of a continuing relationship makes effective competition very difficult to maintain. In this setting, the pressures which bear on FP firms will always drive them toward oversupply and, if professional agents mediate purchases, little if any price competition.

Accordingly, FP firms in this ''central core'' of health care are likely always to be heavily regulated. Unfortunately, such regulation will generate its own inefficiencies and is unlikely ever to be fully effective. Moreover, there is a tendency, resulting from the powerful growth dynamic of FP firms, for them to penetrate and absorb NFP or NOFP sectors. Titmuss (1970) has documented this process in systems for collecting and distributing blood and blood products. On fairly general criteria, voluntary blood donor systems are both more effective and less costly, but FP systems are more profitable and tend to drive out voluntary systems unless restrained by public policy. FP private insurance firms, by experience rating and seeking out good risks, were similarly cutting into the market of NFP insurers in Canada prior to the public programs. FP chain pharmacies control a growing share of the dispensing business. And in the United States FP hospitals have shown a dramatic resurgence in the past decade. Health policy toward for-profit firms must then balance the trade-off between the specific virtues and specific vices of FP firms, structuring the regulatory environment accordingly and recognizing their inherent tendency to try to circumvent, or to burst, regulatory bounds. The appropriate balance may be struck quite differently in different sectors; indeed, an argument can be made that present policy is *too* balanced. In some sectors, FP organizations should, by reduced or changed regulation, be allowed to become dominant and left to compete among themselves. In others, they may not belong at all.

PART 3

THE GOVERNANCE OF HEALTH CARE

CHAPTER 11

EVALUATING HEALTH CARE PROGRAMS: EFFICIENCY, EFFECTIVENESS, AND COST

PUBLIC POLICY AND PRIVATE INTERESTS

The discussion thus far has emphasized that one cannot describe, analyse, or hope to understand and predict the behaviour of either users or producers of health care in isolation from the other. But we have also seen the public sector, the state, intervening in a number of ways to influence the behaviour of both. Either directly or through delegated authority, the state regulates access to health care markets by buyers and sellers. It prohibits, regulates, or mandates the sale/use of particular commodities or services, determines who shall and shall not be permitted to offer or provide them, and regulates or empowers self-regulation of the conduct of providers. It provides information to assist decision-making by private transactors through public information campaigns, certification of provider qualifications, product labelling, and providing technical information to providers.[1] It taxes or subsidizes particular forms of consumption or investment in particular types of capacity—grants for construction, training, or research. Some forms of services it provides

---

[1] At present the informational role of the state, like that of providers, is difficult to separate from that of marketing. Warnings on cigarette packages are intended to modify behaviour, not to inform, just as cancer or heart disease awareness campaigns or school dental education programs are intended to encourage increased use of practitioner services. No one has ever launched a campaign saying *"Don't* see your doctor or dentist under the following circumstances."

But in principle, at least, the genuinely informational role of the state could be significantly expanded in support of either providers or individual consumers. Certification of members of occupational groups, for example, can serve in place of licensure by providing consumer/patients with authoritative information about provider qualifications while permitting them to choose whether or not to deal with the uncertified. Licensure prohibits such dealing. "Technological assessment," such as the federal reports on cervical screening and periodic health exam, can improve information available to practitioners on the effectiveness of interventions. More broadly, if future health policy involves the development of alternative systems of care competitive with fee-for-service or hospital inpatient care—Health Services Organizations, Surgicentres, Self Care, Home Care, or Care-by-Parent programs—the role of the state in disseminating, or at least facilitating, the flow of information may have to be greatly expanded.

directly, superseding the market—public health programs everywhere, Canadian hospital and medical insurance, the Saskatchewan Dental Service, the United States Veteran's Administration hospitals, the British National Health Service. No other sphere of economic activity, with the possible exception of defense, is so extensively subject to public intervention, in so many different ways.

In the previous sections, however, we have encountered these interventions as they impinged on the behaviour of users or providers—our focus was on the analysis of these actors. Now we change our perspective, walking around to view the elephant from a different angle, as it were. But we pursue the same approach, regarding government as a behaving entity within society, pursuing various objectives by means of particular strategies and under certain constraints.

In the process, we shall take a rather traditional view of the objectives of government, treating it as an instrument for the furthering of collective, public purposes. Implicitly we assume the existence of some sort of general public interest, with all the problems of identification and definition which that implies. We thus regard the proper role of government as the designing of public policy to serve the public interest.

An alternative viewpoint, which has enjoyed a recent vogue among economists, views government as a transactor in the marketplace cheek by jowl with the others, differing only in that it sells coercively enforced rules of the economic game in return for votes or the wherewithal to buy votes. From this perspective, the public interest is an empty concept; there exist only various private interests which are furthered through private or public institutions. And indeed many of the actions of governments *are* better explained as responses to the interests of powerful private groups, not to broader public interests. Critics of the public interest approach thus refer to the alternative as a "positive" as opposed to normative, analysis of government, returning to Machiavelli's claim to describe what is done rather than what ought to be done (Stigler 1971; Posner 1974).

The study of professional regulation conveniently demonstrates the contrast of approaches. From the public interest point of view, regulation is intended to protect interests which for various reasons would be unduly vulnerable amid the free play of market forces (Trebilcock *et al.* 1979). It responds, or should respond, to specific breakdowns in the conditions under which markets lead to desirable outcomes in terms of resource allocation and/or output distribution. The "positive" theory, however, notes that in fact professional regulation is almost always sought by the profession itself, not by the supposed public beneficiaries. Following Shaw, "all professions are conspiracies against the public," it views regulation as a form of market power, economically advantageous to the regulated, ''purchased'' by them from government in return for various forms of political support.

The process of public economic regulation, as it actually goes on in and out of health care, provides a number of examples which strongly support the ''positivist'' view. Agricultural marketing boards, for example, admit no other plausible explanation. But even the most enthusiastic positivists concede that its predictive power is unsatisfactory—the conspiracy approach explains why all want self-regulation, but not why only some get it. Nor can it explain regulation which the regulated find onerous and energetically lobby against—drug safety testing, for example. And the theoretical models of government as a quasi-economic transactor—buying votes and selling rules or enforcement—suppress significant parts of the institutional reality of political behaviour. If there is a political ''marketplace,'' it is obviously oligopolistic, and economists' efforts to formulate plausible theories of oligopoly behaviour have been notoriously unsatisfactory. Information plays a very different role in this ''market''— to be seen to be purchasing or selling regulation may be very costly to the seller, at least. Overt political bribery can cost votes, and in some forms is illegal. Politics is not just economics carried on in a slightly different language. There *is* a difference between a government and a Mafia enforcement agency, which is what the legitimation of sovereignty is all about.

Moreover, the logical limit of the postivist approach is, in fact, quietism. If all supposedly public policy is simply a collection of private transactions, then there are neither criteria for analysis and criticism nor means for modification. What is, is. The tendency for positivist analyses of government to be associated, in practice, with advocacy of *less* government and more reliance on private market forces is wholly illogical. If one is unwilling to critique extant distributions of wealth or influence or power, then presumably whatever set of markets arises to support economic or political transactions is the best available: Positivism meets Pangloss. As for changing or reducing the role of the state, that will occur, on the positivist theory itself, *only* if it serves the interests of the dominant private interest groups. And the advocates of such policy, in the positivist view, are simply the ''hired guns,'' or public relations arm, of those groups. The development of United States political and academic culture in the 1970s and early 1980s, and the role of positivist economic analysis of public policy in this process, serve to illustrate the argument (Evans 1982*b*).

The public interest approach, however, grounds the analysis of public policy firmly in the normative. Policy *ought* to be devoted to general public ends. In many cases it is not; these are cause for criticism and, perhaps, correction. Perfection is not anticipated, in this life at least, but by assumption a process of analysis, education, and exhortation can lead to improvement. Nor is the policy-maker, the philosopher-king, the only target of this process. "Bad" policies such as professional regulations which benefit only the profession and harm the general public, or similarly, agricultural marketing policies, probably *are* the result of balances of political interests, not ill-informed or stupid policy-makers (Hartle and Trebilcock 1983). In a democratic state, the informational component of public policy analysis extends to the whole society. The analyst of policy from a public interest perspective may better serve, not as advisor to the Prince, but as preacher or teacher to the multitude. But what are the alternatives?

PROGRAM EVALUATION: A GENERAL REPRESENTATION

Accordingly, our perspective on government assigns it the role of choosing among policies and programs on the basis of their consistency with the public interest—cost-benefit analysis writ large.[2] Each possible act has both positive and negative consequences across the society as a whole. The task of policy formulation involves the identification and measurement of all of these benefits and costs, and their aggregation in such a way as to determine whether the policy is on balance good or bad. Designing mixes or "portfolios" of policies, whose effects interrelate with each other, adds an additional level of complexity. In this chapter, however, we will look at the government's problem in terms of a single project or small scale program—an immunization campaign or the funding of a new diagnostic facility—before extending the general approach to such larger issues as public insurance systems, or strategies for research funding or health promotion. In some cases individual projects may form the building blocks for more general programs, in others, universal public insurance, for example, they do not.

The analytic representation of the public sector program evaluation problem is very simple. One has only to test whether:

---

[2]   What follows is not intended to be a comprehensive survey of the now vast field of cost-benefit and cost-effectiveness analysis. Nor is it a "how-to" guide. For more comprehensive treatments of the principles involved see Drummond (1980) and Warner and Luce (1982). Drummond (1981) also provides a catalogue and brief description of evaluation studies in health care.

The treatment in this chapter owes a great deal to discussions with Greg Stoddart, David Sackett, and other members of the Department of Clinical Epidemiology and Biostatistics, and to work by George Torrance, all at McMaster University. None of them should be in any way implicated in remaining inadequacies or distortions.

$$\sum_{i,k,t} \left[\frac{P_{ikt} B_{ikt}}{(1+R)^t} \right] - \sum_{j,k,t} \left[\frac{V_{jkt} C_{jkt}}{(1+R)^t} \right] \gtrless 0 \qquad (11\text{-}1)$$

If the expression above associated with a particular project or program is positive, then it should be carried out; if not, not.

As is typical of economic decision rules, however, the formal correctness of an expression is not much help, except perhaps as an organizing framework for future work. The really interesting issues, and the difficulties, arise when we try to give content to the various symbols above, to define and measure them, and to deal with the complications when this proves impossible.

To begin, however, we must define the symbols themselves. B and C are the measurable impacts or results of a particular program. The benefits B might be measured in terms of lives saved, days of ill-health averted, or disabilities reduced by a health program, or they might be extra tons of grain produced by an irrigation project. Costs, C, on the other hand are the things used up by this project—human time, energy, and skills, physical resources, capital equipment services—which are therefore unavailable for other purposes.[3] The pattern of benefits and costs, B and C, generated by a project is also a description of the project itself in technical terms, whether the technology be engineering, agricultural, or clinical. If resources of C are applied in the manner described by the project, desired outcomes B will result.

But neither resources used nor benefits generated are uniform, homogeneous entities. Thus they are indexed, in three different dimensions. The subscripts i and j run across the different forms of benefit and cost. A project with several different types of benefit would have them measured, in some appropriate unit, as $B_1, B_2, B_3 \ldots, B_i$, and the corresponding different types of costs or resources used up are $C_1, C_2, C_3 \ldots, C_j$.

The benefits and costs also, however, impinge on different people or groups, and the evaluation process may have to be sensitive to these distributional questions. Hence both B and C are indexed over the people in the relevant community; B_{ik} represents the kth person's receipt of an amount B of the ith type of benefit.

Finally, projects have a time dimension. Most commonly, though not necessarily, costs tend to be higher at the beginning of a project, and benefits come later. In any case, it matters at what time period costs and benefits are incurred or received, and thus C_{jkt} represents C units of a cost of type j, incurred in period t, by person or group or agency k.

---

[3] The similarity of this discussion to the general description of economic analysis in chapter 1 should be apparent.

The definition of the *B* and *C* patterns associated with a project embodies a critical step, which is all too often passed over unconsciously. The state of the world in the absence of the project has simultaneously been defined as a situation in which particular consequences *do not* occur. In general, it is desirable to specify this alternative explicitly, since otherwise the project being evaluated may be compared with an irrelevant or implausible baseline. And one must specify *all* the project consequences, intended or unintended. Particularly common in health care are claims that particular projects, seatbelt use for example, or home care of potential hospital patients, or new diagnostic interventions, will pay for themselves by dramatically lowering costs in some other area of care. Implicitly this means that suppliers of these competitive forms of care will be put out of work and will leave the industry. If that is not, in fact, anticipated, then full specification of the *B* and *C* for the project must include some description of what is likely to happen to redeployed substitute resources, and the costs or benefits of their new activities. If, as is frequently the case, new projects merely add on to existing activities for which they are nominally substitutes (cimetidine *plus* antacid therapy, CT scanning *plus* other imaging techniques, long-stay or day surgery beds *plus* a maintained level of inpatient activity), then there will be no cost offsets. And the benefits of the new activity must be measured relative to what was previously occurring, not a zero base line.[4]

In aggregating these benefits and costs across the whole society, one must employ various weighting factors to add up the apples and oranges involved. These weights are in the form of prices, converting units of measurement to units of account, and are represented by the P_{ikt} and V_{jkt}. In a society using dollars as currency, it is natural to think of P_{ikt} as the

---

[4] Cost offsets can lead to a technical problem, though they need not. If a new project leads to cost-savings elsewhere in a system—real ones, not just redeployment of resources—then it obviously makes no difference whether such savings enter the first term of equation 11-1 as a positive benefit, or the second as a negative cost. But in some applications a benefit/cost *ratio* is defined, the first term divided by the second, and this ratio *is* sensitive to how cost offsets are classified. A program with (present value of) benefits B, direct costs C, and cost offsets K has a present value (PV) of $B - C + K$ but a benefit-cost ratio of either

$$\frac{B + K}{C} \text{ or } \frac{B}{C - K}.$$

Shifting K between numerator and denominator cannot move the ratio from above to below unity, or conversely, so the absolute (un) desirability of a project is unchanged, but if the *relative* values of projects, their priority ratings, are based on the ratio, then the analyst can fiddle the rankings. If the budget for all projects is constrained such that not all positive PV projects are possible, the better procedure is to choose a project "portfolio" of maximum PV subject to the budget constraint, not to rely on benefit/cost ratios to set priorities.

dollar value per unit assigned to benefits of type i, accruing to individual k, in time period t, but any accounting unit will do as well. In some cases benefits and costs will have well-defined prices determined in private markets, which may be appropriate for use in equation 11-1. In other cases, particularly in health care applications, there may exist no market for the benefit (*e.g.*, human life), or the market price (volunteer services, professional services if monopolized, subsidized commodities) may not represent the true resource cost or opportunity cost of the commodities involved. The analysis may then require calculation of shadow prices, synthetic values of P_{ikt} and V_{jkt} which attempt to represent their true rates of exchange with other goods or services.

The indexing of P and V across k enables the evaluator also to build in different values for benefits or costs affecting different people. Thus, if some particular groups—low-income people, the elderly, children— are considered particularly deserving, augmenting the P_i and V_j for those subsets of the society has the effect of favouring programs which benefit them. On the other hand, if benefits and costs are to be counted equally "to whomsoever accruing," then P_{ikt} and V_{jkt} will be constant for all k.

DISCOUNTING, INFLATION, AND CONSISTENCY

The time discount rate, R, plays a special role in the aggregation process and interacts with the time-pattern of the P and V in a way which can lead to serious errors of analysis. As noted, the consequences of many projects arrive over time. But one cannot aggregate present and future consequences, even if they are measured in the same units, because as capital markets remind us, time is productive. A dollar now is worth more than a dollar in the future, and the amount of this advantage is reflected in the interest rate, R.[5] If, for example, the going rate of interest on loans for a length of time spanning the main effects of the project in question were currently 10 percent, then $1,000 worht of benefits accruing five years from now could be "bought" with a present investment of:

$$\frac{\$1,000}{(1.10)^5} \approx \$620.92.$$

That sum, invested now at 10 percent (compounded annually) would be worth $1,000 in five years; hence the present value (*PV*) of $1,000 five

---

[5] Strictly speaking, R is itself time dependent, and future effects should be discounted using the time-pattern of R between now and their arrival—preferably in continuous time. But in fact no one forecasts interest rates well enough to justify specifying a function $R(t)$, and benefits and costs tend to be reported by budget year. With increasingly sophisticated cash management the time profile of R will become more important, though not, alas, any easier to predict!

years hence (whether benefit or cost) is $620.92. Present values *are* additive, so we can evaluate a project yielding $1,000 worth of benefit in five years and requiring a current outlay of $600 and say that (at 10 percent interest) it is worth doing. If the current outlay required were $700, it would not be. Furthermore, if interest rates on five-year loans were 20 percent, the *PV* of $1,000 five years hence would be

$$\frac{\$1,000}{(1,20)^5} \approx \$401.88$$

so the project would no longer be worthwhile at $600 outlay.

Failure to discount future benefits, or cost offsets, can be particularly deceptive in the evaluation of programs with long-term effects, such as prevention of handicap. Rubella immunization, for example, or screening for Down Syndrome (*plus* abortion of affected foetuses) may reduce future support costs over many years. But to add up undiscounted cost offsets as if a dollar twenty or thirty years hence were equivalent to a dollar now, when in fact such a future dollar could be purchased now (in capital markets) for a much lower sum, would grossly overstate the cost offset component of program effects.

It is obviously an abstraction to refer to "the" market rate of interest, there being a wide array of such rates; and there has been extensive debate over the appropriate choice for public investment projects. Moreover, while financial flows, or flows of benefits or costs which (like tons of grain or man-hours) have well-established money prices, must be discounted at some rate, the case for discounting non-traded or non-tradable things such as human lives or illness states is less clear. One cannot trade present for future lives, either directly or through some intervening financial market, as one can trade, for example, wheat. The person whose life is lost now is *not* compensated by the saving of one, or even 1.5, lives some years hence. We will return to this point below.

What *is* clear, however, is that whatever discount rate is chosen, it must embody some treatment of inflation, and thus must interact with the time-pattern of P_t and V_t. Market interest rates are nominal rates; they include an estimate of the rate of inflation over the relevant time period. The faster money falls over time in purchasing power, the higher must be the nominal rate of interest to compensate for this. If $R = 20$ percent, but prices are rising at 12 percent per year, the true or real interest rate is only 7.14 percent.[6] Real resources given up now can be traded for only 7.14 percent more resources next year, even if for 20 percent more money.

---

[6] The inflation-adjusted or real rate of interest is calculated from the *ratio* of the nominal to the expected inflation rate, thus

$$\left[\frac{1.20}{1.12} - 1\right] = 7.14 \text{ percent.}$$

The subtraction approximation of $20 - 12 = 8$ percent becomes more inaccurate as inflation rates rise.

Thus the value chosen for R, and the values assumed for P_t and V_t, must be consistent. If one chooses a 12 percent discount rate, which would have been reasonable in mid-1984 based on then current market interest rates, one must keep in mind that this embodies an expected inflation rate of about 6 percent. Accordingly, the values of P_{it+1} and V_{jt+1} should be about 6 percent above P_{it} and V_{jt}, for all t. If inflation is implicitly in the denominator of equation 11-1, as it is when one uses a market interest rate, then it *must* be built explicitly into the numerator. Of course one may believe, for various reasons, that particular P_i or V_j will rise faster or slower than the general price level. But to fail to escalate them at all, and then to use a market discount rate, amounts to assuming that the prices of B and C will remain steady in nominal dollars while everything else rises in price at the expected inflation rate built into the market interest rate. In inflationary times, this creates a serious (and erroneous) bias against projects with long payoff periods and high initial costs.

One can, of course, ignore inflation in the numerator of equation 11-1 and then discount by a real rate in the denominator, *i.e.*, a market rate reduced by expected inflation. One might, for example, compare current (annualized) inflation rates with long-term government bond rates to estimate (on the assumption that current inflation rates are expected to persist) the current real rate of return. Such a procedure emphasizes the inherently uncertain nature of returns on all non-indexed investments. One cannot define real returns without assuming (guessing at) future inflation rates.

Such rates on, for example, long-term bonds, have historically tended to fall in the 2–4 percent range, well below the 8–12 percent used in official cost-benefit guidelines. Short-term fluctuations may move well outside this range—real rates were negative for part of the early 1970s and in the early 1980s reached 8–10 percent—but these were temporary aberrations. Few professional investors have consistently earned 4 percent real over long periods of time, let alone 10 percent. Anyone recommending 10 percent as a discount rate for public projects, without inflating the numerator, should be invited to try running a portfolio![7]

COSTS AND BENEFITS TO WHOM? WHERE YOU STAND DEPENDS ON WHERE YOU SIT

This way of setting up the program or project evaluation problem is sufficiently general as to be merely a particular representation of the rules

---

[7] There is, as always, more to the story than this. Private-sector returns on capital (after-tax, risk-adjusted) run well above 4 percent. But governments do not borrow at such rates.

of rational behaviour. It is a framework for identifying all the consequences, good and bad, of an activity, reducing them to a common metric (dollars) by weighting factors (prices) which reflect their differences in time of occurrence as well as intrinsic characteristics, and then adding them up to see whether or not the good outweigh the bad. The evaluation of public projects is in this respect no different from that of private projects. The individual firm or consumer in economic theory is represented as going through a precisely similar calculation.

The private firm, for example, evaluates a production decision or a long-term investment project in terms of the stream of saleable outputs, goods and services, which will flow from it, the B_i, and the costs in terms of productive resources which will be used up in the process, the C_j. It then estimates the prices at which the B_i can be sold, P_i, and the prices V_j which it will have to pay for the C_j, and adjusts for the time-pattern of receipts and expenditures. Equation 11-1 represents the firm's net revenue stream, or its profits from the activity. Assuming profit-maximizing behaviour, the firm chooses to carry out only those projects for which 11-1 is positive.[8]

Similarly the rational consumer, in allocating her budget over consumption alternatives, present and future, or more generally in choosing patterns of resource supply (allocation of productive time and skills, as well as other owned productive assets) and commodity consumption, is modelled as carrying out a utility-maximizing process in which the B_i are commodities consumed, the C_j are resources supplied to the market, and the P and V are composed of market prices and personal marginal utilities or disutilities.

The principal difference from the evaluation of public projects, however, is that in the private calculations $k = 1$. The private firm or consumer calculates costs and benefits to him/her/it alone, disregarding "external effects" or consequences of the project, positive or negative, which fall on others. If it is indeed the case that B_{ik} and C_{jk} are very small or zero for all k other than the decision-maker, then clearly private and social decision processes would give the same result. But if there are many k for which B and C are significant, then obviously calculations made over only a subset, or one, of the relevant k can be erroneous in either direction. In such cases, as discussed in chapter 3 above, private markets lead to faulty resource allocation decisions and public programs develop to respond to this market failure. Thus public projects frequently involve calculations of effects over a large number of people or institutions.

Accordingly in any cost-benefit analysis it is critical that one be clear

---

[8] Complications arise as projects can be carried out at different scales, different projects interact with each other, and the P and V may be functions of the B and C, often negative and positive respectively.

about the perspective chosen—*whose* benefits and costs? Health care programs, for example, will affect patients, providers of care, public budgets, and taxpayers. Particular individuals may play several of these different roles. And a program or project may, frequently will, serve to redistribute costs and benefits among members of society as well as to generate them. A successful project to shorten hospital stay, for example, might serve to lower hospital costs and thus benefit governments who pay such costs—and through them, taxpayers. But if it generated significant costs in the home for patients, it might in fact raise costs overall. Similarly, a government which negotiated a reduced fee schedule for physicians in return for permitting extra-billing of patients would have lowered costs in the public sector and presumably benefited taxpayers. Patients, of course, lose; providers gain (insofar as fees plus extra-billing exceed the fees they would otherwise have received) at least on average, and at the society-wide level the whole transaction may wash out as a pure income redistribution, depending on whether or not actual patterns of care utilization are affected. Full evaluation of any project thus requires the identification of all costs and benefits, wherever they impinge or accrue.

But it is often useful to identify also the partial sums across k, the subgroups of winners and losers. It is frequently the case that one man's cost is another man's benefit, and much conflict over program evaluation has its roots, not in disagreement over society-wide effects, but over partial distributions of gains and losses. A program which involves increased demand for the labour and skills of particular types of workers will be viewed favourably by the owners of those skills, even though from a society-wide perspective the using up of those scarce resources of time and skills is a cost. Cost to society is income to the resource owner.[9]

We have seen this phenomenon above in several contexts. The overhead cost of a universal public health insurance system is known to be much less than that of multiple-source private insurance, but higher costs are the revenues of private insurers. A public dental service for children using dental nurses is, from a society-wide perspective, much less costly than public or private insurance for private dentists' services. But the costs of the latter program are dentists' incomes.

---

[9] If input markets were perfectly competitive, then resource owners could all sell their resources of labour, skills, or capital to any one of a large number of potential buyers at "the" going market price. They would be undetectably affected by the presence or absence of any one program. This discussion therefore rests on an assumption of imperfect competition in the relevant input markets, monopoly power as well as quasi-rents to investment in industry-specific skill acquisition. A perfect competition assumption is wholly out of place, and a policy analyst who relied upon it would get some nasty surprises!

Hence programs which seem obviously efficient from a society-wide perspective are frequently blocked because they impose losses on a powerful subgroup whose interests cannot or will not be compensated, while other programs whose costs viewed globally seem clearly beyond their benefits are adopted because of their partial payoffs. The cost-benefit analyst may treat all winners and losers equally; the political system does not.[10]

PRICELESS DOES NOT MEAN VALUELESS: SHADOW-PRICING LIFE AND LIMB

In addition to their impact on a range of different people, whose interests pro or con are often difficult or impossible to represent in a market framework, public programs frequently involve benefits, and sometimes costs, which are very difficult if not impossible to represent in a common metric of dollars, or anything else.

The framework of equation 11-1 assumes that a P_i or V_j can be identified for each B_i or C_j, such that costs and benefits can be summed and compared. This process is straightforward if B_i and C_j are traded in well-functioning markets where their relative prices are established. This will be true, for example, of the costs of new construction associated with a public project, which can be contracted out to the private sector or organized in-house, but in either case at well-defined dollar costs. Similarly the benefits of a land irrigation project may be identified in terms of increases in yield of particular crops, which will in turn be sold at clearly identified prices.

Somewhat more complex are the cases in which prices or costs of inputs and outputs are available, but are systematically distorted from true resource costs or market values. A public program might receive administrative or building services from some other branch of government, at no budgetary cost. Yet building space and administration use up real resources, so the evaluation process would have to use a "shadow

---

[10] It is possible, as noted above, to vary the P and V in equation 11-1 explicitly across k so as to weight differentially the interests of particular people and groups. Projects would be favoured which paid off to those groups. While logical, this approach has not been widely used. Its weakness may be that while formally and overtly we would all wish, and wish our political system, to assign high weights to the disadvantaged, poor, elderly, in practice program choices frequently follow the interests of the wealthy, highly organized, and politically powerful. The most potent combinations are programs which appear to, and perhaps do, benefit the disadvantaged, while also providing payoffs to politically powerful interest groups. There are also, however, social costs which result from making redistributional processes, in whichever direction, too overt in operation.

price'' reflecting the true cost of such inputs. An irrigation project might increase output of a commodity for which there was a price-support program; a government agency might be accumulating surplus stocks to hold market prices up. In this case, the apparent market price overstates the value to society of more (surplus) output. A hospital might receive donated equipment or space, or use volunteer labour, which was ''free'' in its budget, but such inputs are clearly costly, resource-using, from a society-wide perspective, and should be shadow-priced.[11] In general the particulars of how a program is financed, from whose resources, should not affect the society-wide evaluation of its costs and benefits, though clearly the interpersonal pattern of gains and losses will be affected.

The problem of shadow-pricing, however, shades into that of evaluating costs and benefits which have no obvious financial metric at all, conceptually or in practice—the ''life-and-limb'' problem. Shadow-pricing assumes that a conceptually appropriate price for each of the consequences of a program exists, though it happens not to be reflected in existing market prices or budgetary entries and must therefore be calculated directly. For consequences involving life and death, pain and suffering, physical, psychological, and social functioning, it is not obvious that any shadow price exists.

Yet it is clear that programs with mortal and morbid consequences must be evaluated. The human life may be priceless, but it is not infinitely valuable—we implicitly assign it a finite value in any number of settings. Individually we drive cars (or worse, ride bicycles), ski, climb mountains, smoke, thus trading life expectancy for other satisfactions. Collectively we establish policies on factory, highway, or product safety, knowing that risk-reduction is costly and can only be pursued up to a point. On the other hand, lives are not valueless either, nor is the avoidance of pain, suffering, or grief. To leave them out of an evaluation process because their values are ill-defined is bad economics as well as bad policy.

The life-and-limb issue has been addressed in two distinct ways. The

---

[11] Volunteer labour presents a special conceptual problem, which illustrates the concept of opportunity cost. The argument for shadow-pricing such labour in any particular program is that, if not used in this program, it could have been used elsewhere. Just like wage labour, volunteer labour has a cost in terms of other productive opportunities foregone and its V_j value should reflect this. If volunteer labour substitutes for a category of wage labour, the market wage for that category would be an appropriate shadow price. On the other hand, it is conceivable that the volunteer is willing to serve only in one capacity. A parent on a care-by-parent ward is there to look after his/her child, and no one else's. The volunteer is, of course, foregoing other earning or leisure opportunities, but presumably the satisfaction of looking after one's own child outweighs these costs (or the child would be placed in a regular ward). Thus one should not shadow-price the one-activity volunteer—the opportunity cost is zero—but should shadow-price *e.g.*, the members of a religious nursing order.

first is to try by a variety of techniques to calculate shadow prices for life and limb. Since all actual program decisions which involve life and limb implicitly place values on them, it is argued that better, or at least more rational, decisions could be made if the values used were explicit and consistent. It is not difficult to show, for example, that at present public program decisions are quite inconsistent. In some fields (airline safety) resources are used to save lives or prevent deaths at a much higher cost per life saved (at the margin) than in others (highway safety). If all saved lives (or averted deaths) are equally valuable regardless of the nature of the threat, then we could be better off, so goes the argument, if we redeployed our lifesaving resources.

The alternative approach is to abandon efforts to evaluate life and limb explicitly, as productive of more confusion and misinformation than enlightenment. Cost-benefit analysis, as represented in equation 11-1, in which all components are weighted in dollar terms, is replaced by cost-effectiveness analysis in which some at least of the consequences of a project are measured only in terms of their natural units. The transition from cost-benefit to cost-effectiveness analysis in the United States was most clearly demonstrated outside the health care field when program evaluation techniques were extended from water-resource projects to weapons systems. Payoffs to irrigation activities—increased crop yields, flood control, recreational benefits—can be calculated using market or shadow prices. But the dollar value of megatonnage delivered to downtown Moscow is difficult to measure in any meaningful sense.[12] Cost-effectiveness analysis takes the objective as given—extending lives or terminating them, and measures the relative costliness per unit of desired consequence from alternative projects for achieving the same or comparable consequences. Such alternative projects might be different approaches to the same problem—submarine versus land-based missiles, school immunization campaigns versus subsidies to private physicians— or they might be different scales of operation of the same program.

VALUING LIVELIHOODS: ESKIMO ECONOMICS

Attempts to identify explicit shadow prices, money values, for life, disability, pain, and suffering began from the human capital view of the person as a set of productive capacities whose value was represented by earning power. A life cut short before its normal time is a loss of economic product, equal to what that person would otherwise have earned (on the

---

[12] Whether its value is positive or negative is also rather sensitive to whether or not the evaluator is a Muscovite.

assumption that markets ensure that a person's earnings equal the economic value of her production) over the remaining expected life, discounted back to its present value at point of death.[13] Lives saved by a project are then valued at the present value of their possessor's subsequent expected earnings. Disability costs can be measured the same way, by the present value of economic output lost if the disabled person must take a lower-paying job, or none at all.

This "value of livelihood" approach has the advantage of yielding concrete results, apparently firmly grounded in economic reality.[14] But it is now largely discredited among students of program evaluation because of its fundamental inadequacies in both theory and application.[15]

The decision rule implicit in the value of livelihood measure can be summarized as "Eskimo economics," embodying the priorities (alleged to be) characteristic of pre-contact Inuit culture. When the game fails, and starvation threatens the community, the elderly population must be sacrificed. If conditions remain bad, the children go next, followed by women, and then men in reverse order of hunting prowess. The best adult male hunter is the last to go, as he has the best chance of finding food for whatever is left of the band—in the end, him.

These are precisely the priorities of the human capital approach to project evaluation. The elderly, living on pensions and other assets, have no earned income and are worthless. (They may be credited with some non-market production of rather ill-defined value in a more sophisticated analysis.) Children are worth something, but their future product is discounted back to the present and thus, for very young children particularly, becomes very small.[16] Earnings of women, in most cultures, are below those of men, so the value of saving a woman's life is correspondingly lower. Unemployed time is worthless, so value of life must be adjusted for expectation of employment. In the United States, blacks earn less on average than whites, so black lives are worth less. Specific examples of

---

[13] It is only the person's earned income, from labour and skills, which is counted. Income from other assets such as bonds or buildings is unaffected by the death; it is simply transferred to someone else.

[14] It also requires a number of intricate and sophisticated calculations, largely impenetrable to the user of evaluations, which is an advantage for analysts.

[15] Yet particular program evaluations relying on this measure continue to turn up. Erroneous analytic techniques, like inefficacious surgical procedures, take time to work through a group of practitioners!

[16] Thus we find calculations of the "costs" of thalidomide which assign a negative value to phocomelia equal to the present value of the stream of (lost) market earnings of the disabled newborn—which of course does not start for about twenty years! If in addition one overstates the discount rate as described above, the costs of disabling conditions in the disabled newborn become almost trivial. It is best to put such calculations in an appendix.

these powerful value judgements, masquerading as objective quantitative analysis, can be found in the cost-benefit literature.

But these priorities do not in general govern resource allocation in our society. The elderly and/or disabled receive a far higher share of health care (per capita) than do the general population, largely because they are sicker. The classic dictum of the lifeboats is: "Women and children first." If we, as a whole society, lived on the margin of subsistence, we might follow the same rules as the Eskimo did. We do not.[17]

The difficulty with the human capital approach is that, when capital assets have zero or negative present value, they are not repaired but scrapped. Indeed some versions of the livelihood approach take it to its logical conclusion, and measure value of life by the individual's net production, earnings less consumption, adjusted for taxes and use of public services, and for gifts and bequests. Does society, *excluding* the individual in question, profit (in dollar terms) from that individual's existence? Obviously, this figure is negative for almost all retired persons, indicating that a low-cost euthanasia program, not just for the terminally ill, but for all the retired, would be the highest valued public health program one could mount.

At this point one can insert an embarrassed footnote that of course other considerations apply, which they certainly do, but the absurdity of the conclusion is *not* simply an unfortunate result in a particular application. It arises from the fundamental assumptions of the technique, which are themselves absurd. For in fact, human capital is *not* indifferent to being scrapped; lives are of value to the living person, as they are to his or her relatives, friends, associates, and in general (in decreasing amount) to a wide ring of those who are aware of the life. In the same way disability, pain, and suffering, or rather their absence, are valuable and valued independent of their economic consequences. Loss of the left hand may have devastating consequences for the earning power of a pianist or surgeon; little or none for that of a (right-handed) academic or hospital administrator. Yet it does not follow that the latter would be indifferent to such loss, or what is the same thing, would place no value on saving the hand. And the individual sufferer in question is one of the k in equation 11-1. Her preferences matter, even if no one else cares (which in general they will, only less).

In theoretical terms, equating value of life with livelihood is erroneous because, as we recall from chapter 1, the economic value of anything is defined in terms of what some individual or group is willing to give up

---

[17] Where resource constraints are absolute, *e.g.*, in the case of a life-saving technique in fixed supply and excess demand, allocation rules may be used which are based on age, family situation, etc. But these are related only indirectly to the present value of the expected earnings stream, and as discussed below have other and better bases.

in return for it. In a competitive market, under various stringent conditions on demand and supply, this value will tend to be equated with cost of production, *i.e.*, what must be given up to produce the commodity. But there is no competitive or any other production of lives, independent of the people concerned. My life is unique, no other lives compensate me for the loss of it.

In a slave society, the market price of a slave would tend to equal the present value of net earnings, production less consumption, and in long-run equilibrium this would in turn equal the cost of producing slaves of a given age and skill, in accordance with the value of livelihood model. But the slaves would not be counted among the k of equation 11-1, and their asset values would tell us nothing about the proper value of *masters'* lives.

YOUR MONEY OR YOUR LIFE? WILLINGNESS-TO-PAY AS A SOURCE OF SHADOW PRICES

Efforts to value life and limb explicitly have therefore shifted to attempts to measure willingness-to-pay for life-saving consistent with the basic concept of value in economic analysis. Such approaches encounter two problems immediately: (1) whose willingness-to-pay? and (2) for what?

The first is usually answered in terms of individual choice, the potential sufferer. There have been some suggestions that value of life, or pain and suffering, might be inferred from decisions by legislatures concerning public projects with mortal or morbid consequences (positive or negative) or damage awards by courts, but it is generally recognized that this is a circular procedure. Such agencies look to analysts for guidance as to the values *they* ought to use. The inconsistency of their decisions is a principal justification for efforts to find an explicit monetary value by quantitative analysis.

But if the individual potential sufferer is to be the source of information, it is clear that the problem must be posed in statistical terms. Faced with the certainty of life or death, the individual's willingness-to-pay is bounded only by her wealth, plus whatever she can beg, borrow, or steal. The proponents of this approach have focussed on individual valuations of *probabilities* of death. One can explore how much an individual would pay to avoid a 1 percent chance of death over the next year, for example, and then sum over a hundred such people to determine what value the group would place on saving one (expected) life.

The willingness-to-pay approach opens up a number of interesting research possibilities for determining individuals' values. Life insurance purchases were suggested, and quickly rejected as reflecting the individual's estimate of her financial obligations, not value of life. Wages paid in hazardous occupations, explicitly as hazard pay or implicitly as above-average wages, can be compared with the degree of hazard to calculate the implied value of life. But this assumes full information and perfectly competitive labour markets, which students of labour economics find implausible; further if people differ in their valuations one would expect to find those with lowest life values (or least information!) in hazardous occupations. Thus generalization is suspect. Other measurements have been based on seat-belt use, balancing estimated values of time against risk. Still others try questionnaires.

Apart from the intricate problems of measurement, however, it is clear that this approach raises some deeper problems. First, individual valuations are not linear. If I will pay $1,000 to avoid a 1 percent chance of death in the next year, but not $1,001, it does not follow that 10 percent is worth only $10,000, still less that I would prefer certain death to paying $100,100! Thus whatever results emerge for a particular risk level cannot be generalized to other levels.

This fact has been given a rather peculiar twist in discussions of prevention versus cure. It is sometimes alleged that individuals will forego relatively cheap preventive activities, yet spend very large amounts to save or prolong lives *in extremis*, thus valuing lives or years of life very differently in the two settings. This apparent inconsistency, however, can be "explained" in terms of standard consumer theory. When one has many (expected) life years ahead the marginal value of life years in terms of "other things" is less than when one has very few. Hence it is "rational" to spend little on prevention and much on cure.

This argument has a number of problems, including the facts that information about the efficacy of prevention is notoriously poor even among specialists in the field, that expenditure on terminal care in every country is covered by public or private insurance, and that death is a discrete event. Groups have life expectancies, individuals have lives, and when the current life year is given up, the rest go with it.

But on its own terms, the argument illustrates a problem of micro-rationality leading to macro-irrationality. Suppose a group of people, a society, make their allocations between (efficacious) prevention and cure on the basis of individual marginal rates of substitution. By spending less on prevention, and more on cure, they may as a group have both shorter life expectancies *and* higher expenditure on life-prolonging care. (Any parallel with United States health care is accidental, though the micro-rationality argument does come from the United States.)

If an investment decision presents itself strictly in terms of statistical lives, the individual willingness-to-pay approach may be useful. But health care problems rarely present themselves in that form. There is usually a stage in the illness process in which sufferers are known, flesh and blood individuals, and the project decision will take the form of whether or not to care for *this* person in *these* specific circumstances. At the theoretical level it can be shown that *ex ante* optimal decisions are not necessarily optimal *ex post*, and conversely (Evans 1983); in practice, it is obvious that people who have made a particular decision as to the value of statistical lives will wish to recontract when the time comes.

Nor will those around them be keen to enforce the contract. Apart from the inherent unpleasantness (in most cases) of letting someone else die, still more of expediting the process, there is the difficulty that lives are of value to other than the individual concerned. And the individual willingness-to-pay criterion, like market processes generally, provides no way of taking those preferences into account. Each of us is, to a greater or lesser extent, a public good (though Donne said it rather better).

As a further complication, individual valuations of lives will of course be very sensitive to individual income or wealth levels. If public program evaluations are based on individual preferences, they will favour life-saving for the wealthy. One could, of course, average values across society, but this undercuts the theoretical basis for the individual approach.

Finally, recent psychological research on decision-making under uncertainty has cast serious doubt on the empirical validity of the expected utility model. Decisions in uncertain situations seem to be quite sensitive to the setting or framework in which the decision is taken; changes in this setting which are formally irrelevant to the payoffs available can lead to reversal of choices (Schoemaker 1982).

COST-EFFECTIVENESS ANALYSIS: LET THE OUTCOME STAND FOR ITSELF

For all these reasons, and perhaps others as well, most people evaluating health care programs have abandoned the attempt to establish explicit monetary values for life and limb, pain and suffering. It remains true that any program decision, go or not go, implicitly places a value or at least a one-side bound on the values of such consequences. But cost-effectiveness evaluations do not attempt to build such values into the analysis, rather they confront the decision-maker with a menu of costs and consequences, relying on the political process to yield the "right" choice.

The cost-effectiveness approach to evaluation is most straightforward to apply when a choice is to be made between two alternatives whose consequences are equivalent. Given that, for unspecified or unevaluated reasons, a certain level of megatonnage is to be delivered, which system gets it there at least cost? Two forms of health care, inpatient and day-care surgery, for example, may be therapeutically equivalent for a particular set of conditions which, it has been determined, are to be treated.

This form of evaluation is really only a cost analysis and comparison, measuring the second term of equation 11-1; the decision to do something has already been taken.

In this comparison, different programs may be essentially similar in process, or radically different in concept and activity. Dietary versus surgical approaches to heart disease, for example, or prevention of rubella syndrome by either mass inoculation or "rubella parties" to ensure that female children have the disease before child-bearing age, or prenatal (or even pre-conception) dietary supplementation versus neonatal intensive care, each represent totally different activities. But the intended results of each are the same, and they can therefore be compared in cost and reliability of achieving that result.

Measurement of project effects is necessary in the more general case, however, in which either no action is a possible option, or projects have different scales of operation. ("Do nothing" is simply operation at zero scale.) In these cases, project consequences in physical terms must be compared directly against costs: X lives saved for Y dollars, $X + A$ lives saved for $Y + B$ dollars. The outcomes are in commensurate physical terms, but the judgement as to whether X lives are "worth" Y dollars, or if they are, whether A more lives would be worth an additional B dollars to scale up the project, is ultimately, in this context, a political choice. In general one expects that, following Figure 1-3, projects of particular types will show diminishing returns. The dollar cost per life saved will rise as the program expands; $Y/X < B/A$. But if there is always some possible project with a potential positive effect on health status, then as in Figure 1-3b, the person or body with decision-making responsibility will have to set a cut-off value for lives.[18]

---

[18] A classic example of the scale problem, and the importance of marginal analysis, is given by Neuhauser and Lewicki (1976). A very inexpensive test for occult blood in the stool will detect a pre-cancerous condition, but it has a false negative rate of about 5 percent. To reduce the chance of missing a "curable" case, one can perform the test several times. The clinically recommended technique of performing the test six times reduces the probability of failure to find a true positive case to $(.05)^6$, and still represents a relatively low cost of testing per person tested. But the probability of finding a case on the sixth test, which was not already found during the first five, is $.95 (.05)^5$, so the cost per *new* case found, on the sixth test, would be $1 \div [.95 (.05)^6]$ or 3,040,000 times the cost per test. The marginal cost per case found, on the sixth test, could easily run into the tens of millions of dollars. Maybe six times is too many.

The stool guaiac test studied by Neuhauser and Lewicki has since provided a second lesson. Their analysis rests on the assumption that a true positive finding, at whatever cost, leads to an effective intervention—"cure." But as of early 1984, research currently underway suggests that intervention is *not* effective, and contrary to previous belief has no effect on life expectancy (David Sackett, personal communication). If so, then the test has no value, the optimal number is zero, and cost data are irrelevant.

Still more difficult is the case of multiple types of non-monetary consequences—projects which influence the full spectrum of lives lost, temporary or permanent disability, and pain, fear, and suffering. Consistent with the basic concept of cost-effectiveness analysis, the analyst can then only present the alternative menus of differential miseries associated with different activities and let the politician or administrator choose. But obviously the possibility of informational overload grows with the complexity or ramifications of projects.

A number of attempts have therefore been made to find ways of combining the diversity of dimensions of project outcome into a single index, an explicit "health status" measure, which could serve as an ordinal or even cardinal measure of the total payoff to a particular program. More ambitiously, such an index could even measure the progress of a population and its health status through time, or permit inter-regional comparisons. But while, as discussed in chapter 1, such a concept seems to be implicit in all health policy, its explicit representation is fraught with conceptual and measurement difficulties (Culyer 1978; Berg 1973).

A LIFE AFFIRMED, A DEATH CONFRONTED: LIFE YEARS AS OUTCOMES

A promising solution to this problem, within the context of cost-effectiveness analysis, begins from the observation that while we speak loosely of life-saving projects (probabilistically or with certainty) the brute fact of existence is that we can do no such thing. The most solidly established regularity in epidemiology is that one out of one dies (known also as the Law of Competing Risks). Death can be postponed, but life cannot (at least by non-spiritual means) be saved.[19]

If death is postponed, however, then *years* of life are saved, and this represents a natural physical unit in which to measure outcomes. It is consistent with our general sense that saving the life of a child is in some way more significant than terminal care for the elderly. This sense is sometimes expressed in equity terms—the child has not had a chance to live—but also reflects the obvious quantitative comparison of life expectancies.

The significance of different sources of mortality is dramatically rearranged by a refocussing from lives to life years; cancer becomes much

---

In this case, better data on therapeutic efficacy have dissolved what appeared to be a "grim trade-off" between lives and dollars, providing an illustration of the general point made previously. Too much fascination with the philosophical and political issues in such trade-offs distracts attention from the possibilities for unambiguous improvements in efficiency.

[19] Sadly, as the military examples show, deaths or megadeaths *are* well-defined consequences.

less significant because it usually strikes late in life, while accidents which carry off the young represent a much higher cost in lost life years. Even if cancer were to vanish completely, life expectancies in North America would rise by only 2–3 years (and presumably mortality from heart disease would leap upwards).

Measuring the physical consequences of health programs in life years may lead in some cases to results which parallel those of the livelihood approach, since the present value of one's expected earning stream, like one's life expectancy, falls with age. Both will tend to give less weight to programs benefiting the elderly. But there are several very important differences.

First, and most obviously, the value of life saved does not fall to zero at retirement. The livelihood approach values the life of a sixty-four-year-old man who happens to earn $50,000 a year at $50,000; next year when he retires, he is worthless.[20] But the life-year approach merely subtracts slightly less than one from the stock of expected remaining life years represented by that person, when he ages by one year.

At the other end of the scale, a child's life saved now represents a large number of added life years. The present value of livelihood for a child, however, is substantially reduced by the discounting process—earnings will not accrue until the child grows up and enters employment. Thus the life-year approach increases the weights at the high and low ends of the age spectrum—precisely where health spending (per capita) is in fact greatest.

Finally, the life-year approach does not weight by earning capacity. One person's life year is as good as another's. The fact that women or members of some ethnic groups have in North America lower average earnings than white males (which may reflect either lower economic product or discrimination—or both) is not built into the process of project evaluation so as to assign lower values to projects benefiting them. As a practical example, the estimated relative payoffs to screening for breast cancer, hypertension, and tuberculosis will differ significantly according to whether one values outcomes by life years or by livelihood.

But the focus on life years raises an awkward point concerning cost offsets which can more easily be neglected in the "life-saving" context—the living use more health care than the dead. The person whose life is saved today lives to grow old, or at least older, with increased probability of using health care later on. The anti-smoking campaign which saves lives and costs of treatment for lung cancer is generating future costs of heart disease, as well as treatment for senility. A quick and fatal heart

---

[20] The present value of income net of consumption for a sixty-four-year old is already large and negative; his consumption during retirement is counted as a net loss to the rest of society.

attack at sixty-two is, in the long view, cheap, not only in saving future pension costs, but also in "saving" future health care interventions which the sufferer might otherwise have needed over the next twenty years.

This is *not* an argument for euthanasia. Life is, we strongly believe, better than death,[21] and is worth paying for. But consistency in project evaluation requires that we record and cost *all* consequences. And if a program saves life years now, those years have cost implications in the future which must also be recorded.

How they should be treated in decision-making is, however, another issue. Stason and Weinstein (1977), for example, take a "hard-nosed" view that all subsequent health care use by those kept alive through a particular program should be included in the costs of that program. And certainly anyone responsible for health care planning or delivery should take account of the additions to later utilization which will result from a successful "lifesaving" program. But the proper treatment of health costs in subsequent years, when evaluating that program, is ambiguous.

It is clear that, at one extreme, a successful program addressing a particular condition which requires interventions for that condition in each subsequent year of life should have the costs of those interventions included in program costs. On the other hand, a "one-shot" successful program which extends its beneficiaries' lives will still require that they eat over the years of subsequent life. Such eating uses up resources which might otherwise be "saved," yet we do not include it as a cost of the lifesaving program. (Unless we are taking a purely instrumental view of the person; Stason and Weinstein do not.) At what point do particular forms of resource use during the added years of life cross over the line and become program costs? If all health care costs are included, then the evaluation of a particular program becomes sensitive to patterns of cost and effectiveness over the rest of the health care system; it is no longer being evaluated solely on its own merits. Accordingly, most analyses have tended to exclude from costs subsequent health care use during additional life years gained from a particular program, which is not directly related to that program.

QALYs: NOT ALL LIVES ARE WORTH LIVING

Life years are, moreover, themselves seriously incomplete as a measure of consequences, as they fail to take account of the impact of health care programs on morbid but non-mortal conditions. Further, lifesaving may have very different morbid *sequelae*; a life year as a quadriplegic or on a renal dialysis machine is not quite the same as a year of complete health,

---

[21] Despite absence of evidence.

defined either in some absolute sense or as normal for one's age and situation.

The concept of the quality-adjusted life year (QALY) has been developed in response to this inadequacy. Weighting factors (between zero and one) are attached to years of life in particular states. If a program keeps one alive but bedridden and/or in permanent pain, those years of life are "marked down" to represent a smaller number of QALYs before being compared with the outcome of some other program which restores its beneficiaries to full health. Programs dealing with non-mortal problems can also have their outcomes measured in QALYs; improved states of physical function or shortened periods of pain or disability represent increased QALY values for the same expected life years. QALYs thus represent the value or utility of the health status outcome of a program to its beneficiaries; evaluation using such measures is known as cost-utility analysis.

To illustrate, suppose two hypothetical programs are each expected to save ten lives a year. But one benefits children (average age five), the other elderly people (average age seventy-five) and life expectancy is otherwise eighty-five. Furthermore, the program for the elderly leaves them alive but permanently bedridden, and this state is judged only 60 percent as desirable as full health. Comparing lives saved, the two programs are equal, but in life years the first saves 800 and the second only 100. In QALYs, the comparison is 800 to 60.

The politically responsible decision-maker must still determine how much a QALY is worth, and is under no constraint, logical or otherwise, to apply common dollar values to QALYs in different settings. The calculation does, however, assemble information on the physical consequences of programs in a way which seems more consistent with overall social preferences and behaviour than do the livelihood or individual preference approaches.

The measurement of outcomes in physical terms does, however, raise questions about the appropriateness of discounting over time. These arise in two ways. The outcomes of projects or programs arrive over time, so that a particular payoff which represents a life or life-year saving may occur at some time in the future. In addition, an outcome occurring now will have, if its effects are measured in life years, consequences accruing over the expected lives of the present beneficiaries. Is keeping one person alive for the next ten years "worth" as much as keeping ten people alive over the next year, or should the future QALYs be discounted?

If there is a consensus among analysts, it appears to be in favour of discounting, on two lines of argument. First, it is obvious that economic resources, costs, must be discounted because markets exist which generate well-defined prices for future resources in terms of present, and conversely. If one can also trade resources for life years in both the present and the future, through varying the scale and scope of "life-saving" programs, it follows that an indirect market exists in which present and future life years can also be traded, at the same relative price. So one should discount future life years. Second, individuals clearly display time preference—in concrete (and informed) situations they indicate a willingness to trade expected life years in the future for years now at more than one to one. Cancer victims, if allowed to choose between surgery and radiation therapy, place more weight on short-run surgical risk and less on five-year survival rates than they would if indifferent to time (McNeil *et al.* 1978).

Against discounting, one might note that while particular investments in health care, now or in the future, may in fact represent the trading of lives for dollars, or conversely, that is a far cry from a well-developed futures market in life years. And the life years accrue to different people; a discounting of future life years relative to the present represents a weighting of different people's life outcomes. If the world were fully known, continuous and twice differentiable, all such discrimination could be compensated. In practice it will not be. Moreover it is difficult to separate time preference from diminishing marginal rates of substitution in the interpretation of individual behaviour, again because, for better or worse, one cannot choose to live either five life years next year or one each over the next five years. Life years may be a measure of outcome, but they are *not* commodities, and differ from such in crucial respects. (If you miss this year's life year, you've missed them all—*pace* Hotblack Desiato.) If there is time preference in individual cases, it is not clear that it should necessarily be reflected in social decision-making (though in the cancer case, since the alternative techniques affect the same individuals, the case for reliance on individual preferences is much more compelling). And in any case, the absence of the necessary direct markets in physical outcomes implies that (real) rates of interest set in financial markets have no particular privileged position as discount factors, if such are to be used.

There is a more fundamental problem, however, with the QALY approach to program evaluation. Where do the weights come from? While it seems beyond dispute that health is better than illness, and some forms of illness or disability are more serious than others, the use of these insights in project evaluation requires their quantification. How does one determine the relative valuations which people attach to life years spent in different circumstances?

One can construct hypothetical scenarios, explain them to subjects, and ask them which situations they would prefer. There are, of course, a number of difficulties with such techniques, including identifying "representative" subjects—patients with the condition to be studied, providers of associated care, M/WITS?—and ensuring that the respondent has sufficient information to respond. Alternative techniques include the time trade-off, in which subjects are asked to indicate how many years of life with a particular condition (from the present) they would regard as equivalent to a standard number of years of normal health (followed in each case by painless death). Standard gamble techniques confront subjects with a choice between a particular condition (for a specified period) and a gamble between present (painless) death and normal healthy future life. The odds in the life/death gamble are adjusted until the subject is indifferent between the choices; the higher the acceptable risk, the worse the condition.[22]

Such techniques are still in the experimental stage. So far they have shown some promise, but are far from representing a finely calibrated tool of measurement. Certain interesting regularities seem to emerge, however. Sufferers in a state of illness seem to regard it as less bad than non-sufferers, suggesting either that anticipation is worse than reality, or that people adapt. To which preferences should cost-effectiveness analysis respond? Moreover, some states appear *worse* than death (severe graft versus host disease following bone marrow transplant, for example). Clearly one should mark down the effectiveness of a program, one of whose possible outcomes is that "beneficiaries" would rather be dead, and an arbitrary cut-off of weights at zero would over-estimate its benefits.[23]

PRIOR CONSIDERATIONS: IF THE PROJECT DOESN'T WORK, EFFICIENCY IS NO HELP

Cost-effectiveness and cost-utility analyses share with cost-benefit analyses the characteristic that they take as given the sets of B_{ikt} and C_{jkt} associated with a project under study. The economic dimension of project evaluation, like economic analysis generally, assumes that the technical, engineering, or clinical work has all been done, and that full information on the technical transformation of inputs into outputs is available before the economist arrives on the scene. If any concession to incomplete information is made, it is in the form of an assumption of probabilistic

---

[22] The evaluation of states of ill-health will generally vary from person to person, though if the approach is to be convincing they should be roughly consistent. Weights used in a project evaluation will have to be some average of those of the people questioned. The same aggregation problem, of course, arises with efforts to monetize the value of life and limb; measurement is taken over a population which may not accurately represent the population at risk.

[23] It is not inconsistent with these findings that people in such circumstances continue to live. The act of terminating life, one's own or others', is "costly" in utility terms, so that one might perfectly consistently wish to be dead yet refrain from suicide.

outcomes, in which the range of possible outcomes and their associated probabilities is well known, and various sophisticated techniques for decision-making under uncertainty can be applied.

But as the evaluator of real-life projects rapidly learns, this idealized situation is very far from the norm. The specification of a project, in terms of what is to be done and what are the expected outcomes in physical terms, frequently proceeds in parallel with the economic evaluation, though it is logically prior. This process can be represented by the triad of concepts, efficacy, effectiveness, and efficiency, which, while most readily applied to drug trials or other well-specified clinical interventions, can be used without too much stretching in the more general world of project evaluation.

Efficacy refers to the impact of an intervention under ideal or laboratory conditions. It is related to the economist's *ceteris paribus* assumption. If all confounding influences are held out of play, and if the drug is administered correctly or the project managed competently, will the desired result be achieved? In our terms, is it possible that a particular set of resources C_{jkt}, manipulated according to present best practice, could yield amounts B_{ikt} of a specified set of benefits? If not, then no further analysis, economic or otherwise, is needed. Projects which do not work are not worth doing at any (positive) price. (Recall the stool guaiac example).

But the point is far from trivial, for two reasons. First, though logically there is no point in the economic evaluation of a project for which efficacy has not been established, in practice the available information is usually rather fuzzy. The range of positive (and negative) effects of a program, and their quantitative significance, will all be open to a greater or lesser degree of doubt, and the economic analyst will frequently have to evaluate (or seek help in evaluating) the quality of the technical data as well. Evaluation may have to be conducted for several possible outcome scenarios, not just for "the" B_{ikt} "known" to be the project result.

Second, attempts to explore the bases for efficacy estimates frequently reveal alternative or additional objectives for a project or proposal. Not infrequently, a project is advocated by a particular group, either because they expect to benefit from it, or because they have views as to the interests of the wider society which they feel those responsible for funding public projects may not share. The project is then justified in terms of alleged benefits, efficacy, which if taken at face value by the economic analyst might well satisfy equation 11-1 or its cost-effectiveness equivalent. But a certain amount of probing of the bases for efficacy estimates can often reveal inconsistencies or unjustified extrapolations or interpretations of existing technical data. While this may not be within the sphere of economic analysis narrowly defined, there is no point in carrying out elaborate analyses on unsound or non-existent efficacy foundations. A little checking helps, and the economist or any other analyst who goes into program evaluation without some understanding of the technical aspects of the project is at risk of looking rather foolish.

Effectiveness extends the concept of efficacy from the laboratory to the field. Efficacy is a necessary, but not a sufficient condition for effectiveness; a program or intervention which will work under ideal conditions or with ideal management may simply be unworkable under field conditions. While efficacy is in principle a purely technical issue, effectiveness has an economic dimension in that one may make more or fewer resources available for program implementation. Two different immunization programs might be built on equally efficacious interventions—both using the same vaccine, for example, which has been demonstrated under controlled conditions to confer a specific immunity—but in terms of achieving a particular percentage of population immunity, or drop in the illness rate, one program might be effective and the other not. The difference might be simply one of resource input, effort level, or it might be a difference in organization and approach. The effectiveness of clinical programs, in particular, depends on the extent of patient compliance with therapeutic recommendations, as well as on the success with which the target population can be located and assembled. It is not uncommon in health care to find that better organized programs can be both more effective and less costly. As in the case of efficacy, however, an explicit focus on effectiveness forces one to address the question—effectiveness for what?—and can smoke out a number of collateral or alternative objectives which may be smuggled in along with the ostensible benefits of a public program.

The efficiency component of the triad should be self-explanatory; it has been the subject of most of this chapter. Once efficacy and effectiveness have been established, the B and C patterns specified, then various forms of economic analysis can be applied to determine if the project is worth doing. Such cost-benefit, cost-effectiveness, or cost-utility analyses, however, form only a part of the overall program evaluation problem, and particularly in the health care field one can argue that the problems of efficacy and effectiveness evaluation are at least as challenging. If we know whether the program does what it was supposed to do, the economic analysis is often fairly straightforward. But the clinical and epidemiological problems of establishing what works, under what circumstances, create the real difficulties.

When the appropriate cost and outcome parameters of a project are, as is usually the case, shrouded in uncertainty, the recommended response is sensitivity analysis. The doubtful parameter or parameters are assigned a range of values plausible to the investigator or her expert advisors. Benefits of type i, for example, accruing to people k in time t may be doubtful, but firmly believed to be no lower than B^-_{ikt}, and no higher than B^+_{ikt}. Is the project present value positive at $B_{ikt} = B^-_{ikt}$? Or negative at B^+_{ikt}? Or the discount rate may be varied from 2 percent (or zero) to 8 percent—does the project pay off (or fail to) for all values?[24]

If moving from "best guesses" to "plausible ranges" for program parameters fails to modify an initial go or no go finding, then obviously one can be more confident about the robustness of the decision with respect to uncertainty. On the other hand, if the evaluation turns out to be very sensitive to the assumed value of a key parameter or parameters— project payoff or input requirement, shadow price, or discount rate— about which there is substantial uncertainty, then obviously one's findings are correspondingly doubtful. The response may be to invest more effort and resources in establishing the value of the crucial parameter(s), but if this is not possible, then the appropriate decision rule is, "When in doubt, don't." If the project is to go ahead, it must be on the basis of some other considerations.

Such "other considerations"—the need to be seen to do something, continuation of past practices, the desire to generate earnings or to display professional prowess, perhaps above all the need to *act* in unsatisfactory situations—seem to underly a remarkably large part of health policy as well as health care services. While formal project evaluation has made enormous strides in the past decade in both methodology and range of application, there remains a great gulf between what is learned from such analysis and what is done.

Not least, of course, this is due to the fact that such analyses are threatening to clinicians, administrators, bureaucrats, and politicians alike. They call into question existing patterns of activity and raise embarrassing questions, not only from outsiders, but in one's own mind. Accordingly, while there are some clear cases—hypertension screening, for example— in which formal evaluations have given clear-cut answers that are translated into clinical practice, more generally the results of project evaluation, at least in health care, are ignored or resisted.

And a large proportion of health care interventions are innocent of any

---

[24] Sensitivity analysis on a parameter-by-parameter basis is of course a crude version of the more formal analysis with explicit probability distributions. As outlined, it assumes rectangular and independent distributions on each parameter, and fails to consider the implications of joint probability distributions even in the independent case. What if several uncertain parameters *all* take extreme values? A formal analysis of probability contours in a multi-dimensional parameter space would be much more elegant; it is also very uncommon. The reason is only partly that analysts (to say nothing of their readers or clients) are not familiar with the necessary "statistical tap-dancing"; there is also a strong (and probably correct) feeling that our relatively crude knowledge about the values of the components of equation 11-1 does not justify the extra effort.

formal or scientific evaluation at all, not just of efficiency, but even of efficacy. It is remarkable, and may be without parallel in human activity, that so much effort and resources are devoted through public or private channels to health care whose effectiveness has not been conclusively demonstrated, at least for the purposes claimed, either in the setting of application or at all. Odd.

CHAPTER 12

PUBLIC INVESTMENT PROGRAMS IN PREVENTION AND RESEARCH

INVESTMENT ACTIVITIES WITH DIVERSE AND NON-MARKETED BENEFITS

Many of the general issues outlined in the previous chapter emerge in specific, and particularly intractable, form in the fields of illness prevention and health care research. Both represent investment activities, in that resources are given up in the present, in anticipation of future benefits in the form of either reduced incidence of illness or injury, or enhanced capability of responding to them. And a special public interest is recognized in each of these fields. Public health activities and public subsidy to, as well as actual conduct of, health care research, predate public intervention in the financing and delivery of health care generally, and remain largely independent programs.

Canadian public health and research activities in 1982 accounted for $952.8 million and $327.1 million respectively, or about 3.2 percent and 1.1 percent of total health spending (Canada, Health and Welfare Canada n.d. [1984]). Public health activities, however, are not restricted to prevention, nor is prevention solely the province of public health. Indeed it is somewhat difficult to establish a precise definition of preventive activity, since both curative and to a lesser extent "carative" services may not only alleviate a present situation but also prevent it from deteriorating. Research activity is also included in other sectors of the health economy. A component of prescription drug prices covers the costs of research by private firms, and research and development expenditure by private equipment manufacturers similarly enters the prices of their products, which in turn show up in expenditures by hospitals, private practices, or other providers who purchase the equipment. And of course research outside the health care sector itself, in universities, government, or private industry may have significant effects, intentional or otherwise, on the health care system.

Going beyond Canadian health care expenditures, research in other countries generates new knowledge available in Canada, external effects across national boundaries, such that the link between resources *devoted* to research in Canada and new knowledge *available* for use in Canada is rather tenuous.[1]

The arguments for public intervention in the funding and direction of prevention and research follow the same lines as the general arguments for public intervention in health care developed above, though they have some distinctive features. First and foremost, as illustrated by the permeability of national boundaries in allocating the output (as opposed to resource input) of research activities, is the significance of external effects. Costs incurred by particular individuals or groups for both prevention and research generate benefits some or most of which accrue to other members of society, within or beyond national boundaries. Private decision-makers will (quite rationally) fail to take account of these external benefits; they will forego those investments for which (in terms of equation 11-1) costs exceed benefits when summed over a single value or subset of k, but benefits would exceed costs if all k were counted. Accordingly, optimal levels of activity require that the state either subsidize the private decision-maker—lower costs to the subset of k thus represented—or carry out the privately unprofitable activity.

As noted in chapter 3, this is the most ancient of the justifications for public intervention in health care, arising particularly in the context of contagious diseases. It underlies not only public immunization programs, which amount to lowering the cost to a private individual of activities with more general public benefits, but also compulsory regulation of private actions, paternalistic or otherwise.[2]

THE "NEW PERSPECTIVE": A PUBLIC INTEREST IN PRIVATE LIFESTYLES?

Beyond the field of communicable disease, however, the externality justification for preventive programs becomes much more questionable.

---

[1] This cross-national issue arises to a much lesser degree in prevention, but Canadians did benefit from the WHO program to eradicate smallpox. The risk of contracting the disease fell from very low to zero, and preventive activities in Canada, such as immunization, ceased to be necessary. Successful prevention elsewhere in the world thus yielded domestic benefits which could not have been achieved with any amount of local effort.

[2] Compulsion is paternalistic to the extent that it requires people to do what others think is good for *them*, as well as for their neighbours. This would include, for example, a requirement that all female children entering high school be immunized against rubella. But non-paternalistic compulsion would cover quarantine or other specific disabilities imposed on the ill for the protection of others. In terms of equation 11-1, public subsidy or provision seeks to lower the private costs of socially beneficial activity while relying on private decisions; paternalistic regulation responds to different shadow prices, P and V, on the consequences of the action and compels the individual to act as if she

My immunization status may influence your risk of infection, but my hardened arteries do not affect your risk of heart attack. Yet the focus of preventive activity has largely shifted, within the last decade, from communicable disease to problems of the hardened artery type. The *New Perspective on the Health of Canadians* (Lalonde 1974) assembled extensive data on mortality and morbidity patterns, showing that the most serious threats to health are now illnesses associated with particular unhealthy lifestyles and environments, against which the effectiveness of clinical intervention is distinctly limited (and very expensive). This document was part of a general shift in attitude, a great resurgence of interest in preventive activity in the broadest sense, as likely to be of greater effect than attempts at after-the-fact care in dealing with heart disease, accidents, or cancer. But this shift also undercut the traditional justification for public intervention in preventive activity. If my lifestyle affects my health, what concern is that of yours? Indeed, one can construct fairly elaborate formal economic models of the consumption of preventive services as a purely private activity. Such models are distinctly implausible, and seem to miss most, if not all, of the interesting policy issues surrounding prevention. Nevertheless, they raise an important question, to which there are several different answers: Why is prevention a public issue at all?

One set of answers involves a reinterpretation of the external effects involved. In motor vehicle accidents, as obvious examples, one person's behaviour significantly affects the health of others. Public programs to encourage safe driving, by exhortation, regulation, or punishment, thus fit comfortably within the externality framework. The linkage is directly from A's behaviour to B's health, not via A's health as in the communicable disease case, but it is no less strong for that.[3]

Environmental hazards to health similarly fit into the external effects category, insofar as the activities of one person, group, firm, or industry generate threats to the health of others. The role of the state in controlling environmental hazards is a natural extension of its responsibility in the

---

held these different values; non-paternalistic compulsion may overtly recognize that the preventive behaviour is undesirable for the actor but require it in the interest of others.

[3] In theory, an individual suffering damage from the actions of another can claim redress through the courts. An ideal and costless tort system would internalize external effects and thus remedy a major source of failure of private market systems. It would also eliminate a principal justification for public intervention. In practice, however, the problems of establishing liability, both fact and quantum, in addition to the sheer administrative inadequacies of the tort system (Dunlop 1982), make this prospect as illusory as the parallel interest in professional quality assurance through malpractice insurance rather than licensure.

field of communicable disease, except that in the environmental case the polluter is usually a net beneficiary from the process of hazard creation. Thus prevention of illness arising from unhealthy environments will typically involve public regulations or clean-up projects which may be globally beneficial but will impose net losses on some subset of the population. This may raise difficult issues of compensation. It also generates political conflict at a number of levels—including within the evaluation process itself—which will delay or deflect preventive activity.

A further twist arises in the area of occupational health and safety—the problem of defining the boundaries of "the environment." If one conceives of workplaces as settings which workers enter as part of a fully informed and voluntary decision, explicitly accepting all the positive and negative consequences therefrom, then the health consequences, risk of present accident or future illness or disability, are merely part of the employment contract. Public intervention, by regulation, requires some justification in terms of incompleteness in this contract. Systematic biases in information available to workers, or imperfect competition in labour markets resulting in a restricted range of characteristics of the employment setting offered, may undercut the assumed voluntary and fully informed nature of occupational choice.

Another form of externality is pecuniary, not physical; A's behaviour imposes monetary costs on B insofar as B must share the costs of health care generated by A's illness. For this purpose it is immaterial whether A and B participate in a public health service, a public health insurance program, or a private health insurance program with or without public subsidy, so long as A's behaviour affects B's costs. Collective Bs then have a justification for trying to influence A's behaviour.[4]

Beyond the pecuniary externalities is the more general social interaction, altruistic or paternalistic, which rests on the assumption that members of society care about each other, and about each other's health. Highway safety programs are not indifferent to one-car, one-occupant accidents, and suicide is regarded as something more than an individual consumption (investment?) decision. This argument is particularly relevant to preventive programs directed at children or other persons in a dependent condition; there is a collective responsibility to oversee the

---

[4] In a hypothetical world of perfect information, insurance contracts would be written such that each person's premium reflected all aspects of her behaviour bearing on risk. All costs would then be internalized; A's premium would fully cover the (expected) costs of A's behaviour and B would be unaffected. But the costs of monitoring plus the inadequacy of epidemiological data on risk make this hypothetical situation irrelevant in practice. Private, competitive insurance systems do introduce more premium differentiation than public, on an experience-rated basis, but this links costs to group health status, not individual behaviour.

decisions made by particular others on their behalf. But it applies between independent (?) adults as well; if A cares enough about B, or B's health, to subsidize health care consumption, then presumably her interest is equally legitimately reflected in public programs to influence B's behaviour or otherwise reduce the probability of B's falling ill.

COMMUNICABLE BEHAVIOUR: AN EPIDEMIOLOGY OF LIFESTYLES?

A more sophisticated reinterpretation of the externality argument, however, goes beyond the individualistic postulates of conventional economic theory to observe that (as every advertiser knows) individual lifestyle decisions—smoking, drinking, jogging, dieting—are not taken in isolation. Each individual's lifestyle becomes part of the environment which affects the decisions of others. In part the interaction is psychological— a herd instinct. Most people find it uncomfortable in and of itself to be the only one doing or not doing X. But there are also scale or threshold effects on the costs of particular activities. It is tough being the only cyclist in a city, for reasons which are quite directly physical, not psychological. When the baby boom reached middle age, the quality of jogging shoes rose spectacularly in response to the new market. When a large number of a firm's employees become fitness-conscious, it is worthwhile to provide centralized facilities.

Figure 12-1 (from Schelling 1978) depicts this process. The horizontal scale measures the proportion of a population perceived to engage in a particular activity; the vertical measures the proportion willing to do so. If no one else is doing it, a few rugged individualists are still willing to stand out of the crowd. As the activity becomes more popular, "bandwagon" effects develop, and a larger and larger proportion choose to participate. But at the other end of the scale, we find the equally rugged individualists who will not do X even if the whole rest of the world does.

Equilibrium is established where the S-curve cuts the diagonal—desired participation equals actual.[5] But, as shown in Figure 12-1, there may be several such equilibria, depending on how people respond to others' behaviour. Moreover some are unstable—the equilibrium at *B*, for example—and any shift in perceptions will cause a change in behaviour which is self-reinforcing. The *A* and *C* equilibria are stable; a shift in either behaviour or perception is self-damping. But high and low levels of participation are equally stable and equally the result of "individual

---

[5] Since desired participation depends on perceived participation, systematic distortions of perception which do not die out lead to somewhat more complicated equilibration processes.

FIGURE 12-1

A Representation of Interactions Among Members of a Community in Willingness to Engage in Particular Activities

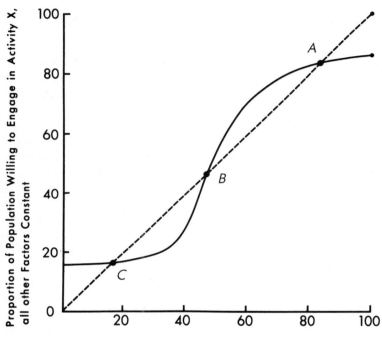

Proportion of Population Perceived as Engaging in
Activity X - Smoking, Jogging, Giving Blood...

choice.'' Private advertising campaigns often focus on shifting perceptions of participation—most people, or beautiful people, or important people, people like you or whom you would wish to be like, are doing X—in order to sell particular products. Public prevention programs may likewise attempt to stimulate ''healthy epidemics''—shifts from high to low equilibrium levels of use of products which are harmful to health. The creation of smoke-free areas, for example, serves not only to protect the non-smoker from the smoker, but also to symbolize and reinforce the anti-social nature of smoking. Publicity campaigns serve not only to convey information about hazards—which after all are widely known—but to shift people's perceptions of what others do or approve. The tendency of smoking behaviour to begin among children in response to media and peer group pressure, and then to become addictive, emphasizes the inadequacy of the individual choice framework and the significance of external effects.[6]

But the informational aspect of prevention cannot be wholly discounted. The extent of current information as to the links between illness and either individual behaviour or environmental characteristics is woefully inadequate even among specialists in such fields, and *a fortiori* among the population as a whole. A public role can thus be justified both in supporting or conducting additional research in this field, and in disseminating information on the positive and negative effects of different activities or products. If the benefits of such research and dissemination could be captured by private individuals or firms in the process of selling particular products or services, then the public role might be redundant. In practice, however, prevention seems more often to involve *refraining* from use of particular goods and services Moreover, the problems of imperfect information severely limit the effectiveness of the market response. The strong positive demand, willingness to pay, for prevention in a broad sense is indicated by the rapid growth in the last decade of sales of health and fitness products. But while in some cases (*e.g.*, jogging shoes) there has been a dramatic increase in the quality and quantity of technical and performance information available to users, and corresponding product improvements,[7] in others—health food stores—the result has been the promotion of consumption of peculiar chemicals and dietary supplements whose effects on health are at best questionable.

Indeed private markets, being neutral on issues of health, lend themselves as readily to the promotion of unhealthy products and associated lifestyles, tobacco being the leading example. If a principal justification for public preventive activity is the need to remedy imperfect information and enable people to make more informed judgements as to the consequences of their actions, how can this be reconciled with the continued promotion of pathogenic products? Obviously, health promotion (and

---

[6]   Apart from the obvious evidence of advertising campaigns themselves, anti-smoking campaigns among school children have found that non-smokers and smokers together greatly overestimate the proportion of children in their schools who smoke. Thus the perception of peer pressure is accentuated. ("Come on, *everybody's* doing it!") And as Figure 12-1 emphasizes, it is *perceived* collective behaviour which matters. Actual behaviour generates external effects of this form only insofar as it affects others' perceptions of prevalence. Pressure to keep certain forms of behaviour unobtrusive or even secret may therefore shift the curve in 12-1 and affect actual patterns. "Coming out of the closet" can affect actual patterns of behaviour, as well as perceptions.

[7]   Though the most widely used source of such objective information ceased to publish it between 1981 and 1982, and reverted to a "popularity poll." Magazines must respond to the interests of their advertisers, which may call into serious question the potential for information generation and dissemination by private, for-profit firms in a competitive marketplace. Magazines like *Consumer Reports* and *Canadian Consumer* accept no advertising and are non-profit—and one to a country.

consistent policy) give way to political feasibility. The illogicality of giving tax deductions for the promotional expenses of tobacco companies and subsidies to tobacco farmers while funding public anti-smoking campaigns illustrates the fundamental importance of defining the standpoint in any process of program evaluation—*cui bono*? More generally, the pathological agents who are the targets of preventive activity are commonly people and organizations with political influence, politically potent pathogens (Evans 1982*a*). The micro-organism or cell which is the target of clinical interventions may have a variety of weapons, but at least it does not advertise on its own behalf, vote, or make campaign contributions.

FROM LIFESTYLE POLICY TO HEALTH CARE EXPENDITURE: LONG CHAIN, WEAK LINKS

The difficulty of evaluating programs, or of making policy, in the area of prevention may be shown by considering explicitly the steps in the argument which lead from exhortation to expenditure. It is frequently suggested that a particular program—an anti-smoking campaign, a seat-belt law, dietary education in school programs—will lead to reductions in health care expenditure, and thus pay for itself, saving money as well as improving health. Advocates of expanded preventive services often point to the present very large expenditures on cure or care, relative to prevention, as an irrational allocation of effort—an ounce of prevention being worth a pound of cure.

The links in the chain run from a policy—advertisements, regulations, changes in physician fee schedules to make preventive interventions more rewarding, to a change in behaviour—people stop smoking, exercise, buckle up, eat less fats, see their physicians for check-ups, etc. This behavioural change is then supposed to lead to better health, lower rates of morbidity and/or mortality, which in turn are expected to lead to reduced health care utilization. And that, finally, should lower health care costs. Schematically:

Figure 12-2

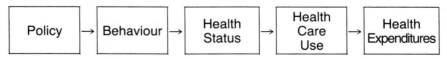

Isolating each separate step of the process demonstrates the number of causal links which are necessary to support the argument for prevention as a cost-saving strategy, and the points at which it is vulnerable to attack.

Policy interventions include information or education campaigns, regulations, and taxes or subsidies on particular activities. It appears that when a form of unsafe behaviour can be narrowly targeted, regulations and tax policies are effective in modifying behaviour. When regulations on seat-belt use and driving speeds, or immunization requirements for school entry, are established and enforced, behaviour responds in a significant and measurable way. Similarly, taxation of tobacco and alcohol appears to have measurable and substantial effects on use levels. Determining the effects of educational or facilitational campaigns, however, is much more difficult. Dissemination of information does not necessarily induce behavioural change, and from the point of view of the health care system, knowledge enhancement is not an end in itself.

Nor does participation in particular activities, such as fitness programs, necessarily serve as a measure of behavioural change. To determine that an employee fitness program has changed behaviour one must know the pre-program activity levels among participants and non-participants, and the amount by which each changed when the program was introduced. To attempt to infer program effect by comparing activity levels of participators and non-participators would probably result in a serious upward bias in assumed effect—participators being almost certainly more active to begin with.[8] Determining the effects, if any, of a policy intervention requires a certain amount of sophistication in evaluation design—simple comparisons can be seriously misleading for a variety of reasons.

If it is established that policies are available which can modify behaviour in desired ways, it is yet another matter to show that the behaviour will in fact have the desired effects on health status. Again, in narrowly defined areas like driving behaviour or tobacco use, the linkage from behaviour to health status is well defined. Speed kills, seat-belts save lives, smoking causes cancer, and water fluoridation reduces tooth decay—uncertainty remains only out on the lunatic fringe. But the linkages from exercise or stress to heart disease are at best observed correlations whose causal significance is still questionable. It may well be true that physically active people have less heart disease than inactive, but then sick people do not exercise much. A relationship between dietary cholesterol and heart disease has similarly been inferred for many years from correlations and speculation; not until early 1984 did experimental findings confirm the causal linkage.

The same problem of establishing causality applies to the dietary,

---

[8] The same criticism applies to reported savings of sick time and absentee rates generally, or of higher employee productivity and morale, from fitness programs. It seems very probable that such programs differentially recruit the healthier, fitter, more company-minded employees. Ideally, one would like to assign people randomly to participation and control groups and compare the performance of each; failing this, paired before-and-after comparison would probably be conclusive. In either case, though, the non-participation group might conceivably be contaminated by ''halo'' effects.

occupational, or environmental correlates of cancer. And trying to control morbidity or mortality by influencing a risk factor which is not causally connected is like trying to cool a room by putting ice cubes on the thermometer.[9] Unfortunately, the present state of knowledge appears to be insufficient to establish hard and fast causal links between behaviour and the major lifestyle-related sources of illness, cholesterol being a very recent exception. In this situation, the payoff to preventive programs is inevitably rather difficult to establish.

PREVENTIVE SERVICES IN THE CLINICAL SETTING: PROBLEMS IN ASSESSING EFFICACY

Clinically focussed preventive programs are subject to the same sort of problems. If one thinks of willingness to undergo screening procedures as a form of behaviour which can be promoted by exhortation, subsidy, or regulation, then the linkage from that behaviour to health status is increasingly questioned. It seems now generally agreed that routine ''annual physicals'' for the population at large are ineffective, and that screening should be targeted only to pre-selected high-risk groups (Canada, Task Force on the Periodic Health Examination 1980).

There are numerous specific traps in the determination of efficacy of clinical preventive manoeuvres, arising from the incompleteness of the underlying knowledge base.[10] Early detection of illness, in a pre-symptomatic stage, is preventive only if intervention is more effective or less costly at an early stage in the evolution of the condition. If the outcome of therapy is measured, however, by survival rates, after, say, two, five, or ten years from date of diagnosis, as is the case for cancer, then early detection may artificially raise measured survival rates by bringing forward the date of diagnosis even if the course of the disease is unaffected. The patient is actually made worse off, by spending longer in a ''labelled'' condition of pre-symptomatic illness, without gaining any corresponding benefit from therapy. In evaluating the benefits of early diagnosis and intervention, one must be sure that survival rates are measured from when the illness would have been identified in the absence of early detection, but this may not be known. If an early detection program is associated with increases in measured five-year survival rates, but also with an increase in population-wide prevalence of the condition, and no change

---

[9] If the thermometer happens to be part of a thermostat, the consequences are still more awkward.

[10] This section in particular leans heavily on the work of Sackett and others at the Department of Clinical Epidemiology and Biostatistics, McMaster University, who are however in no way implicated in its inadequacies.

in mortality rates, one must suspect that its influence is only on date of diagnosis.

A similar problem arises in the case of false positives. Few tests are absolutely precise in distinguishing pathological conditions; most are calibrated to trade off type I and type II errors. Some cases of "illness" will be missed, false negatives, and others wrongly diagnosed as ill, false positives. But if treatment is initiated for all positives, then the success rate will be contaminated by the false positives who will presumably show up as "cured." In the limit, a totally ineffective therapy will have a "success rate" equal to the ratio of false to total positives in the testing process which diagnosed the condition. If early detection programs lead to pre-symptomatic intervention, they may raise the proportion of false positives treated, and hence the "success rate," even if the therapy is totally ineffective. This problem is particularly likely when early detection identifies prior conditions—"silent" gallstones, carcinoma *in situ*—whose probability and time path of transition to a symptomatic condition are uncertain. The positives are not exactly "false," but a large number of people may be "successfully treated" who would never have become symptomatic in any case. Again, the proper approach is to identify population-based experience and compare it with controls—if the preventive program results in an increase in therapeutic intervention, an increased "success rate," but little or no change in morbidity or mortality in the target population, then the payoff to intervention may be illusory.

The point is not that clinical or other preventive interventions never "work" nor that reliable evaluation is impossible. Techniques of evaluation design and statistical analysis exist to surmount these problems, and to identify the critical gaps in knowledge. That is part of what epidemiology is about. But casual approaches to evaluating efficacy of preventive interventions are even more subject to bias and error than clinical interventions generally. The simple faith that "an ounce of prevention is worth a pound of cure" will be misleading if we do not in fact know how to prevent, and naive evaluation can easily hide our ignorance from us.

The uncertainties associated with links one and two in the chain in Figure 12-2 are sufficient to undermine a very popular argument for prevention, based on gross spending levels. It does *not* follow that just because much more is spent on cure or care than on prevention, therefore preventive activity should be expanded. The key questions are the marginal ones: What will be the payoff, in terms of health status, if more resources are added to either prevention or cure? What is the slope of the curve in Figure 1-3 with respect to these alternative activities? If preventive activities are ineffective, then no amount of spending on cure (or good intentions by their proponents) justifies their expansion.

Of course in practice the situation is more likely to be that such activities have not been *demonstrated* to be effective, but they might be. Under these circumstances, one must choose between investing resources in a program of uncertain payoff, or investing in research to make the payoff more certain. To this dilemma there is no general answer; presumably the choice depends on the urgency of the situation, the degree of uncertainty, and the cost and expected payoff of research. But as a generalization, "hoping to goodness" is likely to be expensive as well as theologically unsound.[11]

HEALTH STATUS AND THE LIFE CYCLE OF CARE USE: DEAD MEN USE NO SERVICES

The marketing of preventive services as a method of reducing current levels of health care expenditure, however, also depends on the next two links in the Figure 12-2 chain. These are prone to failure for reasons unrelated to imperfect information, but rooted in the structure of the health care industry and in the human condition itself.

It is regrettably not true, in general, that improving health status lowers health care utilization—it may or may not. The ambiguity is partly a result of the distinction made by Thomas (1971) between half-way and decisive technologies, and partly stems from the inevitability of the aging process itself. The development of polio vaccine was clearly an example of a decisive technology which both contributed to health status and lowered health care utilization. On the other hand, seat-belt use shifts the whole distribution of injuries so that some are alive who would otherwise be dead. It is a researchable question, whether the totality of health services used by accident victims is higher or lower when seat-belts are used; the answer cannot be given a priori. Similarly, hypertension screening and drug therapy create a population of regular users of physicians' services who would not otherwise be symptomatic or labelled "ill." The incidence of stroke may fall as a result, but whether utilization of health services by stroke victims falls by enough to compensate for the increase in use by hypertensives under care—keeping in mind that

---

[11] It is sometimes argued that it is unfair to subject preventive programs to rigorous standards of evaluation which have not been met by the vast majority of curative and carative interventions. Yet the ultimate objective is surely not one of fairness to different providers or balance among unproven techniques, but of benefit to patients and taxpayers. If resources are being wasted in one area, it is not obvious that waste in others is thereby justified. On the other hand, if some degree of waste is inevitable, perhaps a balanced service offering does require symmetry of evaluation standards. Certainly the status quo should not be exempt from scrutiny.

strokes may be fatal—cannot be answered a priori.[12] (But it *can* be answered, as the seat belt question can, by analysis of utilization data).

Apart from the problem of identifying the impact of a successful preventive intervention on utilization patterns, by the target population, of care related to the intervention, there is also the issue of unrelated care. Everyone dies, and in our society, most people become aged. In the process, various biological systems fail. Medical, drug, and particularly hospital utilization rise sharply with age. Preventive interventions which lengthen life also increase the number of years spent in the high use period. The overweight smoker who dies on the street of a coronary at age sixty-two will generate no further utilization; the energetic jogger who lives to be ninety-two will probably require a substantial amount of maintenance care in the final thirty years.

Or she may not. It is possible that improvements in health status resulting from adoption of healthy lifestyles may extend the horizon of good health and reduce the needs of the elderly at any specific age. The well-preserved seventy-year-old of the future, if prevention works, may display the utilization patterns of today's fifty-year-old. But at present we do not know. The case can be argued either way (Fries 1980; Schneider and Brody 1983), and the jury is still out. It would therefore be unwise to assume away the possibility that preventive services, if effective, will actually increase per capita health care use. In any case, age-specific use rates among the elderly are now rising, not falling and have been for a number of years (Evans 1984) but factors other than health status may be at work.

SAVINGS AT WHOSE EXPENSE? THE INCOME-EXPENDITURE IDENTITY AGAIN

Finally, even if a preventive program is able to thread its way through the causal chain in Figure 12-2 and actually serve to lower health care utilization by its beneficiaries, it does not follow that health care costs will fall as well. As emphasized above, health care expenditures are by definition also the incomes earned from the health care sector. Thus a policy which is successful in limiting expenditures must also lower incomes—again by definition. If British Columbia's compulsory seat-belt

---

[12] The hypertension case adds an extra complication. Case-finding *labels* people as "sick," leading to real psychological costs for the patient as well as, in some cases, behavioural changes with measurable (negative) economic effects. But not all patients will comply with therapy. Those who do not are clearly made *worse* off by the case-finding intervention (Haynes *et al.* 1978). The same is true for patients labelled by a screening process, for whom therapy turns out to be ineffective (earlier detection of an inoperable cancer).

law were really to save $120 million in health costs, as claimed when it was introduced, that $120 million must be made up of reduced fee income of orthopods, fewer nurses hired, hospital beds closed—resources either withdrawn from the production of health care, or paid less for their services. If neither of these happens, then no money is saved.

In practice, however, the influence of care providers over their own activity levels is such that resources do not go unemployed. The surgeons who are no longer re-assembling accident victims can instead replace arthritic joints; the nurses and beds are not left idle but are used to care for other types of patients. And if workload and incomes do fall in the fee-for-service sector, this translates into increased pressure in fee bargaining. Only if the preventive policy is matched with deliberate independent efforts to close beds, reduce hospital budgetary allocations, and limit the supply of medical practitioners will its effects, if any, on utilization result in expenditure savings.

Of course the redeployment of resources may itself be a gain, depending on what is believed to be the payoff to additional resources in health care. But if public policy generally is struggling with a perceived over-supply of physicians and hospital beds, it is clearly inconsistent to argue for a preventive policy on the grounds that it will serve to make more health care services available for other purposes.

This is *not* to say that such a policy would be valueless. An effective preventive policy which contributes to improved health can be evaluated on that basis alone. But it can easily be misleading to go beyond such health benefits and argue that, in addition, the policy will ease expenditure pressure on hard-pressed governments. When the savings fail to materialize, or are eaten up elsewhere, the resulting loss of credibility may jeopardize all preventive initiatives, effective and ineffective alike.

This possibility is of particular concern in times of fiscal restraint, when it has become increasingly tempting for advocates of health care programs of all types to try to market them as cost-saving, on the basis of evaluation analyses ranging from inadequate on down. New and expensive drugs and high-technology diagnostic and therapeutic interventions are always guaranteed, along with their contributions to patient well-being, to avert other misfortunes or supersede other expensive procedures, such that despite their direct costs, overall costs will fall. Preventive programs often mount the same bandwagon.

PREVENTING POVERTY AMONG PROVIDERS?

Yet a cynical observer might suspect the reverse intention. Recalling the identity of health expenditures and health incomes, much so-called "preventive" activity may be viewed as an effort to expand the scope and intensity of health care interventions to include the currently healthy population. Curative and carative interventions are to some extent limited by the presence of pathology in a population, and their effectiveness can be judged relative to that presence. But prevention is a completely open field; there is no limit on the amount of potential evil which one might hope to avert. And after the fact it is very difficult—impossible at the level of the individual—to determine if the prevention was effective.[13]

Thus prevention serves as an excellent way of absorbing the energies of an expanding health labour force in activities which probably do no harm, may do some good, and offer the psychological rewards of the celebration of wellness. Moreover, since the range of alleged, and possibly valid, preventive techniques extends well beyond the conventional health disciplines, prevention creates a point of entry for other practitioners into the very favourable regulation and reimbursement structure enjoyed by health care providers. Not surprisingly, reimbursers and currently approved providers find themselves allied in opposition to this expansion in the supply of health care incomes.

But the preventive interventions which *have* been proven effective in improving health are largely or wholly outside the clinical field. Tax and regulatory policy have been shown to be effective (and cheap) in controlling smoking and drinking behaviour and seat-belt use; efforts to influence such behaviour in a clinical setting have yet to be shown effective and are certainly more expensive. Fluoridation of water supplies is very effective and cheap; prevention in the dental chair is of much less effect and relatively expensive. Mass immunization campaigns are cheaper and more effective than initiatives by private physicians. There may, of course, be exceptions to this generalization—hypertension control and prenatal care being possible examples of effective forms of clinical prevention. (More generally, see Morgan 1977.) But there does appear to be a trade-off, both in principle and in practice, between the interests of the community in cost-effective prevention, and those of health providers in expanding the markets for their services. There is a real danger that the health care industry may find itself allied with other interests in the community which are threatened by effective preventive interventions, in the promotion of expensive and ineffective clinical alternatives. As an example, responding to lung cancer by more cancer research and by radiological and surgical interventions, rather than by controlling smoking, serves the economic interests of scientists, clinicians, and tobacco producers. But it is an expensive way of not achieving the allegedly desired result.

---

[13] Most of those who undergo a preventive intervention would not suffer the evil in any case, and even if the intervention is effective, some of its subjects may still fall ill. Efficacy can only be determined at a population level, often over a long period of time.

On the other hand, the inadequacy of the economic self-interest model in explaining professional behaviour is clearly shown by the universal support of dentists for fluoridation of community water supplies, a highly effective preventive intervention which directly substitutes for clinical services, both restorative and preventive.[14]

HEALTH CARE RESEARCH: WHAT IS THE PUBLIC INTEREST, AND HOW IS IT BEST PURSUED?

Health research, like prevention, displays two faces. On the one hand, it represents a form of social or private investment in the acquisition of new knowledge, which can improve the effectiveness and/or efficiency of the health care delivery system. In terms of Figure 1-3, the curve linking health status to resource inputs should be shifted upwards and to the left by successful research. On the other hand, research and the technological innovations it makes possible are frequently criticized as contributing to the escalation of health care costs—presumably by shifting society out along the relatively flat section of Figure 1-3, or even into the negative slope—and reducing the quality of care by dehumanizing and mechanizing it—losing the carative dimension—without corresponding gains in curative effectiveness.

In principle, research activity can be fitted into the cost-benefit framework of equation 11-1, and there are some examples of studies which measure the costs of and payoff to particular research efforts. One can add up, suitably priced and discounted, all the resources devoted to achieving a particular piece or collection of new knowledge, and compare these with the benefits in terms of reductions in other health expenditures, increases in productivity of those spared, or cured of, particular illnesses, and the overall value of lives extended in quantity and improved in quality.[15] These benefits are available to the community as a whole, assuming the results of research are widely disseminated, and private individuals or groups undertaking research will thus bear all the costs but reap only part, perhaps a small part, of the benefits. Research will, in general, be underfunded unless the public sector provides some sort of support.

There is substantial choice, however, as to the form of support; and the relative effectiveness of different approaches, for different types of

---

[14] It is conceivable that, by postponing or preventing tooth mortality, fluoridation might increase dental service utilization on a lifetime basis—the edentulous have little need for care. But to suggest that such expectations explain professional support for fluoridation seems not only cynical, but silly.

[15] Weisbrod's (1971) work on polio research demonstrated the evaluation of a clear-cut research success, whose costs and benefits could be identified and compared.

research, is itself an under-researched topic. The state can conduct research itself, as through the National Research Council or the Defense Research Board or agencies in particular Ministries. It can make grants to not-for-profit agencies or their employees—universities, research institutions, hospitals—as does the Medical Research Council or the National Health Research and Development Program. It can let research contracts to private for-profit firms selling research services. It can grant special tax treatment or other forms of public subsidy to the exploitation of new research information. Or it can grant patent protection to private firms, or give them privileged access to government purchasing programs, thus increasing the commercial value of their in-house research.

The inclusion of patents in the spectrum of public policies in support of health care research may seem somewhat unusual. From an economic perspective, however, a patent right is an asset, with an economic value, conferred by the state. The state creates and maintains, by coercion if necessary, a monopoly position for the patentee which enables him to ''tax'' purchasers of the patented product by charging them a price above production cost, and above what a competitive market would establish. It is thus like an agricultural marketing board, a delegation of the state's taxing power to a private entity for its own benefit.

The purpose of such delegation is twofold. First, in the absence of patent protection innovators would have an incentive, where possible, to keep secret the results of their research. The resources thus devoted to security, and by their competitors to industrial espionage, are a dead-weight loss to society as a whole. Moreover, insofar as innovators are successful in maintaining security, they retard the dissemination of new knowledge and lower the rate of technical progress generally. But if security is weak or impossible, then successful research conveys no commercial advantage because it can readily be copied by competitors, and no one firm will find it worthwhile to undertake.[16] The level of investment in research will be too low. Patent policy thus becomes a delicate balance between providing too much protection, such that the monopoly power granted to innovators imposes excessive allocative and distributional distortions on the relevant industry, and not enough, such that the rate of innovation is too slow and/or the level of effort in industrial security is too high.[17] But it parallels the political questions of how much to spend

---

[16] In some fastmoving fields copying may be too slow, and market power depends on speed of innovation. In others, production-specific ''know-how'' may be difficult to transfer. In these situations, patent policy may be relatively unimportant.

[17] In a static equilibrium world, the optimal patent life is zero, as is the technical progress rate. Patent policy presupposes a trade-off in terms of welfare losses, departures from Pareto optimality, at each point in time, in return for a faster growth rate over time. Optimizing across this trade-off is a social, not an individual, problem since the requisite state power is collectively held.

on in-house, or grant to "out-house" research; in each case the state must, by using the direct or indirect taxing power, balance present resources used up or benefits foregone against future benefits gained.

CONSISTENT MANIPULATION OF UNKNOWN QUANTITIES: THE ECONOMIC ANALYSIS OF RESEARCH

The difficulty with cost-benefit or cost-effectiveness analysis in this context is that, while it can in some cases be done after the fact, it is notoriously difficult to do in advance. It is painfully true that "if we knew what we were doing, it wouldn't be research." Of course, in some areas the nature of the objective may be well specified. The substantial amount of research carried out by private firms is generally focussed on a particular product—a drug or machine—whose desired effects or operating characteristics are relatively well defined. There may, however, be substantial uncertainty about the time and effort required to develop them. For more basic research the eventual payoff, if any, may be very difficult to predict and may occur in fields apparently quite unrelated to what the researcher or supporter had in mind. It is in just these areas, where some participants feel the highest long-run benefits may lie, that the necessity for public support is greatest. But since the B values of equation 11-1 are almost totally unspecified, if not unspecifiable, the potential contribution of economic analysis is distinctly limited. And its limited contribution is primarily negative, in that it can clear away some of the fuzzy thinking surrounding research policy and reveal the problem in its full intractability.

In the first place, economic analysis emphasizes, as always, the essentially marginal nature of the policy problem. The issue is not whether a society should support health-related research at all, but whether the $327.1 million reported as spent in Canada in 1982 was too much or too little.[18] And was it spent in the areas of greatest probable payoff? The rhetoric of technical progress or regress too often seems to be devoted to maintaining that research is a GOOD THING, which no doubt it is, but so are many other things. The whole of the GNP should not be spent on health research, nor even half of it, but what criteria can one apply to set a level? The judgements of professional researchers about appropriate funding levels overall are obviously unreliable, both because researchers are far from disinterested, and because they lack either the professional expertise or the political legitimacy for making such balancing decisions. They may, however, on the basis of their expertise

---

[18] An additional amount was spent through the prices of health products, particularly prescription drugs and some hospital equipment, but this research was almost all conducted outside Canada and is not an object of Canadian policy.

advise as to the outcomes to be expected from different effort levels, and on the mix of activities or appropriate targets.

Secondly, there is no automatic linkage between appropriate research levels and the economic or human magnitude of a health problem. The efforts by the Ontario Council of Health (Fraser *et al.* 1976) were an interesting exercise, but provide little guidance for recommendations on research funding. As in the case of prevention, the fact that much is spent on curative or carative activities does not, in and of itself, indicate that more should be spent on research (or, for that matter, less). "Magic ratios" of 1 percent or 2 percent or whatever of health spending to be devoted to health research, have unfortunately no rational basis beyond the aspirations of researchers. The key question is not simply, "How big is a particular problem? but "What probability is there that a particular research effort will actually contribute to the solution of a problem large enough to justify the effort?"

Estimates of the costs, direct or indirect, associated with a particular class of problems may have negative significance—a small problem obviously does not warrant a large research effort. But the converse need not hold. For example, the finding by the Ontario Council of Health that diseases of the teeth and supporting structures generate a relatively large direct economic burden is not an argument for more research in oral biology. As noted above (chapter 7), a large proportion of this cost is a result of technical inefficiency in the delivery of dental service, over-utilization of dentists instead of dental nurses to carry out restorations, a result not of lack of knowledge but of professional self-protection. An additional component results from incomplete application of well-established efficacious prevention—community water fluoridation. If new knowledge cannot be expected to lower costs, whatever other benefits it may entail, then high costs cannot be an argument for more investment in research.

"FREE RIDING" VERSUS NATIONAL PRIDE: OR DR. BANTING, MEET MR. PODBORSKI

Nor is a higher level of research effort in other countries an argument for more research effort in Canada, quite the contrary. The more other countries spend on research in a particular area, *ceteris paribus*, the *less* we should spend in Canada, because the more likely we are to benefit from others' work, and to find that our own is duplicated. We should concentrate on areas that others have left alone. Of course, the *ceteris* are not *paribus*; it may be that others have left an area alone because they judge the expected payoff to research there to be small. But for a wholly self-interested small country in a large world, the optimum research strategy may be none at all—better to ride free on the product of others' efforts.

There are, of course, other considerations. "Free riding" carries a mildly offensive connotation, however rational it may be. Canadians' self-image, of themselves and their country, may be enhanced by a feeling of doing their share on the world scene. Supporting research efforts, and perhaps Nobel Prize winners, is a source of collective satisfaction akin to supporting Olympic medallists or downhill racers, or beating the Russians at hockey. Most Canadians take vicarious pleasure in, and are willing to pay something to support, such achievements. But there is no necessary reason why such support should be particularly for health research.

One can also make a sort of "infant industry" argument, that support for research can help to develop high technology industries in Canada, with consequent benefits in jobs, skills, earnings, and profits. But this is not an argument particularly for health research, and insofar as it does bear on health research, it is only as a means to production and sales, not as a way of improving health care. Assisting the development of Connaught Labs as a multinational pharmaceutical firm, for example, may or may not be a proper part of Canadian industrial policy, depending on the expected net payoffs, but it has nothing at all to do with health policy. In fact, the effects may be negative if the Canadian health care system is viewed as a protected market for the domestic development of exportable health care products whose health benefits are at best marginal. Industrial subsidies become hidden in health budgets. The profitability and growth of health care suppliers and the cost-effectiveness of the health care system may, as noted in chapter 10, be in direct conflict.

On the other hand, new knowledge does not always arrive neatly packaged on the shelf. Domestic skills may be needed to adapt new information, and these skills may be maintained only within a domestic research program. When a new drug is made available in Canada, its effective utilization does not depend on whether it was developed in Toronto, New Jersey, Belgium, or outer space. But new therapeutic techniques or management systems may require localized expertise for their adoption. The hard-nosed free-rider policy may lead to a country's being slower to adapt new knowledge because its providers are unaware of its existence or significance, or simply have to learn how to use it.

And the use of research, the delivery of care, may not be separable from the research process itself. Opportunities to advance human knowledge, or to satisfy their curiosity, form part of the professional self-expression of some at least of the best clinicians. Just as high quality university teaching requires the presence of active researchers, so it is argued that the maintenance of clinical standards, striving for excellence, may depend on the proximity of an active research environment. Otherwise professionals will migrate to foreign research centres, or to the ski hill.

Finally, health-related research spans a continuum from the "hard end"—physics, chemistry, or biochemistry—through the biological sciences to the social and managerial disciplines. Results from the former know no national boundaries, but the latter are culture and system dependent. Health care system research in the United States or Sweden may have some implications for Canada, or it may be completely irrelevant, depending on the extent of similarity of the institutions or behaviour studied. We each have to do our own research on our own health care systems, if the results are to be helpful in addressing our problems.

These are all rather general considerations, which do not provide much concrete guidance to issues of research funding and priorities.[19] And that is probably inevitable. If the expected benefits of reseach are intangible and highly uncertain, the techniques of economics are singularly weak. At the very least, however, one can ask advocates of increased research funding—whether in the form of grants, favourable tax treatment, or increased patent protection—to come up with some plausible estimate of the resulting benefits.[20]

And it is certainly important, as in any public or private expenditure

---

[19] Though the easier importability from other countries of research results at the "hard end" would suggest that rational policy for a small country in a large world is to concentrate on social and managerial research—health systems and delivery—not basic science. In particular it casts doubt on the widsom of devoting resources, either directly or through the patent system, to encouraging domestic pharmaceutical research by multinationals; this is the easiest of all research to import.

[20] The suggestion, for example, that Canada modify or end its program of compulsory licensure of the importation of patented drugs, in return for increased research spending by drug companies in Canada, represents a transfer of funds from Canadians (and their governments) as drug buyers to pharmaceutical manufacturers for research purposes. Whether this would lead to increased research worldwide is unclear, though presumably Canadians would regard increased domestic employment as a benefit. But the results of such research, though supported by Canadians through higher prescription prices, would remain the property of the companies concerned. Canadians would have no privileged access to the information generated by such research, whether or not carried out in Canada, even though they had effectively funded it. The proposal would in essence be equivalent to a job-creation program run by private companies with federal grants raised by a tax on particular pharmaceuticals, without any effective linkages between the size of the grants and the number of jobs created.

A policy of selective public assistance to pharmaceutical research as part of a long-run strategy of "Canadianization" of pharmaceutical production, or at least the development of one or two world-scale Canadian-based producers (Gordon and Fowler 1981) raises more interesting issues both pro and con, but they are beyond the scope of this work.

program, to scrutinize carefully the results of such efforts. (They may not be what was expected, or promised, but there should be *some* results!) In the end, though, it is undoubtedly worth supporting a certain amount of "pure" research, whose expected payoff is totally beyond quantification. How much, is essentially a political decision. Economics may help to clarify some of the issues involved, but cannot add much to the final answer. How much was Expo '67 worth, or the Montreal Olympics? Our collective judgements on such matters are made, albeit rather imperfectly, through the political process.

THE PROFITS ARE IN "HALF-WAY" TECHNOLOGY: PROBLEMS OF MOTIVE

In the special context of health economics, however, there is an additional consideration. Thus far, as in most discussions of research activity, we have implicitly assumed that new knowledge was always a positive good. If so, the payoff to research is always non-negative. A good program produces a lot of new knowledge for the money, a bad program little or none. But one cannot be worse off, as unhelpful new information can always be ignored.[21] Yet in health care, it may be that valid research can have harmful consequences. In the first place, as noted in chapter 10, the economic incentives which bear on the choice of research programs are predominantly towards cost escalation.

Consider Lewis Thomas's (1971) three-stage characterization of health care technology. The first stage, palliative care for an illness whose course cannot be influenced, is usually cheap and ineffective (though becoming less cheap). As knowledge progresses, we learn to deal with the consequences of the illness—iron lungs, organ transplants, renal dialysis—to keep the patient alive and perhaps functioning better. This "half-way technology" stage is partially effective and very expensive. Finally, when knowledge advances to the point that the disease process itself is fully understood and controllable—the real high technology stage—the decisive intervention is again cheap but now effective.

Thomas's argument leads toward more "basic" research in biology and biochemistry, in the hope of reaching stage three, rather than "applied" research, which focusses on specific problems at the stage two level. The argument is attractive, though it does not tell us how much basic reseach to support—or who to ask for the answer. From a private

---

[21] Of course, research may lead to erroneous findings. The hard sciences have relatively effective ways of cleaning out bogus results fairly quickly. But at the other end of the spectrum, misleading results from, for example, bad economic research can have powerful negative effects. Most people, including economists, would agree with this statement, but would disagree over what was bad research—which makes the point.

economic perspective, however, stage two technology is the profitable level to address. Expensive half-way technology yields sales and profits. Decisive technology removes the problem—and the market. Indeed, it is a positive (commercial) advantage that, for example, micro-organisms become resistant to antibiotics—there is always a market for new drugs.

This rather macabre perspective should not be interpreted as imputing malevolent motives to individuals or firms; it merely addresses the obvious. Profits are earned by selling things, not by not selling them. It follows from this that research directed to producing high sales will have a large expected payoff, and that profit-oriented firms will, quite rationally, tend to support that sort of research. Moreover, insofar as the adoption of new technology by providers of health care is biased toward that which is complementary to their skills, enhancing their sales potential, and away from that which substitutes for their services and is cost-reducing, this will further bias the research process toward the development of cost-enhancing technology.

This points up the weakness in the argument that technology per se is neutral and that problems arise only from the way in which health care providers use new information. If technological advance is associated with cost escalation and ineffective utilization, that is the fault of the workman, not the tool. But the argument is too simplistic. Insofar as research is conducted by for-profit firms, it will be focussed differentially on those developments which are most likely to be overutilized—overutilization translates into sales volume—and the promotion of products embodying new knowledge will similarly encourage use separately from efficacy. Hence, the frequent observation of unquestionable technological breakthroughs which improve the effectiveness of care, and in a particular context lower its cost, but which tend to be used far beyond their range of demonstrated efficacy, with corresponding cost-escalation effects. The research process itself is not, cannot be, neutral; much less the process of diffusion of new knowledge into practice.

AFTER SUCH KNOWLEDGE, WHAT FORGIVENESS?

Finally, on a still more difficult level, health care is not motivated solely by efficacy considerations. The sense of having "done everything possible" for the patient is itself of value to providers and relatives, if not necessarily to the patient herself. The significance of the desperation reaction in technological diffusion (Warner 1975) may be partly based on the same feeling—if the outcome was not satisfactory, at least nothing was left undone.

In this context, new knowledge may simply add to the range of things which should not be left undone. The tendency for new diagnostic techniques to be applied along with those they were expected to replace appears to be an example of this phenomenon. And it is not merely a matter of provider uncertainty. For the patient and the wider society as well, unavoidable evils are easier to bear and less productive of distress or outrage than those which might possibly have been avoided—if someone had done something.

In a fully rational world, of course, people would make judgements about expected payoffs, would decide who should and who should not be treated, and would then go home and sleep well (or suffer in silence). In our world, however, the development of new technology with very high costs and low but non-zero benefits may well make people worse off, in that now more decisions to withhold treatment must be made— or else costs must be allowed to escalate. In terms of Figure 1-3, an increase in diagnostic or therapeutic knowledge which increases the slope of the curve from zero to some very small positive value is by no means an obvious gain in well-being. Such new knowledge, while privately profitable, may carry negative externalities—be a public "bad." But does that mean we should try to suppress it, assuming that we could?

CHAPTER 13

HEALTH MANPOWER POLICY—LEADING THE HORSES TO WATER

PUBLIC INVESTMENT IN PRIVATE CAPITAL

Boulding (1968) finds "the whole manpower concept repulsive, disgusting, dangerous, fascist, communistic, incompatible with the ideals of liberal democracy, and unsuitable company for the minds of the young. (It) is basically . . . an engineering concept, and one of the main problems of society is to keep engineers in a decently subordinate position." Without pretending to do justice to his subsequent argument, we may note that the concept of manpower[1] explicitly categorizes people, as well as their competence and intellectual development, as objects of analysis and inputs to production processes, means to some external ends, rather than as ends in themselves. It is in direct defiance of the categorical imperative.

Yet the manpower concept, like engineers, turns out to be unavoidable and often quite useful. The survival, let alone growth and development, of all organizations depends on the availability of human resources, time, effort, and skills, to carry out their activities. Governments may refer to manpower policies while private firms speak of personnel policy, but each must consider the nature, numbers, and source of the trained personnel needed for or implied by its other objectives. As in so many other areas, it is impossible *not* to have a policy, although the actual policy may be more or less explicit, consistent, or farsighted.

Nor can the manpower concept be blamed entirely on the engineers. Economists have quite happily developed the concept of "human capital." The time, energy, and other resources spent by a person in acquiring skills or abilities, or by others in inculcating those skills, are thought of as an investment in the creation of an intangible form of capital equipment which increases the productivity of the trainee, just as time and effort might have been devoted to creating a piece of machinery, physical

---

[1] Or worse, ill-conceived neologisms such as personpower.

capital, for her to work with.[2] And almost all economic analyses of labour markets or production processes explicitly treat labour as a commodity, an input to production or an object of exchange, differentiated, if at all, only by its admixture of ''human capital'' services.

Boulding is not the only one to object to the notion that this ''commodity'' can be manipulated separately from its human or social context. Unemployment is not simply an excess inventory of labour input, like a pile of coal, nor can human capital be ''scrapped'' on the basis of the same calculations as an obsolete blast furnace or a damaged automobile. But such concerns have troubled economists little, if at all.

They do, however, create an important distinction between the manpower policy of the state and the personnel policy of a private firm. Unless it is very large or highly specialized, the individual firm's decisions do not determine the market for labour. In acquiring skilled services, it can choose to hire or to train internally, and its ''de-hiring'' decisions, while potentially traumatic to an individual, do not in themselves foreclose other employment opportunities. The manpower policy of the state, however, is defined over the whole labour market (abstracting from immigration) and is thereby more constrained. If a public program or policy, such as the expansion of the health care system, requires more skilled personnel than are available, or different ones, educational programs must be established or expanded to train them, and the time required may influence the timetable of program introduction. Moreover, educational programs in general have been accepted, in Canada as in most other countries, as a public responsibility separate from the particulars of health policy. Manpower issues thus cut across two conceptually separate areas of social policy whose co-ordination has been somewhat less than perfect.

On the other side of the coin, and perhaps more relevant to present Canadian conditions, the ''de-hiring'' decisions implicit in public programs may affect entire markets. If the expansion of the hospital sector is curtailed, while training programs continue to turn out nurses with ever more extensive and expensive training, some at least of the newly manufactured ''human capital'' will be idled. Similarly, medical schools,

---

[2] Nor need the ''human capital'' represent specific skills. Health and general education spending have often been advocated as ''investments'' which increase the subsequent productivity of the labour force. Healthy educated people represent more ''capital'' in the sense of ability to do work, than ill or ignorant ones. The heavy concentration of health spending on the elderly or chronically ill, and the significant consumption aspects of education, weaken this argument somewhat. It can be restored by expanding the concept of ''human capital'' to include sources of direct satisfaction to the holder— the stock of ''health capital'' as both an object of investment and a source of future benefits, for example. But despite its theoretical elegance, this approach appears to have generated more confusion than clarity.

whose throughput now appears sufficient to keep the physician-to-population ratio climbing at least to the year 2031, create enormous stresses for provincial governments and medical associations trying respectively to limit the escalation of medical costs and to maintain their members' incomes. The state as reimburser for, if not operator of, health programs has an implicit responsibility to provide employment for the "human capital" which it has encouraged and assisted individuals to acquire; surplus capital cannot be stockpiled or scrapped. Whether or not this responsibility is explicitly accepted, the political process will ensure that it cannot be entirely escaped. Thus the manpower decisions of the present set many of the parameters for delivery systems in the future, over as long as a generation. And the program constraints imposed by the skilled people who are not now available are much less serious and long-lasting than the constraints imposed by those who are.

A POLAR CASE: PATTERNS OF MANPOWER ALLOCATION IN PURE COMPETITION

These constraints arise from the regulated and subsidized nature of the health care system itself; there are similar problems in other regulated occupations such as law. It is worth recapitulating how a hypothetical perfectly competitive and unregulated health care system would deal with manpower issues, not in order to suggest that such a system would be more appropriate, but only to indicate how the key issues of manpower policy derive from the peculiar nature of the commodity "health care" itself, and the peculiar regulatory and financing structures which this makes necessary. "Market failure," and public intervention in the production and distribution of the product, leads to "market failure" in the process of human capital production as well, and the need for further intervention at that level. Failure to co-ordinate such intervention can lead to dramatic and costly problems in the delivery system.

If the production and distribution of health care were not regulated, but governed by the laws of the free market as they exist in economics texts and editorials in the business press,[3] there would be no need for public "manpower policy." Privately owned firms, probably incorporated, would own and manage hospitals and medical clinics on a for-profit basis, competing for customers by some combination of (real or perceived) quality differentiation, promotional advertising, and competitive pricing. The "product lines" of such organizations, the range of services they chose to provide, would be determined by what they felt to be most profitable. Individuals could enter this market freely, as employees or self-employed practitioners, without the need for licensure,

---

[3] Though perhaps nowhere else.

though they might well seek some form of public or private certification in order to communicate their skills to potential customer/patients in a convincing manner.

The manpower mix in this imaginary health care system would be governed by the hiring decisions of producer firms and by the ability of self-employed practitioners to find a clientele. In particular, profit-oriented firms would hire the least-cost combination of personnel necessary to produce their products. The constraints on any resulting quality dilution would be, not licensure or regulation, but the refusal of customer/patients (assumed fully or adequately informed) to patronize low quality establishments. This might be backed up by regulations to prevent false advertising or other forms of consumer fraud, as in any other retail business, and perhaps also by some enforcement of minimum standards of product quality or safety, as in the food industry. Further, customers could use the tort law system—malpractice claims—to recover for bad outcomes traceable to producer fault. But *process* of production would be unregulated, and inter-provider competition would ensure that the least-cost mix of personnel, which might or might not be the least ''human capital intensive'' process of production, was used. Pharmacists would no longer find employment moving pills from large bottles to small, dentists in drilling teeth, or physicians in performing well-baby checks.[4]

In this world, the relative demand for and earnings of different types of personnel would be derived from consumer demands for the services they produced, relative to the numbers of people offering such services. The ''net advantages'' model of occupational choice predicts that informed persons choosing careers will treat training decisions as an investment in which current earnings are foregone (and perhaps extra effort required) in order to acquire skills which will command higher earnings later. These later earnings may be in money, or they may be in the form of desirable employment characteristics—pleasant surroundings, flexible hours of work, ''respect,'' self-determination. Net advantages refers to both. As in any other investment, the stream of future net advantages must be discounted back to the present, and compared with the training cost. Thus the *i*th career choice has a present value:

$$PV_i = \sum_{t=0}^{N^i} \left[\frac{Y_t^i - \overline{Y} - E_t^i}{(1+R)^t} \right] \tag{13-1}$$

Here *t* refers to years from the present ($t=0$) to retirement after $t=N^i$

---

[4] Actually, this is an overstatement. Some consumers may derive direct satisfaction from being cared for by the ''high priced'' help; others may treat excess or underutilized human capital as a signal for superior quality, despite the absence of supporting evidence (and the presence of contrary evidence). If so, some providers will find it profitable

years—self-employed occupations permit more latitude in choice of N.
Y_t^i is the earnings plus other advantages (which may be negative) in year
t for occupation i, while $\overline{Y}_t$ is net advantages of some reference occupation
requiring no training. E_t^i are direct training costs in year t for occupation
i. The rate at which the individual discounts future benefits, R, should
be equal to the real rate of interest set in the capital market, expected to
hold over the period $0 \leq t \geq N^i$.[5]

The free market would apply also to training institutions and processes;
thus E_t^i would reflect the full costs of providing training for occupation i
in year t, and Y_t^i would be small or zero in the early years of a career
with extended schooling. $(Y_t^i - \overline{Y}_t)$ represents, abstracting from its
net advantages aspect, the foregone earnings associated with training in
career i.[6]

In long-run equilibrium PV_i will be equalized at zero across all i; no
one occupation will command any advantage over any other in life-time,
discounted net advantages. If it did, informed entrants would differentially
select that occupation, leading to a fall in its members' incomes. Similarly, underpaid occupations would fail to recruit entrants, supply would
fall, and earnings rise.[7]

---

to offer services using more expensive personnel—at a higher price. Consumers will
be able to select from different levels of input capital intensity, but therapeutic equiv-
alence. The market provides Cadillacs and Chevrolets, Toyotas and Mercedes, but all
will take you where you are going.

[5] Obviously the model should allow for uncertainty with respect to earnings, interest
rates, maybe even success of entry attempt. Furthermore, individuals have inherent
differences in physical and intellectual endowments which affect their expected payoffs.
These complicate the conceptual model, without changing its implications. They do,
however, severely inhibit empirical testing. But then, most testing is in practice carried
out in terms of explicit earnings, which amounts to the assumption that "net advantages" are always proportionate to money income. The implausibility of this assumption
means that empirical rate-of-return calculations across occupations can only be indicative at best.

[6] The U.S. educational system displays some of the characteristics of a market, but
relatively few. A number of professional training schools are moving toward, or have
established, full-cost tuition charges, and U.S. governments, federal or state, do not
have the same degree of influence as Canadian provincial governments over number
and capacity of training programs. But the *supply* side of professional education bears
no resemblance to a competitive market, with free entry of (possibly for-profit) training
institutions designing their programs to provide whatever the market is willing to buy.
So long as public or delegated regulation controls the qualifications required to enter
a profession, it simultaneously controls "approved" institutions and curricula. To
observe a genuinely competitive educational system at work, one must go back to pre-
Flexnerian days. Starr (1982) provides a first-class description and analysis.

[7] The equality of present values holds *at the margin*. People whose inherent abilities are
matched to a particular occupation will find that they can earn a positive, perhaps very

Of course *annual* earnings are not equalized; occupations with long training periods will yield higher annual earnings during the (shorter) working period, as they should and indeed must to attract recruits. But inter-occupational earning patterns will (abstracting from other advantages) bear a determinate relationship to each other—high earning occupations over a lifetime yield a surplus just large enough to repay (with interest) their training cost (direct and foregone income).

In this environment, "manpower policy" is unnecessary. A shortage or surplus of a particular class of personnel, resulting from shifts in consumer tastes or producer technology, will be reflected initially in the bidding up or down of the incomes of those types of personnel. The income changes will result from rising or falling prices for the types of goods or services which these personnel participate in producing. The particular mix of skills embodied in a given class of personnel will be determined by producing firms—large corporations or self-employed practitioners, according to the dictates of least-cost production. As incomes in different occupations shift, the *PV*'s of career decisions rise or fall, and recruitment patterns follow. Eventually, supply responses (or shifts of personnel from careers with low *PV* to those with high) will re-establish equilibrium and will equalize *PV*s once more across all occupations.[8]

THE PRINCIPAL CHANNELS OF PUBLIC INFLUENCE OR CONTROL

Of course, the above scenario does not describe health care delivery systems or the processes of personnel recruitment anywhere in the world,

---

large, *PV* in that occupation relative to the next best opportunity—the Wayne Gretzky effect—because these advantages, being unique, cannot be competed away. The equalization of *PV*s occurs after adjustment for "rents to abilities"—which further inhibits empirical testing. Equalization also depends on a continuous distribution of abilities; "holes" in the distribution may lead to unequal *PV*s.

[8] Eventually. But as is well known, the fact that a static equilibrium may *exist* is no guarantee that dynamic processes will get you there quickly—or at all (Nelson 1981). Working off a surplus may take half a generation—it depends on the relative sizes of stocks and flows of personnel and the magnitude of necessary adjustments. Furthermore, new entrants must be fully informed, not only about current and future demands for personnel, but also about supplies, which will depend on the decisions of other potential entrants. They need to know what everyone else is going to do in order to make their own decisions optimally. This interdependence can lead to dynamic over– or under-shoot, depending on how entrants assess the behaviour of other potential entrants. And the existence of an eventual equilibrium a generation or two hence is small comfort to those who guess wrong—in the long run we are all dead.

and has not for at least a century—if ever. Public intervention, to encourage or restrain, is pervasive and, in principle, almost universally accepted.[9]

This intervention takes place in three primary ways:

1. The use of state authority to regulate occupations, either directly or more commonly by delegation to private professional bodies;
2. The provision of subsidies for educational costs, and the determination of how much and what kind of training capacity will be made available; and
3. The structuring of public delivery or reimbursement systems to determine how many of what classes of people shall be hired to provide, or reimbursed for providing, which kinds of services.

There exist, of course, a variety of other public policies which also affect manpower availability or use—legislation governing malpractice liability, for example—but the above three are the big levers.

The process of occupational regulation is of fundamental importance insofar as it determines which combinations of skills and capacities can be assembled in particular individuals. To pursue the "human capital" metaphor, the productivity-enhancing "machines" which are embodied in trained individuals can be assembled in a wide variety of different ways, with a broad or narrow scope or range of functions, and with deep or superficial competence. A very extensive training program can turn out an elaborate and costly piece of "human capital" capable of performing many functions and dealing with problems of great complexity or sophistication; a less extensive and costly program will produce "capital equipment" with a more limited range of functions, whose possessors must refer complex problems to another provider. This is, of course, merely another way of looking at the issue of alternative types of health care providers, addressed in chapters 6 and 7 above. The point here is that the public regulatory structure defines the boundaries between occupations, determining who may do what, and thus regulates which bundles of capacities shall be assembled together and which kept separate. It further determines what bundles of capacities shall be required to perform which functions—as emphasized above, self-regulating groups

---

[9] There are a few economists still out growling in caves in the woods somewhere that the whole system would function better if the state withdrew entirely, but they are not taken seriously even by themselves. The real policy issues, as recent U.S. experience has made clear, are: "Who shall control the state's interventions, and for what ends?" For tactical, political reasons, some forms of intervention are sometimes referred to as "de-regulation" or "free enterprise"; the deception is probably deliberate.

tend to require that licensed providers possess all capacities before exercising any, thus "overcapitalizing" beyond what is technically necessary. Finally, the regulatory structure determines the "process of production" of human capital, the educational steps necessary to acquire and use (legally) the capacity to provide services, as well as prescribing (and proscribing) particular activities of its possessors.

From the point of view of manpower policy, then, the state at the most basic level determines by regulation what the categories of manpower shall or shall not be, and how the bundles of capacities which they represent shall be acquired and used. It is of central importance to realize that these are regulatory decisions; they are not pre-determined by technical or market considerations. The occupational structure, and its educational requirements, are matters of policy choice, and the consequences of those choices are extremely far-reaching.

Yet these issues are frequently neglected in discussions of manpower policy, which usually take existing occupational definitions and divisions, and thus educational requirements, as given data. This is probably because governments tend to take their decisions in these matters with closed eyes, pretending to themselves and others that no decision is being made. The delegation of state authority to private provider associations, which then perform the regulatory functions and delineate occupational roles, permits both parties to disclaim responsibility. Provincial governments can claim that, having once delegated regulatory powers to "expert" external bodies, they are no longer responsible for the consequences, while private regulators disregard (or even deny) the fact that their authority is entirely derivative from the state. Neither claim has a shred of legal validity, being radically inconsistent with the fundamental constitutional principles of parliamentary sovereignty. But politically, the "separation" may be very convenient.

Moreover it can be reinforced by the assumption, often implicit in defenses of occupational regulation, that the existing allocations of functions and required training patterns are in some way predetermined by underlying technical necessity. Regulatory requirements are treated as if they merely reflect the only way people *can* be trained or services provided. The variety of regulation and experience across jurisdictions, however, and the experience with alternative practitioners of various types— different ways of designing and assembling "human capital"—suffice to refute this assumption when it is made explicit.

Any analysis of public manpower policy, therefore, must start with the regulatory structure, or else the largest part of policy is left unexamined. Within that structure, however, the state also plays a fundamental role, through its funding and subsidy policies in determining how many people, and of what types, will be trained. Almost all funding for post-secondary education flows through provincial governments; and while

universities exercise independent control over their curricula and programs, a public decision to expand or contract facilities cannot be ignored.
The offer of funding for a new professional school, or for a major expansion, represents more temptation than a university, however highly
principled, is likely to be able to resist. A denial of funding, of course,
is decisive. Moreover, although direct charges for education are relatively
small in Canada, especially in the health occupations,[10] public subsidies
may be paid directly to students in particular programs in the form of
grants or low interest (perhaps forgiveable) loans. At a later stage, the
direct funding of training positions such as hospital residencies may be
used to influence numbers and types of specialists. And tax legislation
or fee negotiations with providers, or public service salary and benefit
policy, may be used to influence the costs or economic benefits of continuing professional education.

Of course the educational policies of individual provinces may be
undercut by interprovincial migration, either in or out, emphasizing the
need for cross-provincial coordination.[11] At the national level, migration
considerations have at various times been an important part of physician
manpower policy, but not of policy toward the other health occupations.

The rate of physician in-migration seems to be very sensitive to the
"point" value of the occupation for immigration purposes. When it was
classified as a shortage occupation in the late 1960s and early 1970s,
immigration nearly matched domestic production of physicians. When
this status was withdrawn in 1975, immigration fell by about three-
quarters. Later in the decade, physician out-migration to the United States
became more rapid, and was argued by some to impose constraints on
public policy—especially fee-setting—in that if physicians were dissatis-
fied, they would all leave. Increasing saturation of the United States
market, combined with the observation of continually increasing physician-to-population ratios in Canada, has muted this point, but international
migration remains a potentially significant aspect of physician manpower
policy. In particular, public (federal) policy can alleviate a perceived

---

[10] In Canadian universities, program fees charged to students vary much less than program
costs, so the proportion of program costs which are subsidized, though very high on
average, varies greatly over programs. In general, the subsidy rate is highest on the
most expensive programs, which also lead to the highest paying careers, and are lowest
on the least costly and least economically rewarding (to the individual). Justifications
for this pattern are not immediately apparent.

[11] Alternatively, provincial regulations may, as is all too common among professionals
generally, limit the transferability or reciprocity of licensure. This seems far too high
a price to pay for any effect it might have in improving the effectiveness of provincial
manpower policies. The advantages of professional "Balkanization" from the point
of view of professionals in migrant-attractive provinces are obvious. But it is offensive
from every other perspective.

shortage of physicians quite swiftly (and cheaply) by re-opening immigration. A surplus, however, is quite another matter—it seems unlikely that a policy of inducing out-migration would be politically viable.

The payment mechanism is also a critical part of manpower policy: "Who supplies what?" is closely linked with "Who is paid for what?" Most obviously, the right to bill the provincial insurance program for services rendered to patients is of great value to the various self-employed health professions. The decision by a particular province to issue billing numbers to members of a particular occupational group plays a critical role in encouraging the expansion of that occupation. On the other hand, as noted in chapters 6 and 7, the refusal to reimburse services of particular intermediate-level personnel, either in self-employment or as employees of other "approved" professions, will result in professional "still-birth" regardless of the availability or technical competence of such personnel.

More subtle problems arise in those areas where two different occupations share overlapping competences—should the reimburser pay each the same? In some cases, ophthalmologists and optometrists providing refractions, for example, the anwer has been "yes." On the other hand, general practitioners and specialists are paid different fees for the same services in all provinces but Quebec. "Cost of production" and "equal pay for equal work" fee setting are difficult to reconcile—economists instinctively reject the former. But if two different professions—optometrists and ophthalmologists, for example—are reimbursed at the same rate, and the patient perceives the latter as representing "more"—at least a broader range—of human capital than the former, will this not give the latter a marketing advantage, even if the former are less costly to train and equally effective? Yet differential reimbursement for equivalent services is difficult to justify on equity or efficiency grounds. In designing reimbursement systems, it appears advisable to think through their implicit manpower policy content, and be sure that one is happy with the results—accidental policy is not necessarily optimal.

INFORMATIONAL AND INTERACTION PROBLEMS IN PUBLIC MANPOWER POLICY

Working through these three main channels, government establishes health manpower policy either consciously or by default. It is simply impossible to have no policy, though fragmented, inconsistent, ill-considered, and excessively costly policy is all too possible.

Of course, deliberate policy, even if coherent and well thought out, is always vulnerable to unforeseen shifts in demography, technology, and social "tastes" in the broadest sense. Canadian policy toward physician manpower in the 1960s is a classic example. The population forecasts of the Hall Commission missed completely the "great obstetrical contraction" of 1965 and its aftermath (as did everyone else), so that by 1981 they were too high by about five million people, or 20 percent. The effects of such an error on manpower requirements estimates are, of course, massive; the resulting overestimate led to the putting in place of the present excess physician-training capacity.

The problem, however, is not merely that the future is inherently unknowable and that all forecasts are erroneous—barring blind good luck. The error in the demographic forecasts was observable as early as 1966, and the new trend was clearly established by 1970. But instead of re-thinking domestic capacity, which would have threatened jobs and careers in universities particularly, policy makers and forecasters made efforts first to rationalize away the new demographic reality as a short-term aberration, and then to justify the resulting dramatic increases in physicians per capita. Even in the mid 1980s, the nettle of manpower limitation has yet to be firmly grasped. It is much easier, politically, to gear up then to gear down.

The lesson, then, is not so much the difficulty of forecasting and planning, but that of acting on certain kinds of forecasts. The policy response is biased according to the type of information generated in the planning process—for good, sound economic reasons. One must therefore strive to improve, not merely the quality of planning information, but the incentives on decision-makers to use it—to confront the obvious. In any case, failures of rationality do not establish a positive case in favour of confronting the future in ignorance or absence of mind.

The public manpower planning problem can be thought of, without doing too much violence to reality, as a very large cost-effectiveness problem. From this viewpoint it can be fitted into the conceptual framework of chapter 11. Alternative types of manpower can be thought of as different investment programs in the sense that they represent the commitment of resources in the present to yield future benefits consisting of their contribution to the health and well-being of the community. At a very abstract level, human capital, physical capital, knowledge or research capital, or "capital" in the form of enhanced resistance to disease or injury resulting from preventive programs, all represent alternative ways of trading present resources of human time and effort, and physical inputs, for a stream of future health benefits.

Investments in manpower, however, add significant complexities to this analysis. Apart from the very large number of alternative "investment programs" available, and the difficulty of identifying and measuring the future benefits, two additional problems stand out.

First, the investment is a joint one—the public at large and the individual choosing a career are both involved. There is no point in setting up training programs, however cost effective, in which no one wishes to enrol. For most of the health professions, over most of recent history, this has not been a problem. The relative financial rewards of the health occupations have been such as to lead to a substantial unsatisfied demand for entry, so that manpower policy can operate by direct rationing of access. But this need not be true in general, especially in those occupations such as nursing in which large numbers of qualified personnel choose not to practice. A policy of subsidizing entry to an occupation in which conditions of work are insufficiently attractive to hold the labour force is equivalent to keeping a sieve filled by adding ever more water— possible, but peculiar.

Second, and very important, the payoffs to the various "investment projects" are non-additive. For simplicity, we assumed in chapter 11 that the streams of costs and benefits associated with particular projects were independent of the type and scale of other projects underway, so that the measurement of cost-benefit or cost-effectiveness balances for any one project, or decisions to include it in a public agency's "portfolio" of projects, need not depend on what else is going on.

In general, however, this assumption will not be valid. The payoff to research on respiratory disease will be influenced by the effort and success level of anti-smoking campaigns. But it is dramatically falsified in the manpower field, where many of the principal issues revolve around who does what. Particular types of personnel are substitutes for, or comple- ments to, others. We have emphasized the substitution relations above, because the policy-induced distortions in those relationships seem so severe and costly. But obviously surgeons and anaesthetists, or surgeons and hospital ward staff, represent complementary inputs whose numbers require some sort of balance. Manpower planning for one occupation cannot be done in isolation from the rest.[12]

AN "ACTIVITY ANALYSIS" PLANNING FRAMEWORK

Manpower planning frameworks can be appallingly complex in the abstract, reducing to depressing simplicity, if not triviality, in application. One way of setting the problem up, however, which is based on Leontief's Input-Output models of the general economy, has the advantage of bring- ing out a number of the awkward assumptions involved in conventional methods.

First, hypothesize a population, P, which represents the target group— people of Canada, people of a particular province—for whose benefit the planning exercise and its *sequelae* are being carried through. We can then

---

[12] This statement is obviously false. Of course it can, and usually is. The results, however, tend to be rather unfortunate.

subdivide P into categories P_i, in which i indexes the amount and pattern of health services needs of different members of the population. Thus we have a vector, $[P_1 \text{ --- } P_i \text{ --- } P_n]$, such that summing over all P_i yields

$$P, \sum_{i=1}^{n} P_i = P,$$

and within each group P_i, people are believed to be more or less homogeneous with respect to their expected service needs. A very common way of doing this is to let i index age-sex categories, but depending on the data and research effort available one could also break out separately particular ethnic, geographic, or employment sub-groups, or (at any point in time) people with particular chronic conditions.[13]

Given the population structure, one can attempt to determine, at least on a probabilistic basis, its needs for future services.

$$\begin{bmatrix} S_1 \\ S_j \\ S_m \end{bmatrix} = \begin{bmatrix} e_{11} \text{--} e_{1n} \\ \text{--} e_{ji} \text{--} \\ e_{m1} \text{--} e_{mn} \end{bmatrix} \times \begin{bmatrix} P_1 \\ P_i \\ P_n \end{bmatrix} \qquad (13\text{-}2)$$

where the range of m different health services to be provided is represented by the vector $S_1 \text{ --- } S_m$, and the mxn matrix E, whose elements are e_{ji}, expresses the amount of services of type j expected to be needed by the average individual of type i. Put another way,

$$S_j = e_{j1}P_1 + e_{j2}P_2 \text{ --- } + e_{jn}P_n \qquad (13\text{-}3)$$

and so on for all j. Each person of type 1 requires e_{j1} units of service of type j—tooth restorations? office visits? measles shots?—per time period.[14] And total need for services of type j is the sum of the needs for each of the i different population classes, which in turn is the product of the number of people in that class, P_i, times their average service needs, e_{ji}. The vector S then represents the "shopping list" of services required for population P.

The structure of the E matrix will (or should) embody detailed information about the effectiveness of particular services of the sort expressed at a very aggregate level in the health status curves of Figure 1-3. The

---

[13] The vector of P_i is defined at a single point in time, but obviously manpower planning requires, explicitly or implicitly, assumptions about how P_i unfolds through time. Total population P will (usually) rise, but its proportions will also change, most obviously as its age and sex structure evolves. They may also be endogenous, as levels of service provision at one point affect—positively or negatively—later needs. Neonatal intensive care may increase the proportion of the population with high future needs; particular forms of prevention may reduce it.

[14] Clearly, the S and e must refer to some time period, say a year. Then S has dimension services/year, and e, services/year per person.

appropriate servicing pattern for people of category i, represented by the vector $(e_{1i} - - - e_{mi})$, depends on the illness pattern of people in group i and on the capacity of services of each of the m different types to respond to those needs. The level of e_{ji} should be set such that further services of type j supplied to group i people have a zero, or positive, payoff depending on whether the efficacy curve for services j to people i has a well-defined kink (Figure 1-3a) or approaches the horizontal asymptotically (1-3b). In any case, it is the point of application of social priorities for care.

The specification of $[e_{ji}]$ may be quite straightforward for fields like dentistry, where the range of different services is small and the population can be split fairly neatly into different "need" groups. The optimal values of the e_{ji}—optimal maintenance schedules, choice of restoration technique—may be subject to some debate, but the categorizations j and i are fairly easy. Other health care fields, with a very wide range of different services or fuzzy boundaries between services, may present substantially greater problems of definition. Nevertheless, as we shall show below, if the task is not attempted explicitly, it will be done implicitly, and difficult problems are not necessarily better solved in ignorance.

Given the "shopping list" S, there are a variety of forms of resources—manpower and other inputs—which can be used in their production. We can then specify a technology matrix T, whose elements t_{kj} represent the number of units of resources of type k needed to produce one unit of services j. They are the "input-output" coefficients. We can then write:

$$\begin{bmatrix} R_1 \\ R_k \\ R_q \end{bmatrix} = \begin{bmatrix} t_{11} & & t_{1m} \\ & t_{kj} & \\ t_{q1} & & t_{qm} \end{bmatrix} \times \begin{bmatrix} S_1 \\ S_j \\ S_m \end{bmatrix} \qquad (13\text{-}4)$$

defining the amount of each of q types of resources which must be used up in producing the shopping list of services represented by vector S—if technology T is employed. Each row of the matrix T yields an equation:

$$R_k = t_{k1}S_1 + t_{k2}S_2 + - - - t_{km}S_m \qquad (13\text{-}5)$$

implying that if R_k represents minutes of time of a particular class of personnel, say registered nurses, services of type 1 require t_{k1} minutes each of the time of persons of type k. But R_k can also be non-human inputs, either time of capital equipment, or physical units used up of such things as drugs or film.

Putting all these together, we can write the matrix equation:

$$R = T \cdot E \cdot P \qquad (13\text{-}6)$$

where P is the $n \times 1$ vector population groups P_i distinguished by their differing characteristics related to health care needs; E is the $m \times n$ matrix of elements e_{ji} which convert population numbers to quantities of different services needed; and T is the qxm matrix of elements t_{kj} which express the amounts of each different type of resource input needed to produce each unit of service. E may be thought of as the Epidemiology matrix, and T as the Technology matrix, though as we have noted above, the internal structure of the e_{ji} must embody policy choices as well as epidemiological information. So, as we shall see below, do the t_{kj}.

To derive manpower requirements, of course, we need yet an additional intermediate stage, in which numbers of personnel or other measures of total resources available are converted into working time. Thus a given number of people in occupation q, say M_q, do not necessarily each provide the same amount of physical input R_q. The ratio R_q/M_q may vary with provider age, sex, skill level, training location, geographic site, or form of economic organization. This variation is quite distinct from the variation in *service output* per class of manpower, which may depend on the machinery, assistants, etc. available; rather it indicates the time, effort, and skill *input* to production represented by a particular unit of "human capital" and its attached human being.

If provider personnel of type q are divided into W different categories, *e.g.*, by age and sex, such that the average time, effort, and skill per person differs across categories, then total inputs of services q will be:

$$R_q = r_{q1}M_{q1} + r_{q2}M_{q2} + -- r_{qw}M_{qw} \qquad (13\text{-}7)$$

where r_{q1}, r_{q2}, etc. represent the relative input levels from different classes of M_q. The number of *people* of type q will be measured by $M_q = \sum_{h=1}^{W} M_{qh}$, but unless the *proportions* M_{qh}/M_q stay constant, the number of people required to generate a given volume of personnel services will fluctuate—quite apart from the effects of shifts in the r_{qh} themselves.

"MAGIC RATIOS": THE LIMITING CASE OF ACTIVITY ANALYSIS

Going back to (13-6), it is important to keep in mind that it is a matrix equation, resulting from substituting (13-2) into (13-4) and embodying all the detail of each. Neglect of the internal structure of T, E, and P yields the traditional and much more limited manpower planning approach of "magic ratios." The search for "optimal" physician (dentist, pharmacist, podiatrist—not yet veterinarian!)-to-population ratios continues to be a popular way of trying to sidestep the awkward and demanding T and E matrices. In the magic ratio approach, the P-vector is collapsed to a scalar—total population P. T and E are likewise collapsed to a single number, and the relationship between M and R is assumed to be constant. Combining all these constants:

$$M_q = \Theta_q P \qquad (13\text{-}8)$$

where Θ_q is "the" optimal ratio of providers of type q per capita. Clearly, the task of manpower planning is greatly facilitated.

By contrast with (13-6) and (13-7), however, it is also clear that (13-8) has imposed two different types of drastic simplification, on the M_q and P, and on the T and E.

The assumptions that provider and user populations are homogeneous are serious, but not too difficult to remedy. Obviously "optimal" magic ratios should depend on population structure, the relation of obstetricians to the birth rate, and paediatricians and extended care nurses to the age structure, being fairly clear examples. But extending the "magic ratio" approach to take account of variations in age-sex structure, at least, is not very demanding. One merely chooses age-sex specific values of Θ_q, measures the structure of P, and repeats the calculation.

MANPOWER, POPULATION AGING, AND UTILIZATION: CHICKEN OR EGG?

Alternatively, one can abandon the perspective of "optimality," and merely measure age-sex specific utilization ratios. One can then project changes over time in average per capita and total utilization if these specific rates are held constant while the population evolves. This can be a rather useful exercise. Several such studies have been done for Canada which showed on the basis of mid-1970s population projections that the "great greying" of the Canadian population would not, in fact, have much impact on medical care utilization (an increase of less than 10 percent per capita from 1976 to 2001, and of 15–20 percent from 1976 to 2031 (Boulet and Grenier 1978; Denton and Spencer 1983)). The effects on hospital and other institutional use would be much greater, but even so would represent relatively low annual rates of increase compared with the large changes of the 1950s and 1960s.

When these utilization projections are compared with projections of physician manpower availability based on class sizes, immigration rates, and attrition patterns in the late 1970s and early 1980s, obvious discrepancies emerge. Projected increases in physician supply outrun population growth by 25 percent from 1976 to 2031, yielding population-to-physician ratios around 430. Weighting population growth by changing age structure reduces this to about 18 percent, but leaves the basic conclusion intact.

If current rates of physician manpower production are maintained, either per capita utilization rates (age-sex adjusted) must rise, or physician workloads must fall. In either case, it is also true that either physician average incomes must fall (in real terms) or per capita medical expenditure must rise, with some combination of increasing fees (faster than the general price level) or increasing workload per physician. And these adjustments must continue for fifty years! The glacial effects of manpower policy—slow but devastating—are thus graphically displayed.

The 1976 population projections have been overtaken by an acceleration of declines in mortality rates in the late 1970s which is continuing into the 1980s. This has the effect of increasing both the total projected population and its average age. Thus the oversupply of physicians may turn out to be less severe—relative to current age-sex specific use rates[15]— though the implication of either long-term continuing increases in per capita medical care costs or falling physician real incomes remains.

All such projections, however, refer to potential *future* developments. Changes in mortality rates, even large ones in terms of past experience, affect population structure with long lags. (Becoming is not being.) And the aging of the Canadian population, whether faster or slower than anticipated, cannot by any stretch of the imagination explain or justify the conflicts over resource allocation in the late 1970s and early 1980s; it is on an altogether different time scale. Allegations that Canadian health care is currently either ''underfunded'' or suffering from ''cost explosions'' because of population aging, *i.e.*, demographic shifts combined with a pattern of more or less constant age-sex specific utilization rates, are simply unsupportable from the demographic data. They form part of the rhetoric surrounding a struggle over political priorities—attempts to provide an apparently objective basis for one or other set of interests.

What *is* happening is that age-sex specific utilization rates are themselves changing, in such a way as to increase substantially the *relative* utilization of the elderly. Extensions of technological possibilities and increases in available manpower and facilities translate into increased intensity of health care servicing. And these increases occur to a greater extent among the elderly, as they are on average ''sicker.'' It is easier to justify interventions as the organism slowly deteriorates—there is always something wrong (Lubitz and Deacon 1982; Evans 1984). In the end, the process of dying provides a very extensive field for potential intervention. Rather than health care utilization being driven by ''needs'' associated with an aging population, it may be that developments on the supply side, technology and manpower pressures, are driving up use

---

[15] These should not, however, be assumed to be optimal.

among the elderly. The usual (hypothetical) manpower planning process, as expressed thus far in this chapter, may be standing on its head.

PLANNING WITH MAGIC RATIOS: IMPLICIT ASSUMPTIONS AS TO EPIDEMIOLOGY AND TECHNOLOGY

Age-sex breakdowns of the P-vector, such as underlie the discussion of population aging and manpower "needs," could be supplemented by information on other sub-populations of special need status—high or low—in order to refine the planning process. Birth rates, for example, have shown very large shifts independently of population age structure. With enough data one could also pinpoint and project high-use chronically ill or handicapped groups. Furthermore, cross-regional planning could make much more use than at present of population structure data. It should be obvious that a city like Victoria, B.C., with a large elderly population, needs a much higher volume of hospital and medical services per capita than does a young rural region.[16] Planning processes which try to compare manpower availability (and adjust funding) across regions solely on the basis of undifferentiated capitas will build in obvious inequities.

At the other end of the equation, the volume of resource input represented by a particular person or piece of equipment is not a given constant either. Obviously not all trained personnel are in the labour force at all times; some drop out temporarily or permanently and others work part-time. In the self-employed sector, effort and time levels per practitioner are variable. Age and sex explain some of this variation; insofar as they do it should be possible to define a stock of effective, or standardized Full Time Equivalent (FTE) personnel which would correspond to the R_k values of (13-4). Data for this purpose are less well developed than for population and utilization adjustment, but the conceptual problems are equivalent, and such work is underway.[17]

Much more difficult are the problems involved in determining the internal structure of the E and T matrices. The E matrix summarizes "what is to be done"—how population "needs" are to be defined—and the T matrix summarizes "how to do it." The magic ratio approach compresses the relevant rows of each into the Θ_k parameter, the optimal X/Population ratio. The trick is, then, to identify at this level the optimum or target Θ_k.

---

[16] Though not necessarily as many as it has.

[17] The Health Manpower Research Unit at the University of British Columbia, for example, is preparing detailed FTE stock data by health occupation, and related analyses for physicians have been carried out at the Department of National Health and Welfare and in other provincial ministries.

In practice it has turned out to be quite easy, as evidenced by the large numbers of such optimal ratios available for physicians—all different. The traditional method was to identify a range of Θ values across different geographical regions for a particular class of personnel k. The highest such Θ was then selected as a standard, and manpower "needs" were defined as the number of personnel needed to bring all other regions up to the Θ_k in the highest region. Obviously, such needs estimates could be increased by making comparisons across smaller regions—counties, say, instead of provinces.

Apart from its rather implausible assumptions about where new personnel would choose to locate—why would they not distribute themselves in the same proportion as present personnel, preserving the measured "shortage" at a higher overall level of Θ?—this approach rests on two further and fundamental assumptions. First, whatever services are being provided in the target or standard region are all "needed" and appropriate—overservicing or an inappropriate mix of care is ruled out by assumption. And second, the process of provision in that region is accepted as an appropriate standard of technical efficiency. Since *all* the personnel in the most highly endowed region are "needed," they must all be working as efficiently as can reasonably be expected, and must be providing only care which is needed in the sense of being sufficiently effective relative to its cost to justify its provision. In terms of Figure 1-3, the slope of the curve even in the most highly endowed region (often referred to as most favoured, to drive the point home) is assumed steep enough to justify that level of provision, and providers are assumed to be on (or near) the curve, not below it.

Such faith is touching, and has been strong enough to survive dramatic increases in personnel availability. But it is buttressed by the fact that since the entire E and T structure is compressed into Θ, these assumptions are wholly untestable. Only in the context of a much more detailed analysis of specific services, their patterns of production and provision, can the magic ratio be checked. And although more than enough work has been done on *individual* services to call both assumptions into serious question, if not refute them altogether, such work has rarely been assembled to the level of comprehensiveness that it could guide overall manpower policy.

Indeed, detailed service analysis can be carried out in such a way that it preserves the twin assumptions of the magic ratio. The Requirements Committee of the National Committee on Physician Manpower, reporting in the mid-1970s on physician requirements by specialty (Canada, NCMP 1975), used detailed billing data from the public medical care insurance plans to explore medical care utilization patterns. But it imposed as an assumption that whatever was being done was necessary. Its specialty working parties expressed some opinions (not always consistent) about who ought to do what, and some assumptions were made about technological and demographic factors which might increase future needs, but at root the approach was fully in the spirit of the traditional "magic ratio"—whatever is, is right, or at least is not overdone.

On the technological efficiency side, the committee avoided any serious consideration of alternative forms of personnel as substitutes for physicians. There was some discussion of physician time requirements per procedure, but since these too were based on currently observed patterns, and since it was felt that physicians in general worked longer hours than they should, the result was predetermined that more physicians were needed to produce the same number of services. Magic ratio assumptions were thus preserved over an apparently more sophisticated analysis, to ensure that shortages would again emerge.[18]

DEFINING THE TECHNOLOGY: DIRECT MEASUREMENT OR THE "ENGINEERING" APPROACH

It is much easier to criticize present or past efforts at manpower planning, which are always constrained by available data, time, resources, and conceptual apparatus, than to do the job "right." It is also much less dangerous, since attempts to provide a detailed structure will inevitably lead to many and detailed errors and points of criticism. "Magic ratios" bundle all the individual errors into one large fallacy, which is harder to critique because it is harder to come to grips with.[19] There are two general classes of approach to measuring the structure of the T matrix at least, the "engineering" and "econometric," which arise out of the economic theory of production and which have yielded some useful results (Hadley 1974; Reinhardt 1973).

First, in the "engineering" approach one can attempt to measure the T matrix directly, by observing actual practice data, consulting with experts, conducting experiments, etc. For this purpose, however, the matrix of (13-4) is too restrictive and must be augmented. It embodies only *one* technology, one way of producing each service. Further, that one possible technique is assumed to display constant returns to scale; proportionate increases in all inputs yield an equi-proportionate increase in output.[20]

---

[18] The finding of a surplus would of course, be threatening to practitioners as well as to medical school staff—it raises awkward questions about how practitioners, who are obviously not unemployed, spend their time.

[19] The optimal ratio of people per physician is 612. No it isn't . . . and so on.

[20] The more general economic approach is to express the production relationship as a production function:

$$S_j = h^j (R_{1j} \ldots R_{qj}) \tag{13-9}$$

subject to $\partial h^j / \partial R_k \geqslant 0$

To modify (13-4) we must add additional columns, new technologies, to T, reflecting the fact that there may be several ways of producing S with different mixes of inputs. Some of these alternatives may use inputs—nurse practitioners, denturists—which are not used at all in the other approaches, in which case q is increased to span a wider range of input types, and rows as well as columns are added to T. The result is represented as:

$$
\begin{bmatrix}
R_1 \\
\cdot \\
\cdot \\
\cdot \\
R_k \\
\cdot \\
\cdot \\
\cdot \\
R_q
\end{bmatrix}
=
\begin{bmatrix}
t_{11}^1, \; t_{11}^2, \; t_{11}^3 \; ----- \; t_{1m}^1, \; t_{1m}^2 \\
\\
\\
t_{kj}^p \\
\\
\\
t_{q1}^1, t_{q1}^2, t_{q1}^3, \; ----- \; t_{qm}^1, t_{qm}^2
\end{bmatrix}
\times
\begin{bmatrix}
S_j^1 \\
S_j^2 \\
S_j^3 \\
\cdot \\
S_j^p \\
\cdot \\
S_m^1 \\
S_m^2
\end{bmatrix}
\qquad (13\text{-}10)
$$

where as shown there are three alternative techniques available for producing service S_1, using different combinations of inputs R, and the total amount of S_1 produced will be $S_1 = S_1^1 + S_1^2 + S_1^3$, the sum of the amounts produced using each technique. Similarly there are two alternative ways of producing S_m. The total number of columns of T, and rows of augmented S, will depend on the number of alternatives available for each service, which will vary by service.

This approach enables one to represent opportunities for input substitution within the activity analysis framework, though it continues to impose constant returns to scale.[21] It does, however, mean that resource requirements cannot be determined solely on the basis of technical and epidemiological information, which is as it should be. The optimal allocation of production of each S_j among the alternative technologies available is essentially an economic decision, and should respond to the relative

---

saying merely that the volume of possible output of S_j depends in an unspecified way on the amounts of the different inputs used for j production, and more inputs yield more, or at least no less, output. (13-4) is then a special case of (13-9), since holding all other service levels constant we can solve for S_j as a function of the R_k available (beyond that needed for the pre-set levels of other S).

[21] The isoquants are facetted, not smoothly curved, but if several techniques exist and linear combinations are permissible, plenty of scope for substitution is allowed. Constant returns to scale is probably not too serious a restriction either; apparent scale effects in health care production often turn out to result from product mis-specification.

costs of the inputs R_q. The cost per unit of S_j will be equal to the cost of all the inputs used in its production, and these will in general differ across techniques.

It does not follow, however, that one "best" technique will necessarily dominate all the others, such that only one will ever be used. Since resources come in lumpy units (such as people) which are not freely divisible, and have alternative uses, and since geographic considerations (at least) will constrain the size of production units—the Canadian health care system cannot all be put into one huge building just outside Winnipeg—it may turn out to be optimal to use mixes of techniques, or different techniques in different settings. The point to emphasize, however, is that the analytic framework must embody the *possibility* of substitution, and that economic (relative cost) criteria must enter this process in a central way.

Studies of this sort have been carried out in considerable detail for some sectors of health care. A computerized model of dental practice, for example, has been developed which not only identifies all the specific services of a dental practice but breaks them into sub-functions which may (but need not always) be included, and assigns time requirements for each (Kilpatrick *et al.* 1972). Personnel can be "custom-designed" for the model, in terms of the bundle or package of capacities they embody, and realistic problems of queuing, personnel co-ordination, and transfer from patient to patient can be built in. It is thus a much more sophisticated and realistic version of the above model framework, and can be used to determine global manpower requirements under different assumptions as to practice size, structure, and location.[22] In other branches of health care, the application of this framework has been less detailed, but it has been applied to primary medical care (Smith *et al.* 1972) and at a much more aggregated level, to pharmacy (Evans and Williamson 1978).

The strengths of this approach are also its weaknesses. Precisely because the framework provides opportunities to exploit extensive and detailed information, it also *requires* such information. Measurement of the T matrix has usually been done in one or a few specific sites, whose representativeness may be questionable. Practices or clinics which offer

---

[22] It was used for this purpose, by the B.C. Children's Dental Health Research Project (British Columbia, CDHRP 1975) and demonstrated that a given pattern of "needed" services could be provided in radically different ways depending on how practices and personnel mixes were organized. Total, system-wide costs of most efficient combinations were as much as 40 percent below those of standard practice organizations, and implications for training programs were massive. Not surprisingly, the results were shelved.

themselves for study are unusual by definition. Yet the extent of "engineering" information required makes it unlikely that one could ever apply the technique over a large number of practices "in the field." Measured or estimated T matrices demonstrate what is possible, but not necessarily for everyone or under all circumstances. And one is inevitably left with the concern that the large discrepancies which show up between such studies and actual practice may reflect constraints in the field that the experimental setting has neglected.[23]

STATISTICAL OBSERVATION OF PERFORMANCE IN THE FIELD: THE "ECONOMETRIC" APPROACH

The alternative approach takes as its basic units of observation individual production units, not specific services. Variations in patterns of manpower or other inputs used across medical practices, dental practices, hospitals, pharmacies, etc. are identified and linked to variations in output use. This amounts to direct estimation of the production function of (13-9), relating quantity of output in each practice to the amounts of different inputs which it employs.

Immediately, however, one is faced with the problem of defining output. Equation 13-9 referred to a single type of service, S_j, such as an item in a fee schedule, for which it makes sense to think of one or several alternative, but specific, production processes. S_j measures a quantity of (more or less) homogeneous units. But what is the "output" of a medical or dental practice, or a hospital? Obviously, it is a vector, a range of different services or commodities in different amounts. If each practice, or unit of observation, produced the same range of different services in the same proportions, then we could measure the "output" of each by focussing on its production of any one service—say office visits. But they do not, and such portmanteau concepts as an office visit or a hospital day or stay may conceal a great deal of inter-practice or inter-institution variety.

Given an extremely large number of observations, as well as detailed output information on each, one could probably take direct account of

---

[23] That this may be *possible* does not imply that it can be assumed. Pangloss-style circular reasoning can lead one into the trap of believing that if more efficient manpower use were possible, rational, self-interested practitioners in the field would have discovered and adopted such techniques. Therefore, any discrepancy between the field and the "engineering" analysis indicates flaws in the latter. As chapters 6 and 7 demonstrate, this would be theoretically untenable even if managers in the field were fully rational, fully self-interested, and unregulated—which they are not. There are good economic reasons to believe the models may be right.

this variation in output pattern.[24] Instead, however, analysts use a single scalar measure of practice output,

$$Q^v = W_1 S_1^v + \text{---} W_m S_m^v \qquad (13\text{-}11)$$

where now Q^v and S^v refer to the output index and the services of different types produced by the vth practice or production unit. The weights W_j must be the same for each practice. If each practice faces the same set of service prices—or a common fee schedule—as do medical practices in each of the Canadian provinces, then we may use these fees as weights:

$$B^v = Q^v = f_1 S_1^v + \text{---} f_m S_m^v \qquad (13\text{-}12)$$

Then total practice billings are a proxy for total output, whose usefulness depends on the accuracy with which the f_j, specific service fees, reflect the relative resource costs of the different services—including self-employed practitioner time. In an environment where fees are variable across practices, one must deflate practice billings by some index of the relative fees charged in that practice, if available. Alternatively, one may abandon billings entirely and use one or a handful of specific classes of services (with weights assigned a priori by the analyst) as representative of the practice as a whole, in the hopes that other service outputs will either move more or less in proportion, or be "small."

However the output definition problem is addressed (and like the problem of representativeness of detailed practice data, it can only be addressed, not solved), the analyst assembles data:

$$Q^1, R_1^1, R_2^1, \text{---} R_q^1$$
$$\text{------------}$$
$$Q^v, R_1^v, R_2^v, \text{---} R_q^v$$

on each of v practices, indicating their levels of use of each of the classes of input, and resulting index of output. She then seeks some mathematical formula which will combine the R_k^v in each practice to produce an estimated level of output $\hat{Q}^v$ for that practice. A "good" formula is one which leads to small discrepancies between actual observed Q^v and the $\hat{Q}^v$ given by the formula. A common approach is to try to minimize $\Sigma (Q^v - \hat{Q}^v)^2$ or the sum of the squared deviations between actual and "predicted" output. For any particular formula the analyst chooses, statistical techniques can be used to select parameters to achieve the "least

---

[24] Perhaps instead of estimating $S = h(R_1 \text{---} R_q)$ by multiple correlation techniques, one could estimate $g(S_1 \text{---} S_m) = h(R_1 \text{---} R_q)$ by canonical correlation. I do not know, and do not believe anyone has.

squares'' fit, but the choice of the formula itself, the functional form, is part of the black art of econometrics.[25]

However it be done, the end product is some relationship, say, for example:

$$Q^v = \hat{Q}^v + e^v = A(R_1^v)^\alpha (R_2^v)^\beta (R_3^v)^\gamma + e^v \qquad (13\text{-}13)$$

where A, α, β, γ, are the same across all observed and analyzed practices, and e^v is a measure of the extent to which the formula fails to match the actual output of the practice. Small values of e^v relative to Q^v suggest that the formula is a good representation of the way in which the various types of inputs, personnel, capital equipment and/or supplies, are combined to yield service output.[26]

Such a relationship, once found, is merely one way of expressing the "production function," the relationship between productive resources and outputs of goods and services. The technology matrix T is similarly a production function, or set of them, as is a model of a practice designed for computer simulation. The single equation analytic representation of this relationship is popular among economists because of its compactness and analytic tractability, but it has the vices as well as the virtues of simplicity.[27]

For the purposes of manpower planning, however, an analytic representation such as equation (13-13) can be helpful. It permits us to measure the productivity, in actual practice experience, of different mixes of inputs. In this way, it parallels the type of evidence which arises when specified practices are augmented by additional and/or more highly trained personnel. Letting R_k be some form of intermediate-level personnel, for example, equation (13-13) enables us to read off the increase in practice

---

[25] This is the same process as is carried out in fitting hospital cost functions; see chapter 9.

[26] There is, of course, a good deal more to the story than this. Equation 13-13 is not necessarily the best functional form available, only one convenient for representation. Three classes of inputs involve a disturbing degree of aggregation—physician, non-physician, and square feet of office space, *e.g.*, or dentists, non-dentists, and drills—of inputs which may have widely differing characteristics and capacities. But the data available on each practice, system-wide, is often insufficient for greater detail.

[27] Indeed there is a serious methodological question as to whether such relationships exist in any causal or structural sense, particularly when estimated at the aggregate, economy-wide level, or whether their "estimation" is merely picking up parallel trends in economic aggregation. At the level of more homogeneous activities, primary medical practice, *e.g.*, or dental practice, distortions imposed by aggregation are much less severe. But considerable caution is warranted—a single-equation production function fitted across acute care hospitals, for example, may be more misleading than informative.

output which results from increasing by one the number (FTEs) of such people in a practice for given numbers of other inputs.

The analysis generalizes to multiple inputs, divisible into fractional FTE values. It provides a mathematical representation of the extent to which different inputs—such as professionals and auxiliaries—can substitute for each other. The relationship (in more sophisticated forms than 13-13) can embody increasing or decreasing returns to scale over different levels of output. It will usually indicate declining marginal productivity for a particular input resource; if, for example, professional and auxiliary time were the only inputs in production, then as the auxiliary to professional ratio rose, the contribution to output of additional auxiliaries would tend to fall.[28] But in general a given volume of services may be produced with very different mixes of inputs, particularly manpower inputs.

FOR WHOM IS EFFICIENT MANPOWER USE OPTIMAL?

What is possible, however, is not necessarily optimal. At the level of the individual practice, optimality is achieved when the cost of adding one more unit of an input just balances its contribution to revenue— marginal outlay equals revenue product. (This makes the strong assumption that the practice objective is profit-maximization). If auxiliaries are available in a reasonably free market at a constant wage, marginal outlay equals that wage, plus perhaps some additional administrative overhead. Underutilization of auxiliaries (or any other input) would be indicated if the amount of additional practice revenue which an additional auxiliary would generate exceeds the wage plus overhead cost of that auxiliary.

A number of such studies have indicated underuse in this sense. Using an estimated relationship similar to (13-13), plus information on the relative wage rates of professionals and auxiliaries, one can demonstrate what the optimal mix of inputs would be—optimal in the sense of maximizing practice net income per professional—and thus what the physical output of services per professional could be. The results generally indicate substantial potential for gains in output per professional. Any given level of aggregate output, system-wide, could be produced with fewer professionals and more auxiliaries, and at lower overall cost.

---

[28] Returns *to scale* refers to the pattern of output response when all inputs are increased or decreased in proportion; increasing, decreasing, and constant returns to scale describing greater, lesser, or equi-proportionate output change. Diminishing returns to a single input or factor refers to a tendency for increases in output to become progressively smaller as units of a particular input are added to production, holding all others fixed in supply. A combination of constant returns to scale but diminishing returns to each factor is built into the T matrix, being most pronounced in the expanded form of equation (13-10). Its derivation, however, is a bit more involved.

This leaves an important question as to why the existing system leads to underutilization. This issue has been dealt with from a different perspective in chapters 6 and 7; here our focus will be on the implications of this observation for manpower policy.

One suggestion is that the wage rate understates the cost of using auxiliaries in individual practices because professionals do not like to work with, or supervise, large teams. If so, the underuse represents a form of non-money income or satisfaction for professionals, which their strategic position in the management of provider firms enables them to indulge at the cost of the public generally.

Alternatively, however, one should note that equation (13-13) does not in fact describe the relationship of inputs to practice *revenues*, but only to physical outputs. If one can assume that additional output will be reimbursed at the same price (fee) as current output, then it is legitimate to compare physical productivity, multiplied by those fees, to wage costs. But this assumes that each practice faces infinitely elastic demand at the going price. It may be, however, that increased output must be "marketed." This could be, in the rather implausible neo-classical model, by price-cutting and competitive behaviour. More plausibly, particularly in the Canadian setting where each practice faces the same fixed fee schedule, the practitioner must adjust practice style, recall patients more frequently, and generally invest in expanding utilization to match capacity. In either case, however, costs are incurred which may be monetary, or more likely, direct disutility. "Marketing" and entrepreneurial behaviour generally are considered unprofessional. The net effect may be that for an individual practice, expansion may be "unprofitable" in a total utility sense, even if in purely technical terms, less costly outputs could be substituted for more.[29]

These considerations greatly complicate the manpower planners' problem. The cross-practice studies tend to confirm the non-optimality—

---

[29] In the jargon, practice profits are maximized, with respect to any input, when marginal outlay (MO) = marginal revenue product (MRP). (We assume that as utilization of any input increases, MO is either constant or rising, MRP is constant or falling.) If input markets are competitive, MO = Wage (W)—inputs can be hired at a constant unit price each, however many are hired. If output markets are competitive (or fixed fee), MRP = value of marginal physical product (VMP), and VMP = Price of output (P) times marginal physical product (MPP). Equation 13-13 enables one to calculate MPP, and optimal input is chosen where MPP = (W/P). (As input use increases, MPP starts high and falls). But if P falls as output increases (the practice faces a downward-sloping demand curve for its own output) then $MRP < VMP = P \times MPP$, because increasing output requires price cuts. So $MRP = W < P \times MPP$, and $MPP > (W/P)$—less input will be hired. The same effect will arise if P is nominally constant—fixed fees—but costly marketing effort (in money or pride) must be undertaken to expand the practice.

excessive costliness—of current manpower mixes which emerges from
direct analyses of health care production. Their evidence on this score is
particularly important because the econometric methodology is subject
to severe conservative biases. In particular, it cannot show the potential
for manpower substitution by types of personnel not now in use because
of legal, habitual, or other restrictions. Equation (13-13) reflects only
what is, not what could be. Further, it builds in all the arbitrary behavioural patterns of individual practitioners and treats them as technological
constraints. A common finding, for example, is that differentiation among
different types of auxiliary personnel—high and low skill—does not improve the fit of equations like (13-13), so all are lumped together. Yet
we know that the productivity of these different people is potentially very
different; the problem arises in the way they are being used. Different
patterns of use in the United States of females (nurses) and males (physician assistants) with similar training suggest the same problem. Statistical studies of actual practices thus indicate the bare minimum of
possibility.[30] The activity analysis models, based on identifying patterns
of service needs and the technical capabilities of different types of personnel, suggest that one can go much farther.

THE ONLY THINGS WE LEARN . . .?

But the behavioural and ''marketing'' limits raise the very awkward
question: How? Suppose one had all the data necessary to fill in the
matrices of equations (13-6) and (13-10), and had made the political
decisions involved. Educational programs were then re-ordered to produce
the manpower needed in the optimal mixes and amounts $(M_1 --- M_q)$,
allowing for the differential productivities of the different constituents of
each stock M. What then? If individual provider units make use of non-
optimal mixes of manpower, for (economic or non-economic) reasons
which seem to them good, the results will be under– or unemployed
personnel of some types, and shortages of others. The motivations of
individual decision-making providers may lead to patterns of macro-
behaviour which are globally inefficient, but they cannot be ignored.

The sad history of the nurse-practitioner in Canada illustrates this problem: there is no point in training people, however cost-effective, whom
practitioners will not wish to, or cannot afford to, hire. Of course the
picture is clouded by the excess supply of physicians; a serious policy
of manpower substitution would have cut back on physician supply even

---

[30] Of course if all practices were profit-maximizers operating in a fully informed, fully
competitive (which includes free entry) market environment, such behavioural distortions would have been squeezed out by competition. But if that dream-world model
applied, one would not be concerned about manpower issues in the first place.

as new types of personnel were being produced. If that had been done, the innovation might have had more chance. But one cannot be sure that an attempt to induce a ''shortage'' of medical services under present production patterns would have stimulated a shift to the more efficient model. A number of other responses, less satisfactory and politically more uncomfortable, could easily be imagined.

One is left, then, with the fairly obvious conclusion that manpower policy, however sophisticated, cannot be developed independently of the structure of the delivery system. If changes in type, quantity, and mix of personnel are desired, then they must somehow be fitted in, either to the present or to some modified form of care provision. Hence the monumental stability of health care delivery through decades of apparent change. Present manpower training decisions determine future production choices over as long as a generation, by the ''human capital'' they create. Yet present patterns of delivery severely constrain manpower choices by determining who will and will not be permitted to provide services, in what settings. Manpower policies, other than simply quantity adjustments, require simultaneous planning for and intervention in delivery, if they are to be effective.

Accordingly manpower issues make up the most difficult, far-reaching, and critical of the public investment decisons made in health care. It is no wonder they are so frequently made unconsciously, by delegation, or by default. What is perhaps remarkable is that the results are not worse than they are.

CHAPTER 14

DESIGN OR ACCIDENT IN HEALTH CARE POLICY: THE CHESHIRE CAT

ECONOMIC ANALYSIS TO WHAT (OR WHOSE) ENDS?

Economists analysing the health care industry usually adopt a clearly defined subject-object relationship. The health care system of a particular society is a social system, resource using and commodity producing, which while rather complex and displaying a number of unusual features can nevertheless be studied and evaluated at arm's length (intellectually at least), much as one would any other sector of the economy. The economist is at the eye-piece, the physician, nurse, hospital, reimbursement agency, is on the slide.

Yet it is obvious that the participants in the process view the relationship very differently. Individuals or institutions providing health care regard economic analysis (if at all) as a means to their own ends, a discipline or body of techniques akin to (though generally somewhat less useful than) biochemistry or physiology, which can be used to promote personal or collective objectives defined within the health care system itself.[1] Freidson's (1970) distinction between medical sociology and the sociology of medicine has application to economics as well.

This inversion of perspective has significant implications for economic analysis itself. The peculiar institutional features of health care delivery, if taken as a serious social response to genuine organizational problems rather than a series of accidents or nefarious plots by providers, force one back to a questioning of the usefulness of many of the standard tools and concepts of economic analysis, and a re-thinking of their underlying methodology. More generally, this process exposes the significance of certain fundamental, but rather arbitrary and crude, assumptions about individual and group behaviour which are so basic to economic analysis that it is easy to forget that they were ever made. Having worked so long with one particular map, one may need to be reminded that it is not the territory.

Indeed, this re-thinking of basic assumptions may serve as a road out of the "Pangloss-trap" (Culyer 1984) of "neo-Austrian" analysis. If we

---

[1] Readers of *The Hitchhiker's Guide to the Galaxy* may recall the mice.

believe that all behaviour *and all institutional environments* represent the outcome of optimal responses by individuals and groups to the opportunities and constraints which *they* (not external observers) perceive, then it follows that no improvement is possible on whatever situation now exists—in the private *or public* sectors—whatever is, is right.[2]

The case for amelioration, from left or right, then falls to the ground, as does the very possibility of a contribution from economic analysis. And this appears to include the first of Culyer's suggested escapes from the Pangloss-trap, the "entrepreneurial" role of the economist as educator and mobilizer of public opinion—moulder of perceptions—with respect to particular policies (see also Hartle and Trebilcock 1983). Since the economist is just as much inside the Pangloss-process as anyone else, his activities in this regard are equally subject to "optimizing" determinism and have no greater standing than those of a hired PR firm or habitué of Spouter's Corner.[3]

Culyer's second alternative, which is very much in the spirit of this text, is to apply analysis to proximal objectives defined external to the analysis itself. Of course those objectives may require further justification in terms of general political or social acceptability.[4] But the worst criticism he finds for this approach is that it is looked down upon by economists. Accordingly, this terminal chapter will postulate certain general classes of social objectives which might be sought through public intervention in the health care financing and delivery system.[5] It will then attempt

---

[2] Of course the extension of rational optimizing behaviour from the economic sphere of human activity to all other forms of interaction and institutional design rests on either an unsupported (and unsupportable) quasi-empirical generalization or an empty tautology left over from first-year philosophy. But the difficulty is that economic analysis does not appear to contain within its own methodology any definition of its scope of application, of its appropriate boundaries. (Any resemblance to certain unpopular neoplasms is *surely* accidental.)

[3] It is most interesting that in Reder's (1982) analysis of the "Chicago School" of economists and its tendency to extend its methodology over the widest range of human activities—social (the family, religion), political (law, public regulation), even genetic?—only two areas are excluded. All other forms of behaviour become endogenous and "explained" in terms of economic forces. The exclusions are the preferences of transactors, which if endogenous would no longer support the normative propositions favoured by the Chicago school (as Galbraith makes clear time and again)—and the activities of economists themselves.

[4] Or the willingness of a client to finance their pursuit . . .

[5] It will not provide a detailed critique of economic methodology in the light of its successes and failures in the health care field (though some of this is implicit, and often explicit, in the chapters above). There are two good reasons for this. Such a critique would probably be of interest (at best) to a very few economists and almost no health care people, and anyway the task is beyond me. But it needs to be done, perhaps as part of a more general re-thinking of economic methodology.

(very roughly) to evaluate the current (early 1980s) experience with public health insurance in Canada and its possible future developments. Of course all forecasts will be falsified, just as all generalizations are false. But extrapolating the forces presently at work enables one to sketch alternative scenarios which appear internally consistent and plausible, and to rule out others as inconsistent or implausible.

OBJECTIVES OF HEALTH POLICY: A SUGGESTED AGENDA

As the Cheshire Cat pointed out some time ago, if you don't much care where you get to, it doesn't matter which way you go. If you do, it does. And if we, by doing some considerable violence to the actual processes involved, think of public policy toward health care and particularly toward health care finance as making up a sort of very large scale public program or super-project, then we can discern several different types of objectives which may be thought of as the potential benefits from that intervention (Evans and Williamson 1978, Chapter 1; Barer *et al.* 1979).

The objectives which societies and their representative politicians, administrators, and professionals seek through public health care policy can be divided into two major groups, financial, and "real" or functional. The first class, financial objectives, refer to the patterns of claims over goods and services, of credits and debits, across the members of the society, which arise as a result of the incidence of illness and the response of the health care system. In principle (though not in practice) one could imagine financial policies reshuffling these claims, redistributing the burdens of illness and the costs of health care, quite independently of any impact on the health care delivery system itself. Indeed "idealized" insurance programs, free of problems of adverse selection or moral hazard and embodying no *ex ante* subsidies, would do just that. They would redistribute financial resources *ex post* from those who did not to those who did become ill and use care, without influencing levels or patterns of care utilization or production.

Functional objectives, on the other hand, relate to the actual patterns of care: What sorts of goods and services are produced, in what quantities, how, and for whom? In seeking such objectives, public policy intervenes directly in the process of care provision to modify the behaviour of the health care industry and/or of its customers, relative to that which would have been displayed in a competitive marketplace of (more or less) voluntary exchange.

The financial objectives are primarily, though not entirely, redistributional—"spreading the burdens of care." The economic burdens of illness range from the costs of associated "needed" care, through lost income, to pure loss of life satisfactions (utility)—or life. Most societies attempt to redistribute resources in favour of those with large care costs. Some include public systems of income replacement; none (for reasons discussed in chapter 2) appear to address pure welfare losses. However as chapter 2 also pointed out, *public* redistributional policy as expressed though public insurance programs, generally redistributes *ex ante*, from people with low risk of illness, or at least low expected health care cost, to those with high. Competitive private insurance will handle *ex post* redistribution, if that is a social or private objective, but will tend to charge differential premiums (or build in self-selection mechanisms) according to expected loss or risk status. Public insurance transfers wealth across risk classes.

Of course private insurance systems are not perfect, and market failures may develop in private risk-bearing markets. It is quite possible that persons may find themselves unable to purchase health insurance, even though they are willing and able to pay the actuarially fair premium plus a competitive load factor. This failure can arise either because adverse selection makes it impossible for such persons to identify themselves to policy-sellers—being lost in a crowd of higher risk people—or because scale economies, market size, and selling expense lead to an over-diversified or monopolized supply of policies and correspondingly excessive load factors. In this case, compulsory public insurance can remedy failure in private insurance markets—an efficiency objective—quite independently of any impact on either wealth redistribution or patterns of care delivery.

Further, public policy can and does have a significant impact on patterns of income and wealth distribution between providers and users of health care. If all care were provided by for-profit firms operating under exogenous demand curve constraints in perfectly competitive markets with free entry and no specialized irreproducible inputs, then of course all factor inputs would earn their opportunity costs regardless of how public policy affected the overall size or shape of the industry. But this textbook picture bears no resemblance to any actual health care system. And the incomes of health care workers, relative to the rest of society, are quite sensitive to public policies toward occupational regulation, organization, and payment. The dramatic swings in (relative) Canadian physician incomes under private and public insurance, and the contrasting experience of United States physicians, and of Canadian dentists, under mixed private insurance and self-pay regimes, serve as examples; but so do relative wage patterns in hospitals, or profit rates from pharmaceutical sales. A significant part of public health care policy, particularly as it affects "costs," is in fact a form of industry- or sub-industry-specific income policy serving to advance or to contain the income aspirations of particular groups.

Moving from the financial to the functional side, public policy has historically been divided into regulatory policies—principally delegated to professional groups—intended to affect the pattern or mix of services provided, and financial policies—from subsidies to universal insurance—intended to affect the overall level of provision. The initial emphasis of public insurance was on expanding overall utilization—"reducing the barriers to care"—in whatever way providers thought appropriate. More recent emphasis on cost containment uses the payment system to try to restrict overall levels of utilization—capacity and budget restraints in hospitals, controls on physician immigration and (to some extent) domestic supply—while still relying on providers to determine mix. But it is clear that public policy objectives encompass mix of services—maintenance of quality, suppression of quackery, linkage of provision to "needs"—as well as overall volume. Otherwise the whole apparatus of direct and delegated regulatory authority lacks justification.

These functional objectives of public policy, relating to the volume and the mix of care provided, and the particular recipients, are yet another way of expressing the idea from chapter 1 that the resource/health status relationship of Figure 1-3 is the proper concern of public policy. If the ultimate objective of policy is the attainment of a satisfactory relationship between resources used and health status attained, then it follows that policy must be concerned with amounts and patterns of care use.

But it also follows that the technical efficiency of care provision also is, or should be, a policy issue. And while that theme has emerged frequently in the discussion above, it does not appear to have been a major concern of Canadian providers or users of, or payers for, health care. Somehow efficiency was expected to be achieved spontaneously, as a by-product of the professional process. The initial pressure for public insurance was to provide a means of both increasing utilization by some segments of the population, and redistributing financial resources between low and high users—reducing barriers and spreading burdens. Later it was viewed as a means of containing provider incomes and rationing overall utilization. But the perception that regulatory and payment policies have a major impact, for good or ill, on the actual resource costs of whatever care is provided has had relatively little influence on public debate—except among economists.[6]

COMPETING SOURCES OF LEGITIMACY: POLITICAL, PROFESSIONAL, AND MARKET

With this set of fairly general objectives in hand, and noting that the

---

[6] Everyone agrees, when pressed, that efficiency objectives are very important; but they seem to lack political appeal. People will fight for social justice, equity, liberty, rights to care—but not, alas, for efficiency.

particular expression of those objectives varies over time and persons,[7] we can consider where the Canadian health care system is now, and how it may unfold. In the process we may distinguish three different sources of legitimacy or processes of control—political, professional, and market—which confront each other with competing claims to define and govern the pursuit of these objectives. They represent deeply rooted ideological patterns as well as coalitions of particular interests. Each proposes a set of institutions which will give rise to patterns of incentives and information flows and which in turn will generate outcomes in terms of patterns of resource use and wealth distribution. Each postulates an ideal form (more or less unrealistic) of the health care system organized through its preferred institutions, yet suffers from characteristic vices which are all too apparent to its competitors (Culyer 1982). Public policy (or its absence) emerges from the tension among these three.

At present, Canadian hospital and medical care policy is in a state of tension between political and professional ideologies and sources of legitimacy, with a comparatively small role for market forces.[8] Advocates of the professional view sometimes use the rhetoric of the market—"free enterprise"—in their attempts to influence the political process, but this should not be confused with support for an unregulated delivery system. This tension was built into the public health insurance system *ab initio*, as a result of failure to question the assumptions of the "Medico-Technical" model of health care utilization outlined in chapter 1.

Professional ideology holds that the practice of medicine is the preserve of physicians, or more generally, that professional activities are properly controlled by professionals. Making health a "political issue" is an improper development both in itself and because it leads to poorer health care. There may be some bitter debate from time to time as to *which* particular group of professionals has responsibility for which activities, but it is a breach of professional decorum if this debate should unfortunately spill into the public arena. (Public disagreements also weaken the political position of professions, by undercutting claims of collective expertise.)

Within this ideological framework, professionals not only claim exclusive jurisdiction over *how* medicine is practiced, or health care provided, but also over *how much* care is appropriate. They allege the right,

---

[7] Both medical associations and provincial reimbursement agencies, for example, accept relative provider incomes as a significant objective of public policy. They just attach different signs to its weight.

[8] One might suggest that dentistry is in tension (in most provinces) between professional and market ideologies, with a small role for the political process, and drugs and appliances lie between politics and the market, with some limited professional component. But this appealing symmetry is probably overstated.

on the basis of superior expertise, to determine not only where the curve in Figure 1-3 is located, but how far along it a given society should move. Moreover, though somewhat less confidently, professional ideology holds that professionals should determine their own incomes, relative to the rest of society. This is expressed, not in the form of claims to specific entitlements, but in assertion of the right of the individual practitioner to set her own fees, in a "market" reserved for and closely regulated by the profession itself.

Public policy in Canada has not explicitly challenged these professional claims, but has put in place a financing system which is directly in conflict with them. By centralizing the reimbursement of both hospitals and physicians through budget- and fee-setting negotiations, the state has indirectly entered both the "practice of medicine" and the income-determination process in a major way. While leaving professionals in primary control of how available resources will be used, and (by setting the internal structure of fee schedules for self-employed practitioners) of the relative remuneration of different specialties or patterns of activity, the state in setting overall limits is implicitly (and sometimes explicitly) determining what facilities shall not be available, what services shall be discouraged or not provided at all, and (more roughly) what limits shall apply to practitioner or hospital workers' incomes. Its justification for such intervention can be found in overwhelming public support for the Medicare program, whatever the public may think of the particular governments which administer it.

This conflict of competing legitimacies, expertise versus collective choice, is encapsulated in the "underfunding" versus "cost-explosion" arguments of the early 1980s. "Underfunding" means that the state, or society more generally, is not providing sufficient resources to the health care system, either to provide the level of health care servicing which professionals judge appropriate, or to pay the incomes to which they aspire. For obvious political reasons the former shortfall is more openly alleged, although as noted in chapter 7, the availability of hospital facilities affects provider incomes as well.

"Cost explosions," by contrast, imply the converse, too much servicing, of minimal or no benefit at the margin, and/or provided by people who are overpaid or working inefficiently. If none of these implications is accepted, then an increase in costs is a social gain, not a policy problem.

CONSTRUCTIVE INCONSISTENCY: PAPERING OVER THE CRACKS CAN WORK

The outcome of this tension between ideologies has, so far, been a quite constructive inconsistency. The Canadian health care system scores comparatively well on both financial and functional dimensions. Most of the economic burden of health care expense (though not, obviously, the burden of illness) is distributed across society in relation to taxable capacity generally, as indicated by income and expenditure, and is not related to the actual or anticipated illness or expenditure experience of the individual.[9] Universal coverage ensures that no one will be dropped out of the insurance system as a result of adverse selection.[10] And the direct bargaining between state and providers has placed some limits on the process of wealth transfer from the rest of society to providers, a process which during the 1950s and 1960s was proceeding apparently unchecked. Of these effects, only the public assumption of risk-bearing can be interpreted as an efficiency gain, but the other pattern of wealth transfer—healthy to sick, low risk to high risk, and provider to citizen/taxpayer (at least relative to what might otherwise have occurred)—seems to be in line with general social priorities.

On the functional side the picture is somewhat less clear. A substantial amount of literature (Boulet and Henderson 1979; Siemiatycki *et al.* 1980; Broyles *et al.* 1983) suggests that the public insurance system does serve to redistribute health care in favour of "sicker" as well as lower income users. Its influence on overall use is much more difficult to disentangle from that of the general expansion in hospital facilities during the 1950s and 1960s, and in physician supply during the 1960s and 1970s. On balance, however, it appears that the combination of public control over total resources plus professional control over specific applications—priority setting—has led to a more effective use of those resources than would have resulted either from an attempt at direct public control of utilization patterns (which would probably have been politically, if not administratively, impossible), or from a continuation of pre-Medicare policies which amounted to almost a blank cheque for providers. That is not to say that

---

[9] There are of course in some provinces exceptions to this generalization; extra-billing and user charges, and premiums. Premiums, being unrelated to the insured person's expectation of illness, and *de facto* compulsory for most people, are best thought of as a form of poll tax. They do not relate tax burden to ability to pay, and thus offend against a major principle of tax equity, but they do not link it to actual or anticipated care use either. (They may, however, create problems of access if vulnerable groups become uninsured by dropping out of the premium system, *e.g.*, as a result of unemployment.) User charges and extra-billing are difficult to reconcile with the central Medicare principles of universal, comprehensive, publicly administered coverage. As will be discussed below, they inject a foreign element which could represent a transition stage to a very different type of system. They may also, now that the *Canada Health Act* penalizes provincial governments which impose or permit them, be in the process of disappearing. But that is far from certain.

[10] It may lead to certain people being compelled to accept non-optimal "over-coverage," but this is by no means obvious a priori; see the discussion in Evans (1983).

the present health care delivery system is optimized with respect to effectiveness, but only that the compromise has worked relatively well up to now, especially considering the alternatives displayed in other countries.

Where it has functioned less well is in the area of technical efficiency. As emphasized above, cost-reducing innovations, such as manpower substitution or ambulatory alternatives to inpatient care, threaten jobs which in an environment of budgetary constraint may not be made up elsewhere. United States critics of the Canadian system as "public utility" medicine *do* have a point. Innovation has been blocked, not so much in the cost-expanding technologies, which generate their own constituencies rapidly enough, but in the cost-reducing ones for which no constituency exists. And natural experiments do not occur in a uniform public system. The Canadian financing system has tended to freeze in place organizational structures and modes of care provision and delivery, and so to maintain higher than necessary costs of care.[11]

IF THE CRACKS WIDEN, CAN MORE MONEY FILL THEM?

So far so good, but can the compromise, the unresolved conflict between professional and political ideologies, be maintained? Should it be? If so, how? If not, what are the alternatives and what are their likely effects?

The principal source of concern about the viability of the present structure stems from the level of political conflict which it generates, a conflict which is being only partly moderated by the short-run expedient of allowing the health care share of GNP to increase a bit, and releasing much of the pressure on physician fees.[12] Lying behind this conflict is the longer run problem of manpower oversupply (or at least escalation) noted in chapter 13, and the shifts in demography and technology which exacerbate perceived "needs." Just as provincial governments find themselves under

---

[11] Of course, it is easy to confuse the shadow and the substance. The "blooming, buzzing confusion" of the entrepreneurial U.S. system generates a high volume of innovative ideas, but (thus far) remarkably little real progress in improved global efficiency, as opposed to technological virtuosity.

[12] The most obvious source of conflict is the process of relative income determination for providers. While the pre-Medicare environment of professional control of the "market" and private insurance appeared to place no limit on the escalation of provider relative incomes, the present monopoly/monopsony bargaining environment is believed by providers to place them in an unduly weak position. They can only protect themselves from progressively eroding relative incomes—"exploitation" by government on behalf of the taxpayer—by either strikes or threats to the integrity of the insurance system itself—opting out and/or extra billing.

increasingly acute resource pressures, providers perceive a dramatic expansion in their ability to provide effective therapy—if only resources
were available. If both sides grow weary of the endless conflict, the result
could be changes which could lead to quite a different system.

The simplest response to the "underfunding" claim would be to expand
public funding for health care, either by raising taxes or by cutting other
public programs. As commentators on the "politics of restraint" have
pointed out (Dobell 1983), Canadian provincial governments are struggling with the balancing of priorities, not with an absolute lack of resources. Many, indeed most, other developed countries spend a higher
proportion of their national resources on health; why shouldn't we?

The answer is that quite apart from the question of the efficacy of the
additional services which these resources would buy, the conflict situation
would not in fact be mitigated. As pointed out in chapter 1, only the
"finite needs" model of Figure 1-3a, combined with bounded relative
income aspirations, is consistent with a stable upper bound on health care
spending generated within the health care system itself. In the more
realistic case of Figure 1-3b, or adaptive income expectations (or entry
of personnel in response to incomes), the health system has *no* self-
limiting mechanism. Ten percent of GNP, once established as a norm,
would soon become "under-funding," as would twelve. The experience
of other countries, not just the United States, is that upward pressures
on costs, and political conflict, do not abate at higher levels of spending.
They are only moderated by continuing relative increases.[13] Thus expansion of public spending on health care, while it would undoubtedly lead

---

This "safety-valve" view of direct charges has two serious weaknesses. As a collective tactic it imposes no costs on the profession, unlike a strike which harms both
striker and employer and thus creates incentives for settlement. Secondly, it places
pressure on individual patients in a dispute between profession and government. In a
sense, direct billing is a perfectly flexible strike weapon: refusal to serve if pay demands
are not granted, on a case-by-case basis.

Yet it does respond to a real issue. The present funding system *does* represent a
long-term "incomes policy" for health care workers, administered by a government
which has a direct interest in holding their relative incomes down. Strike threats (or
strikes) in hospitals have thus far maintained hospital incomes, but no satisfactory
mechanism of arbitrating physician incomes has yet been developed. Physicians' principal negotiation tactic has been to threaten to wreck the payment system (and to try
to gain public support for doing so), a threat which must become ever more strident
to maintain credibility.

[13] Ironic confirmation of this was given by the Canadian Medical Association in its
testimony before the Special Committee on the Federal-Provincial Fiscal Arrangements
(Breau Committee) (Canadian Medical Association 1981). Working under the common
handicap of out-of-date data, they argued that 7 percent of GNP spent on health was
far too low, and that 8.2 percent (which looks rather like a half-way point between
the then-available Canada and U.S. rates) should be a target to be reached over about

to increased provider satisfaction for a time, because it would transfer wealth from taxpayers or beneficiaries of other public programs to health providers, and expand health care service output, would eventually lead back to the same situation we now face.

PRIVATE VERSUS PUBLIC MONEY: USER CHARGES, EXTRA-BILLING, OR "PATIENT PARTICIPATION"

In any case, federal and provincial governments appear very reluctant to move in this direction. Accordingly, an alternative proposed by some provider representatives is "diversification of funding sources"—direct charges to patients over and above public reimbursement rates, eventually supported by the reintroduction of private insurance. This evolution, building on a combination of open-ended extra-billing by physicians and direct charges by hospitals, appears to offer both relief for provincial treasurers, by holding down public expenditures for health care, and the opportunity for health care providers to increase their incomes and the level of services they provide.

Direct charges to patients, euphemistically described as "patient participation," are ironically advocated both as a means of increasing health expenditures (by Canadian medical associations and some hospital people) and of controlling or reducing health costs (principally by American economists but also by some private health insurance people, working with an assumption of exogenous demand curves; see chapter 2). They are unlikely to do both, for mathematical reasons which are not very complex. There are many different ways of structuring and administering direct charge systems, but on balance it seems most probable that if such charges are administered by providers at their own discretion, individually or collectively, they will have the cost-expansion effects predicted and sought by their Canadian advocates. The American arguments for cost-control effects rest on rather special assumptions which are difficult to justify (Barer *et al.* 1979).[14]

---

five years. The very next year, 1982, a combination of recession plus increased health spending brought the actual figure to just under 8.5 percent—but the system is still alleged to be "underfunded." The reply by CMA spokesmen that the CMA's target assumed increased health spending, not decreased GNP, is reasonable, except that it shifts smoothly from a relative to an absolute spending standard, and is inconsistent with the 1981 CMA position that as a country becomes richer (GNP rising) its share spent on health should also rise. Not to labour the point, the CMA objective was clearly, and quite understandably from their perspective, "More." The specific numbers were just means to that end.

[14] Indeed the argument sometimes put by advocates of direct charges, that provider discretion will ensure that no one who "cannot afford" to pay (in the provider's judgement) will be charged, and that no one will be denied services through inability

The short-run effects of a shift toward more "private" financing, patient payment with or without private insurance, can be extrapolated from current experience with physician opting out and extra-billing in Ontario and Alberta, and from pre-Medicare experience in Canada and United States experience in the 1970s. But the long-run picture is much less clear, and could involve quite dramatic changes in the whole framework of health care organization. The key question is the extent to which the regulatory framework evolves to permit competitive market forces to influence the process of supply.

These short-run effects would be primarily a wealth transfer from patients to providers—higher incomes for physicians—and perhaps to some extent to taxpayers as well if public reimbursement rates escalated less rapidly in consequence. Moreover these transfers would be quite uneven. Alberta data on extra-billing (Plain 1982) show a very small proportion of physicians making very large earnings from extra-billing, while a much larger number earn small amounts (relative to their reimbursement by the public plan) and serve as political and ideological "spear carriers" for the principal beneficiaries. Wolfson and Tuohy (1980) similarly find the principal effect of opting out of Medicare in Ontario to be elevated physician prices and incomes, with concentration of opting out in particular specialties and regions. Thus the wealth transfers are drawn, not from patients in general, but from patients in particular regions and with particular types of problems. Hospital user charges similarly fall most heavily on a relatively small proportion of the population, as hospital use tends to be highly concentrated among the aged and chronically ill.

In addition to these health-related wealth redistribution effects, direct charges appear to have some impact on patterns of care use. Stoddart and Woodward (1980) found evidence of a negative effect of opting out on use by lower income patients, and the studies reviewed by Beck and Horne (1978) and Boulet and Henderson (1979) clearly support the proposition that direct charges inhibit use by the poorer members of the population. But as noted in chapter 7 (see also Barer *et al.* 1979) it does not follow that overall use falls. The principal effect of charges may be to redistribute care from more to less price-sensitive individuals.[15]

---

to pay, can be translated into the framework of the price-discriminating monopolist of chapter 7, charging different prices to each buyer. Total revenue is thus maximized, while output need not change at all, and the entire effect of the policy is to increase prices and provider incomes. Of course providers have neither the ability nor the desire to discriminate so perfectly, and what someone else "can afford" is a very imprecise concept.

[15] How such redistribution would affect the matching of use to needs is difficult to determine conclusively. But the well-established correlations of age, illness, and poverty should certainly place the burden of proof on advocates of charges. Even if, *at*

Apart from these wealth redistributions, it is difficult to see any clear-cut effects on use of care. It is sometimes suggested that hospital user charges might lower overall utilization rates; but the empirical evidence does not support this hypothesis. As noted above, all analyses of hospital utilization show it as, in total, primarily capacity-driven, at least in a fee-for-service context. If, as some of their advocates suggest, user fees were to *increase* total resources available for care, they might support greater servicing intensity, and perhaps higher physician billings.

The impact of extra-billing or user fees on medical service supply is ambiguous. Their presence or absence is unlikely to affect rates of domestic physician training. If the prohibition of extra-billing led to physician out-migration, this would tend to lower utilization and costs. If on the other hand extra-billing should spread, and fee levels per procedure correspondingly rose, the present physician stock might supply less effort at higher income levels (the income/leisure trade-off). The resulting lower level of servicing could then masquerade as a demand response. But overall, effects on care use are likely to be small.

A Medicare system characterized by a relatively low level of direct charges, as those in several provinces have been *ab initio*, thus appears to score somewhat less well than a comprehensive one on both our financial criteria—risk reduction and equity of burden—and perhaps slightly worse, but not very different, on the functional ones. But precisely because it is *not* very different, such a system does not resolve the conflict between political and professional objectives and authority over the health care system.[16] Direct charges on a limited scale may be ideologically offensive or satisfying, and may create specific cases of hardship and affluence, but they preserve the fundamental tension between political responsibility for global funding (95 percent, if not 100 percent) and professional responsibility for what is to be done. The third or market criterion—individual willingness and ability to pay—is suppressed through the continued agreement by both professionals and politicians that needs should govern use, and that supply should be closely regulated.

DISMANTLING MEDICARE: PRIVATE FUNDING, PRIVATE INSURANCE, AND PRIVATE DELIVERY

If neither increased public funding nor small-scale direct charges significantly modify the existing confrontation, what other alternatives exist?

---

the margin, little or no connection is found between health care use and health, it does not follow that a policy which serves to redistribute care from the more to the less ill should be regarded with indifference, much less applauded.

[16] Alberta and Ontario, where physician opting out and extra-billing is most common, do not have noticeably more amicable negotiating processes.

One possibility is a withdrawal or scaling down of the political role in funding, with or without a major change in regulation, and a reversion to a major role for private insurance carriers. This could come about, for example, if provincial governments deliberately held fee schedule and hospital budget escalation well below the growth of the general economy, and permitted or encouraged physicians and hospitals to bill patients for additional amounts.[17] In this case, the proportion of bills paid out-of-pocket would escalate, and the political feasibility of (and justification for) the ban on private insurance would vanish. Private coverage would, like United States "wraparound" coverage for their incomplete form of Medicare, arise to fill in gaps in public coverage, and depending on premium levels for public coverage (in those provinces levying premiums), some groups of the population could find it preferable to move out of the public program altogether. The dismantling of the "Medibank" program in Australia (Deeble 1982) is an example of such a process, where public program premiums and benefit schedules were deliberately manipulated to encourage middle– and upper-income people to buy private coverage.[18]

Canadian past and United States present experience with multiple funding sources, mixed public and private insurance and self-pay, suggests that such a shift would significantly redistribute wealth from ill to well, high-risk to low-risk people, and patients to providers. It would probably expand the volume of services provided, while making access more dependent on income. The key thing it would *not* do, however, is constrain expenditure. It would not answer the question of how much to spend, other than by the professionals' answer—more.

Thus the professionals' recommendation of diversified funding sources and less government interference appears to be dynamically unstable, and to lead towards the present American situation. There, governments are hard-pressed to meet even their limited share of a rapidly expanding total health bill and, in a fragmented funding system, lack the administrative mechanisms as well as the political will and mandate to establish control. But the cost explosion also places great strains on the business firms and unions funding private insurance. From these, along with government, comes the political pressure to "do something." The response so far has been to increase reliance on market-type institutions, on "competition," in the real sense, not as the words are used by professionals. From

---

[17] Alberta shows some signs of moving in this direction, but no province has openly adopted such a policy, and some have specifically rejected it.

[18] The federal government's attitude toward criteria for cost-sharing would become critical here. The passage of the *Canada Health Act* in early 1984 clearly indicates that, for the present at least, the federal government will *not* permit such an evolution, so this discussion is hypothetical. Whether the Act will lead to the prohibition of direct charges altogether, is more problematic.

insurance markets, privatization spreads (inevitably?) to health care markets themselves.

WHAT HAPPENS NEXT? THE UNITED STATES ALTERNATIVES

But for the reasons analysed in chapter 10, for-profit firms in a health care environment—hospitals, laboratories, pharmaceutical firms, medical clinics—make their profits from sales, not cost containment. The incredibly fuzzy United States thinking which, presumably muddled by ideological symbols, equated private for-profit enterprise with cost control, has begun to undergo reality therapy. The future directions offered seem to be threefold.

One, arising from the "welfare burden" arguments of chapter 2, traces the problem back to excessive insurance stimulated by public subsidy, and offers the hope that the "magic bullet" of taxing employer-paid health insurance premiums in the hands of the employee will lead to reduced insurance coverage and an increase in the numbers of cost-conscious shopper-patients who will impose market constraints on provider behaviour. Since it rests ultimately on the hypothesis of an exogenous demand curve for care, this approach of relying on *individual* self-paying consumers to exercise the ultimate control over how much of what sorts of care should be provided essentially folds back into provider control, for reasons discussed in chapter 4. Reductions in insurance coverage would, however, transfer wealth from ill to well, and perhaps to taxpayers, and make access to care more dependent on ability to pay.

The second, and much more interesting "market" approach has been under discussion for a number of years but was brought up high on the political and intellectual agenda by Enthoven (1980). This plan envisions large numbers of private organizations, Health Maintenance Organizations (HMOs) in the United States jargon, selling contracts to groups of patients at a fixed price per time period which bind them to supply (or pay for) all "needed" hospital and medical services (and drug and dental, if in the contract). Of course the organization, or its contracted physicians, determine "need." The key strength of this approach, in terms of long-run stability of the health care sector, is that competition for contracts among such organizations tends to encourage both technical efficiency and concern for efficacy. As we have noted above, it is already amply demonstrated that such groups do make less use of hospital space and high technology interventions, and more use of intermediate-level personnel substituting for physicians. But these are merely examples of *what* they do. The critical difference is *why* they do it; such organizations differ from every other "player" in the health care system in that they operate under economic incentives (in a competitive environment) to hold down the total cost of the care they provide, not to push it up.

They also, obviously, have incentives for both underservicing and careful selection of clients. To date, most experience has been with large, long-established, and non-profit versions of such organizations, motivated by some combination of public service, professional commitment, and economic survival. And they have been operating in a non-competitive environment where outperforming the fee-for-service "competition" in the cost dimension was not terribly demanding. It may thus be dangerous to extrapolate from past performance how large numbers of highly competitive for-profit HMOs would behave. In any case, a substantial regulatory framework appears necessary for this "competitive" solution to prevent "cream-skimming" and dumping of all the high-risk patients on some insurer of last resort, or diluting quality of care, particularly for the few patients *in extremis* who generate very high costs.[19]

The competitive HMO approach to health care is expanding steadily in the United States, but still covers under 10 percent of the population and has yet to demonstrate a global impact. The "magic bullet" of taxation of employer-paid premiums, if it were politically feasible, should significantly enhance HMO attractiveness. HMOs can typically offer lower premiums and/or more comprehensive services than can insurers reimbursing free choice of fee-for-service physician and hospital.[20]

Much more rapid, however, has been the expansion of the third alternative, "de-regulation" and for-profit supply (Gray 1983). United States corporations appear to be rapidly finding ways around legislative and regulatory restrictions on their activity, with the approval of many in the public sector. And professionals, who have in the United States so long used the "free enterprise" rhetoric to mobilize support against the political system, now find resistance to the market rather difficult ideologically as well as practically.[21] The result may be, indeed on some accounts already is, a loss of professional control over the content of medical practice. Not only the NFP hospital, but also the NOFP medical practice,

---

[19] "Thou shalt not kill/But needst not strive/Officiously/To keep alive." The competitive market for group contracts is supposed to discipline this process. Representatives of employee groups are assumed to be informed buyers on behalf of their members, and to withdraw from HMOs who cut corners. But this does not help the elderly widows or the chronically ill or unemployed. Competitive HMOs appear to offer great advantages for the non-old, the non-poor, and the non-sick. But integrating the people who really *need* care into this sort of system, especially in its for-profit form, is far from simple.

[20] Ironically, a change which the "exogenous demand" school argued would lead to less comprehensive coverage, may in fact lead to more. HMOs typically offer broader coverage with fewer self-pay components, but control costs on the supply side.

[21] The Singapore Syndrome: having one's guns pointed in the wrong direction.

is sliding toward larger scale and FP motivation, and the professionals who work *in* it will be required to work *for* it. If patients' interests happen to coincide with profits, well and good. If not, unfortunate.

But the unbridled competitive market appears to share with the professionally controlled, mixed funding system the problem of long-run instability. Since for-profit (''investor-owned'') hospitals expand their markets and earn their profits by expanding costs, they create ever greater problems for the private insurance industry as well as for the more limited public reimbursement programs which, so far, even the United States right wing has not been able to shed. Their growth may be expected to induce protective responses by reimbursers—California's Preferred Provider Organizations (Trauner 1983) being one example, employer as well as union-sponsored HMOs being another.

Thus the longer term result may well be to speed up the development of organizations standing between providers, for-profit or otherwise, and patients, whether publicly or privately insured. However sponsored, these organizations will offer patients access only to ''needed'' care, as determined by their providers or representatives, and from a limited range of providers—no more free choice of doctor. In return they guarantee a fixed cost per time period to the patient or those responsible for her costs. They will then exercise controls over provider behaviour, to limit costs, in return for granting providers access to ''their'' patients. In a situation of general oversupply, and rapid expansion, of health personnel, plus shrinking public budgets for health, the residual traditional fee-for-service market may get quite tough.

But what, if anything, do the remarkable, entertaining, and expensive thrashings of the United States health care system have to do with Canada? Not too much, it is to be hoped. They do, however, dramatically point up both certain dangers and certain opportunities which may confront us as well.[22]

First, it appears that any attempt to mitigate the professional/political conflict by diversifying funding sources and breaking down the centralized political control leads into a dilemma. Either it merely grafts a small and rather inequitable quasi-market, under professional control, onto a system which remains predominantly public, in which case the confrontation remains, or it moves to an environment in which public control over and responsibility for funding are significantly reduced, at least in proportion, in which case costs escalate uncontrollably and eventually the system fragments and ''de-regulates'' on United States lines. This scenario suggests that having fought off political control, professionals would in due course find themselves confronting the private, for-profit corporations

---

[22] ''Nothing is ever wasted, it can always serve as a horrible example.'' (G.L. Stoddart, personal communication).

which are at present held off by the public regulatory system. The competitive FP system which follows scores relatively badly on all our above criteria, except perhaps technical efficiency, but even that is unclear given the overhead costs of competitive marketing (note the experience of private insurance, chapter 2 and the minimal evidence of lower costs, as opposed to higher revenues, in FP hospitals, chapter 10). And it generates a high rate of technical change, again a distinctly mixed blessing.

Overall, a predominantly FP delivery system would probably display a proliferation of servicing, a linkage of access to willingness to pay rather than needs (for-profit institutions describe this as "moving up-market"), distribution of costs according to use (or expected use) rather than ability to pay, and substantial income gains for those providers least inhibited by professional ideology or scruples. If it sells, do it.

This FP system itself, however, also appears to be unstable, subject to uncontrolled cost escalation. But it is too early yet to tell whether it will in the United States evolve into a system dominated by public and private "HMO-type" organizations acting essentially as patients' purchasing agents to control providers, or whether it will attain stable expenditure and utilization levels by simply withdrawing entitlements entirely, dropping the poor, elderly, and chronically ill out of the health care system. After explosive growth in any industry comes the "shake-out"— but in what form?

A PROFESSIONAL ALTERNATIVE: CONTROL BY CARTEL?

The root problem faced by the advocates of professional control, then, is how to create institutions, other than centralized public budgetary control, which will lead to eventual stability of health sector expenditure. At present every participant, except government, faces incentive patterns which encourage more spending, whether to increase servicing or to raise incomes. Is there any conceivable set of professional persons or groups which could recognize *over-funding* (or at least sufficient funding) for longer than six months to a year, and could act to control funding levels accordingly?[23] If the relationship between resource inputs and health outcomes is of the form of Figure 1-3b, we have argued above that determining "how much is enough" (globally, not in individual cases) is a political, not a professional function. But professionals may not only lack

---

[23] Of course Canadian advocates of "privatization" may take the view "Après moi, le deluge." Short-run gains would accrue, and to those late in career, that may be justification enough. The American physicians who successfully fought off national health insurance are home and dry with their investments; their successors face a very different world.

legitimacy in this sphere, they may be, probably are, simply incapable of making the decision. And understandably so.[24]

In the pre-Medicare days, physician-sponsored insurance plans, which were at one time more or less monopolies, did exercise such restraints, but only over physician fees, on a year-by-year basis. Their market position was eroding by the time Medicare was introduced, but it could conceivably have been legislatively sustained. The difficulty is that these insurers were presiding over a longer term dramatic expansion in physician relative incomes and service costs—a controlled explosion, not control. They showed no sign of being able to impose long-run stability even for physician costs, let alone hospital care. And in the present environment of rapid technological advance and proliferation of profit or income opportunities, against the backdrop of an increasing supply of treatable aged, the prospect that a providers' cartel, even backed by a compliant public regulatory authority, could reach and enforce a consensus on anything but "more," seems remote indeed.

The long-run consequences of a scaling down of the public role in Canadian health care thus would appear to be an intermediate period of cost expansion and deterioration of both the financial equity and the overall effectiveness of the health care system, accompanied by a shift from professional to FP control and a United States-type situation. If this is not inevitable, it is hard to see what present or potential future institutional features of the professional system would prevent it. The consequences of a scaling down of the professional role in the conflict, however, could also be rather unattractive.

INCREASED PUBLIC CONTROL: HOW CIVIL A SERVICE?

One could imagine a scenario in which provincial governments were able to maintain expenditure control over health care by essentially lock-step policies—gearing manpower and capital equipment availability to population growth (possibly age-sex adjusted) and setting fee schedules and budgets such that provider incomes rose in line with the rest of the economy, but taking no further interest in the actual delivery process. It is often alleged, and with some plausibility, that such a "civil service" approach could have an enormously destructive impact on the morale and productivity of health care providers and on the quality of their work.

---

[24] Such a role requires individual professionals to act as agents for both individual patients and the collective society, to balance three (including their own) sets of conflicting interests, not two (Evans and Wolfson 1980). This may not be possible, and in any case has not been part of the traditional professional role. The concept of the "cost-conscious physician" suggests that it might become so, but so far the supporting evidence is absent.

Of course the converse proposition, that to be happy, productive, and constantly advancing quality, health care workers must be assured of a constantly growing share of national resources, is unsupportable, as the trees cannot grow to the sky. But there *are* real dangers in what the Americans call the "public utility" model (with a gratuitous slur on some quite progressive public utilities). If the providers of care lose interest in or commitment to their professions, the quality deterioration could be serious indeed. If external limitations on the health care sector are inevitable, they must also be justifiable and acceptable.

Moreover, if the professional claim to represent the broader public interest is diluted by self-interest and lack of information, the political process is not exactly perfect either. We have already noted that shifting the relative income-determination process from the professionally controlled market to the political arena substitutes a downward for an upward bias (though the interests countervailing this bias are rather more organized and articulate). A public reimbursement authority has an equivalent incentive to keep down servicing levels, in both quantity and sophistication, just as does a United States-style HMO. Whether or not "underservicing" now characterizes Canadian health care, it clearly could do so.

A slightly cynical model of the political process would suggest that public resources will be devoted only to those health care services which a majority of the population either feels that it "needs," either now or in the future, or is willing to support for others. Why waste resources on either invisible or unpopular sub-populations of little political significance, or on meeting "needs" which many people might have (or would sympathize with) but are unaware of? The political agency role is at least as subject to incompleteness as the professional one, and politicans and bureaucrats *have* occasionally been observed to be acting in their own interests and/or those of powerful sponsors, not those of the general public which they serve. Just as above we argued that political intervention was necessary to monitor the performance of the professional agency function, so there is a need for the professional monitor of the political agent. This would be substantially more difficult to achieve in a delivery system, whether a public service or merely a publicly funded one, in which providers had lost interest in their professional roles.[25]

---

[25] Whether the U.K. National Health Service refutes or confirms this concern about professional demoralization and/or imperfect political agency is rather difficult for an outsider to determine. So many images of the NHS have been created for both internal and external political purposes (Culyer 1982) that assessing the reality would be a most complex task. Are or were NHS "refugees" in practice in Canada "demoralized," or did they simply see greener pastures? Is Mrs. Thatcher seeking "value for money," or destruction of the NHS?

BUT WHY CONFRONTATION OVER (ALLEGEDLY) COMMON OBJECTIVES?

There may, however, be an acceptable middle ground between public and professional authority. Both ultimately derive their legitimacy from a claim to represent the interests of the population generally, either as citizens/taxpayers/voters or as patients. And each, as demonstrated above, bases its arguments—underfunding or cost escalation—on an implicit judgement about the resource input/health status relationship of Figure 1-3. Yet governments have done relatively little to substantiate the claim, implicit in their cost-control policies, that the curve is flat or declining. And professionals have thus far rejected any obligation to substantiate their claim of a positive slope or to confront contrary evidence, as if such substantiation (on scientific criteria, not merely assertion of professional experience, judgement or opinion) were inconsistent with professional status.[26]

The solution may lie in the development of more extensive interaction between government and professionals, using evaluation methodology and "technological assessment" to develop diagnostic and therapeutic protocols which can be based on the best evidence available as to effectiveness and efficiency. In this process both sides are at risk. If the evidence clearly shows that a proposed activity or program, new or expanded, is likely to have a significant impact on someone's health, this creates an obligation on government to provide resources. But if evidence of efficacy is lacking, for new or established programs, professionals would then be under obligation to assist, or at least not resist, modification or termination.

And if the process is to function, providers will have to accept that, if Figure 1-3b applies, not all "needs" are worth meeting. They cannot both participate in the allocation process at the expert, professional level, and seek to undermine it through the political or market processes (*e.g.*, by selling additional services on the side).

In this process the utilization data generated by the public insurance programs could be of great use, not only to assist in evaluating the effects of particular interventions, but also in identifying the nature of current practice and the impact of recommendations for change. Individual institutions or practitioners could be monitored to ensure that policies agreed on by government and profession as scientifically justified are indeed having the desired impact on actual practice in the field. If not, corrective action can be taken through the payment process, or otherwise.[27]

---

[26] As Freidson (1970) argues that indeed it is.

[27] This would represent a departure from past Canadian efforts to evaluate medical practice—cervical screening, for example, or periodic health examination—in that the results of such studies would be used not merely to inform those practitioners who

In such a process, the results of United States experience with competitive HMOs, private FP hospitals and clinics, and alternative institutions generally could be of tremendous assistance in mapping out the
range of the possible. While Canadians were among the pioneers of day-
care surgery, for example, American ambulatory surgicenters have begun
to do T. & A.s, and hernia repairs at all ages. And it is the United States
HMOs which consistently show that 40 percent reductions in hospital
use, from current Canadian rates, are possible without apparent injury to
the health of the served population. Information on the therapeutically
possible can come from many sources, and the wide range of different
ways of providing care currently developing in the United States is likely
to throw up a number of alternative possibilities for evaluation.

WHAT TO DO, OR HOW TO DO IT—A ROLE FOR NEW PLAYERS?

There is an important distinction, however, between how we learn
what is possible and desirable, and how we create institutions which will
bring such changes about. Proposals in Ontario for the development of
a system of "public competition" (Stoddart and Seldon 1983) based on
Health Services Organizations empanelling patients and reimbursed per
capita by the provincial government represent an attempt to expand the
role of new types of institutions like the American HMOs whose incentives and constraints will lead them to change current patterns of medical
and hospital use in a direction already known to be possible—less hospital
use. The suggestion that government and professionals attempt to review
the evidence for such possibilities, and modify practice patterns by administrative mechanisms, represents an alternative institutional means to
the same end. What form such collaborative action would take, and
whether it would succeed in the end, is at this point too early to tell.

The "public sector competition" approach has the important feature,
however, that it introduces competitive forces and market institutions into
what is presently a two-sided relationship, without replacing either the
political or the professional roles. HSOs could be permitted to compete
for patients in a variety of ways—premium rebates, for example, or
"free" dental or pharmaceutical services. In regions with significant
numbers of opted out physicians, it is difficult to understand why (from
a public interest, as opposed to professional monopoly, perspective) they

---

read journals, but to monitor and modify actual practice patterns with professional as
well as political support. In U.S. terms, Professional Standards Review Organizations
run jointly by the paying agency and the medical association, with financial and
professional teeth.

should not openly advertise their opted in status. And if their public reimbursement includes not only a fixed dollar amount per patient enrolled, but a share of "saved" hospital costs, these extra resources can be used in competing for patients. In this setting, new, and anticipated more efficient, forms of delivery can expand their market shares, not by administrative or professional fiat, but by the choices of individual consumers. The regulatory environment might require some modification to permit such organizations to communicate with their potential customers, and to ensure that they were not frozen out of the public hospital system by their fee-for-service competitors. But in general such institutions seem compatible with continued public control over global funding, and professional regulation of the content of practice.[28]

Such developments have the feature that they introduce a new class of participant, with different incentives, into the political/professional relationship. In this respect they are paralleled by the experiments currently underway with for-profit management teams contracting to run public NFP hospitals. Again, a new player or transactor enters the system, whose economic incentives may be to control costs, not to escalate them.

The conditional statement is required, because much depends on how the contract is written. As noted above, FP contract management in the United States setting has every economic incentive to *raise* both utilization and prices, and any Canadian provincial government which contracted (or permitted a hospital's trustees to contract) on similar terms should collectively seek psychiatric care. But a contract which related the profits of the management team (inversely) to the hospital costs of a defined group of people—essentially capitation reimbursement—and provided for charging back of costs externalized to the rest of the health care system (or out of it) by management action, plus some monitoring of patient-care outcomes, could create the appropriate form of incentives by, in essence, turning the FP management team into a sort of HMO responsible specifically for hospital services. How, or whether, such an institution would work, is fitting matter for experiment and depends critically on the contract structure and the incentives it embodies. But such managements could conceivably encourage shorter patient stays, more use of

---

[28] Of course professional regulation can be used punitively by a dominant group of providers to discipline or suppress potential competitors. A policy of encouraging competitive forms of delivery which pose a real threat to "mainstream" care markets must therefore include some monitoring and control of the professional self-regulatory process. Similarly, critics of such proposals have argued that they will fragment users by social and economic class, and enable provincial governments to spin off the more politically vulnerable into second-class care. Again the response must be monitoring and control through informed public opinion.

hospital-based ambulatory or home care alternatives, and closer attention to both admission and servicing intensity patterns.[29]

INSTITUTIONS, INCENTIVES, AND INFORMATION

At the end, we come back to the basic theme of chapter 1. Canada, like every other society, has evolved a set of institutions which govern the behaviour of transactors in the health care field, by the creation of patterns or flows of information and incentives. The resulting behaviour patterns lead to overall outcomes in terms of resources used up, types and amounts of goods and services produced, and distribution of services and resulting incomes and costs, among the members of society. These outcomes can be evaluated in terms of more general social objectives of equity, effectiveness, and efficiency, and the trick is to develop institutions which lead to satisfactory outcomes. We have argued in this chapter that behind the current sound and fury over underfunding or cost-escalation; user charges, extra-billing, professional freedom and patient protection; patients dying in corridors or overservicing lies the general problem which we share with all other developed countries. What set of institutions (subject to constraints of political feasibility and cultural continuity) will lead to patterns of transactor behaviour—governments, providers, and users—which yield the best available outcomes in terms of efficient and effective health service provision and fairness of the resulting patterns of economic burden and benefit?

WHAT'S WRONG WITH THE STATUS QUO?

We have suggested that the present confrontation of professional control over the specifics of provision but public control over total resources used, and minimal use of market mechanisms such as direct charges, yields a remarkably good compromise—in world terms—but at the cost of what appears to be escalating political friction, and possibly the beginning of a slippage of cost control. And while relatively cost-effective compared with many other countries' systems, it is nevertheless a good deal less effective and more costly than it could be. The absolute cost amounts are very large.

---

[29] Of course if reimbursed a fee based on service load, *e.g.*, patient days, or proportionate to overall costs, such managements would attempt to induce the reverse effects. But no provincial government would be so foolish as to write such a contract. Defense contracting experience with cost-plus-percentage-of-cost (CPPC), or even cost-plus-fixed-fee (CPFF), contracts is sufficiently well documented, and deplorable (Scherer 1964), and in any case common sense should guide.

Finally, the Canadian health care system embodies a number of forces which appear inconsistent with longer term stability. Most obvious is an implicit expansionary manpower policy, which leads inevitably to either higher costs or lower provider incomes. But there is also concern over the potential for continuing conflict in growing provider frustration which, if not constructively channelled, could lead to demoralization as well as militancy. "Alienated" professionals mean poor overall system performance. At the same time the regulatory and payment structure makes unduly difficult, if not impossible, organizational changes which could lead to improved service efficiency. Changes in *what* is provided take place quite rapidly; in *how* it is provided, much more slowly.

Moreover, the Canadian health care system (like most others) has not developed a satisfactory way of dealing with the really fundamental question of life and death. The official political position is that all "needed" care is to be provided, without charge. And this text has emphasized the range of important and difficult allocation and efficiency questions which can be addressed within that framework. Yet technological change is steadily shifting the resource/health status relationship to increase the economic significance of the ethically much more difficult questions of the "pulling the plug" sort. And politicians find open confrontation of the life and death questions, the decisions not to invest resources in prolonging life, extremely dangerous to their political health. Maintenance of the important illusion that "all needed care" is provided may increasingly rely, as to some extent it does already, on a tacit professional agreement that at a certain stage, "heroic measures" are inappropriate. But a really disgruntled profession, armed with a technology encompassing large numbers of very expensive "life saving" or at least significantly life-prolonging interventions, and willing to go public, might well confront provincial governments with the choice between *real* cost explosions, and loss of public confidence in the whole Medicare program.

Thus far, professionals have played on public fears to try to achieve relatively small changes, a bit more income here, a program expansion there, but have not wished to risk the political fallout from an open attack on the system. Perhaps they never will. But as the reach of technology extends, either the political system must find ways to address overtly (or delegate) the problem of balancing specific lives and dollars, or it must be increasingly dependent on the health care system, physicians in particular, to perform this role on its behalf. And their willingness to do so may not be independent of the level of conflict.

Yet proposals for reassertion of professional control, with or without a vestigial market sector, offer no prospect of a satisfactory or stable alternative either. More extreme proposals for a major shift to competitive market institutions, either directly or after a period of professional control, private insurance, and cost escalation, appear at the moment even less attractive.[30]

Alternative possibilities, suggested above, include attempts to develop and expand avenues of communication between political and professional authorities, on the understanding that neither one is going to, or should, go away. A concern for the provision of services of demonstrated effectiveness, and (less apparently) efficiency, of meeting the most needs possible with the resources available, should provide a common ground. This is not a new idea; such co-operation on a limited scale has gone on constructively in Canada for years. But the inevitably confrontational processes of fee and budget negotiation seem to swamp these co-operative endeavours. And so long as professionals, officially at least, regard the content of care as no one else's business, while governments and administrators regard it as not their responsibility, confrontation seems inevitable. Health care is far too important to leave to professionals, and in any case we cannot afford to do so.[31]

The other possibilities above—"public competition" through HSOs, or for-profit contract management—represent different ways of mitigating the political/professional conflict by introducing forms of provider organization with some incentives to contain, rather than expand, spending. Of course limiting spending to any *particular* level is not an end in itself. But eventually stability has to be achieved through some institutional form.

If improved political/professional co-operation on system management cannot be achieved, and if support cannot be generated for alternative forms of provider organization, then continuation of the present tension may be the best available alternative. Canada's health system is said by some to be "in crisis," but most health systems are "in crisis" most of the time. A system *not* perceived to be "in crisis" might be cause for concern, suggesting that the balance of conflicting forces and interests had broken down. So long as both political and professional agencies maintain their confrontation, and neither side becomes tired of the role,

---

[30] There may be, over the U.S. market rainbow, a world of private for-profit firms providing ever more efficacious care, at the lowest possible cost, to citizen/patients who have adequate personal resources, private insurance, or public subsidy sufficient to get the care they need. But it can be seen only with the eye of faith. The present situation appears to be predominantly wind and rain.

[31] In this context it is interesting to note that dual management, explicitly co-ordinated physician and administrator responsibilities at each level, is a fundamental policy of the largest U.S. HMO (Kaiser), while FP hospitals also appear to give physicians a large role on their boards. And in the U.K., "clinical budgeting" extends the managerial role—and responsibilities—of the clinician. The "two lines of authority" may be drawing together in a number of settings.

the experience of the last decade suggests we may not do too badly. But we could do much better.

And eventually the balance may start to shift. The federal-provincial conflicts of the early 1980s suggest that it has begun to do so; behind the trumpeting and bellowing along the world's longest defended border (between the federal and provincial governments) the Medicare system may indeed be in real danger. The *Canada Health Act* should prevent, or at least inhibit, one form of erosion, (not a trivial contribution) but provides no positive directions. Yet whether Medicare survives in its present or modified form, or starts down the slippery slope of "Australification,"[32] the underlying policy issues will not go away. The considerable international variety of social "solutions" to the problems of health care delivery and finance do yield more and less equitable and efficient results—though efficiency is rather difficult to prove conclusively. But each society continues to find itself struggling with the same issues of what to produce, for whom, and how, and how to modify its institutions to get a more satisfactory result. How you play the game matters, and matters quite a lot; but you cannot end the game, by "winning" or otherwise.

AND A LAST WORD ON ECONOMICS—FOR GOOD OR ILL

The role of economic analysis in this process is to try to clarify the implications of different institutional frameworks and policy choices. Logically it cannot, as the Cheshire Cat pointed out, serve as a source of social objectives or values—though economists (including this one) frequently try to do so.[33] What it can do is to provide a framework for assembling and assessing the available evidence, so as to assist in predicting how particular health care systems, or the transactor of which they are made up, are likely to react to the information and incentives embodied in different policies. Further, it can be used to trace through, in a logical and consistent manner, the interactions among such behaviours and to predict the resulting outcomes in terms of social objectives. Economic analysis can also be used to obscure or misrepresent these processes, to yield results favourable to policies benefiting the analyst or her sponsor. Or, as a result of misreading of evidence or inappropriate choice of analytic framework, suppressing key relationships and responses, and highlighting unimportant ones, it may be irrelevant or simply wrong.[34]

---

[32] Which turns out not to be permanent either.

[33] Reinhardt refers to playing politics in the guise of science as a favourite economists' pastime—see also Evans (1982b)—but as your doctor will tell you, there's a lot of it about.

[34] These are immoral and bad analyses, respectively, and are done by other people.

But used with some care, with as many as possible of the cards on the table, and in conjunction with other disciplinary perspectives on the elephant, the economic framework yields a number of insights which seem to come with great difficulty, if at all, from other intellectual traditions. Occasionally some of these turn out to be useful. If this excursion through an economic interpretation of the Canadian health care system turns out to provide one or two such insights for readers responsible for actually making the system function, in whatever capacity (including paying for it), well, I suppose that was the purpose of the exercise.

DATA SOURCES APPENDIX

Expenditures: Data on health care expenditures in Canada, total and by components, on a current outlay basis, are compiled annually by Health and Welfare Canada and released in occasional publications and unpublished memoranda. The most recent publication is *National Health Expenditures in Canada, 1970-1982* (Canada, Health and Welfare Canada, n.d. [1984]). Earlier data can be assembled from several previous releases, but each publication appears to include some minor revisions from previous data. The most recent and historically continuous source is Fraser (1983) Series B504-B513, which reports total expenditures and major components. (It should be noted, however, that B513, Health Expenditures, Canada, 1945-1975, total, is not a continuous series. From 1960 forwards it reports total expenditures on the National Health Expenditure concept, but for 1959 and earlier years it is simply the sum of hospital, physician, dental, and prescribed drug expenses. These components reported prior to 1960 represent only about two-thirds of the total as measured from 1960 on.) A finer component breakdown back to 1960 is given by *National Health Expenditures in Canada 1960-1975* (Canada, Health and Welfare Canada 1979).

These sources are the basis for almost all tables reporting expenditure data, Tables 1-1, 2-1, 7-3, and 8-1, as well as text references to national expenditures. They are the only source of comprehensive nation-wide expenditure data, across all forms of payment; Ontario (Ministry of Treasury and Economics 1981) has reported independent provincial estimates for 1970/71 to 1977/78.

Manpower: The *Canada Health Manpower Inventory* (Canada, Health and Welfare Canada 1980, 1983*b*) reports total membership in each of a large number of the health care occupations. The data are, in most cases, registry or license-holder data, unadjusted for labour force participation, though for physicians an estimate is made of the active civilian physician stock. This is reported with and without interns and residents; the inclusive data are used throughout this book on the ground that interns and residents are providing medical services, even if their costs emerge in hospital budgets.

Canada Health Manpower Inventory data go back only to 1968. A series for active civilian physicians back to 1935 has been pieced together by Barer and Evans (1983) where sources and methods are described. For other professionals, some data are available from the Hall Commission Report and supporting studies (Canada, Royal Commission on Health Services 1964). These sources are drawn on for physician data used in Table 1-2, for active civilian physicians and licensed dentists and pharmacists reported in Table 7-1, and for physician and dentist denominators in Table 7-3.

The other two sources of manpower data used are the Census, and taxation statistics. The Census surveys establishments—practices, hospitals, pharmacies—and counts workers, rather than using registry data by occupation. It is therefore the only regular source of data on total numbers of workers in particular settings, as opposed to numbers of people with particular qualifications, whether or not working. The Census also collects occupational data as part of the household survey. Table 7-2 and the surrounding text draw on the 1971 Census of labour force by industry (Statistics Canada Cat. #94-740, Vol. III part 4, Census Bulletin (3.4-3), Table 2, December 1974) as well as by occupation (Statistics Canada Cat. #94-717, Vol. III part 2, Census Bulletin (3.2-3), Table 2, September 1974). Census data for 1961 by industry are from Statistics Canada Cat. #94-518, Vol. III part 2, Census Bulletin (3.2-1), May 1963, and by occupation, Statistics Canada Cat. #94-503, Vol. III part 1, Census Bulletin (3.1-3), Table 6, February 1963. Census data by occupation are significantly lower than the *CHMI* counts and, in any case, are available only every ten years. They have, therefore, been used only to derive a (very rough) estimate of the numbers of workers in professional practices who are not of the same profession as the owner(s).

Taxation statistics report numbers of tax returns by self-employed practitioners, full- or part-time, who earn 50 per cent or more of their incomes from professional practice. This represents an estimate of the proportion of licenced members of a profession who are actually in private, fee-for-service practice. But it excludes practitioners working on salary in a group which is reimbursed on fee-for-service. The physician relative income data in Table 1-2 refer to self-employed (taxable) tax-filers, comparing their net incomes with the industrial composite of average weekly wages and salaries, and Table 7-1 reports these data as "Physicians in Fee-for-Service Practice" to compare with the *CHMI* "Active Civilian Physicians" series.

Unfortunately, counts from this source depend on the accuracy of occupational reporting to the Department of National Revenue, and the adequacy of their sampling process. Health and Welfare Canada, Health Information Division, has, since 1972, prepared more comprehensive counts of physicians and dentists in fee-for-service practice. The data prior to 1972 are thus drawn straight from the annual publication, *Taxation Statistics*, of the Department of National Revenue, but subsequent counts are from unpublished data provided by Health and Welfare Canada.

Prices: Physician fee indices are a combination of fee-benefit schedule indices compiled by Health and Welfare Canada, linked to the Consumer Price Index, medical services component, in earlier years, and adjusted (crudely) for changes in collections rates (Barer and Evans 1983). This index is used in Table 7-3 to derive an index of "real" physicians' services output, adjusted for fee change, and is compared with the all-items CPI to show the relative inflation or deflation of medical fees. Table 7-3 uses the dental service component of the CPI for the same purposes with respect to dental care expenditures.

Incomes: Incomes of physicians and other professionals as reported in Table 7-4, and (in relative form) Table 1-2, are drawn from the annual *Taxation Statistics* reports. They are net incomes (after expenses, before tax) of wholly or primarily fee-for-service practitioners, full- or part-time, taxable returns only. This is the only source which provides historical continuity back to the immediate post-war period. But as noted in the text, it is believed by Health and Welfare Canada to be subject to increasing downward biases, at least since the mid-1970s, and they have provided alternative estimates in unpublished data reported in Table 7-4. Whether there are similar biases in other professionals' incomes as reported in *Taxation Statistics* is unknown, since there is no cross-check similar to the provincial insurance plan data. The conceptual problems in measuring physician incomes, and a comparison of some of the data sources, are presented in Wolfson, Evans, and Lomas (1980).

Taxation Statistics report income from all sources, broken down by professional income (fee or salary and sessional) and other sources. Provincial medical insurance plan data report payments under the plan to all practitioners, physicians and others, whether or not "primarily" in fee-for-service medical practice. Thus reports of total medical care plan payments divided by total numbers of practitioners receiving payment represent a serious understatement of average incomes. The data in Table 7-5, drawn from federal compilations of provincial insurance plan data (Canada, Health and Welfare Canada 1981, 1983a) are based on estimates of numbers of full-time-equivalent (FTE) physicians, but refer only to plan outlays. They are reported only in rate of change, not level, form.

Insurance Coverage: Data on the extent of coverage by public and private medical insurance plans prior to the public universal programs in Canada, as presented in Table 2-1 and discussed in the text, are drawn from an unpublished Health and Welfare Canada compilation, "Historical Series on Public and Private Health Insurance Enrollment for Physicians' Services, Canada and Provinces, 1950-1971" (Ottawa 1977). Earlier documentation of hospital and medical coverage is given in *Voluntary Medical Insurance in Canada, 1955-1961* (Canada, Department of National Health and Welfare 1963b). Data on the non-profit sector are reported in Shillington (1972).

Hospital Utilization Statistics: Hospital utilization data are derived from various Statistics Canada publications, all of which are based on the Annual Returns of

Hospitals, HS-1 and HS-2. Unfortunately data tables in these publications change from year to year in title, format, and content. Assembly of consistent historical series, and sometimes even year-to-year comparisons, is thus made both time-consuming and difficult. Fortunately, Fraser (1983) now provides a comprehensive source for hospital capacity and utilization, clearly and consistently identified by type and ownership of hospital, but only for 1975 and prior years. This is the source for the pre-1976 data in the first column of Table 1-2, and in Table 8-2. Most cost and use data are reported either for "public general and allied special" hospitals or for "public general" alone. In both cases, federal, private, provincial mental, and (in earlier years) T.B. institutions are excluded. The "allied special" component is primarily chronic and convalescent hospitals, but also includes maternity and paediatric hospitals providing "acute care" similar to that in a general hospital. Fraser (1983) therefore reports paediatric hospitals in the "public general" category—see note to Table 8-2.

Data from 1976 on, in Tables 1-2 and 8-2, are drawn from *Hospital Statistics Preliminary Annual Report 1982/83* (Statistics Canada Cat. #83-X-202) (Canada, Statistics Canada, 1984). The breakdown by type of hospital (Table 8-2) uses data from the annual publication *Hospital Annual Statistics* (Statistics Canada Cat. #83-232) as available, up to the 1979-80 fiscal year. (Hospital statistical reporting changed over to an April 1 year in 1977-78. Hospital data in Table 1-2 after that date are actually fiscal year, not calendar as labelled.) The 1980-81 and 1981-82 breakdowns in Table 8-2 use data from *Hospital Statistics—Preliminary Annual Report* (Statistics Canada Cat. #83-217) (1980-81 and 1981-82). Hospital index data in Table 1-2 are calculated as reported in Barer and Evans (1983).

General Economic Statistics: The scale of the health care sector relative to the general economy is usually indicated by relating health expenditures to the Gross National Product (GNP) which adjusts for general inflation levels as well as scaling for growth in population and productivity. Specific "prices" such as hospital costs per day or physician or dental fees, have been adjusted for general inflation by the all-items Consumer Price Index. Professional incomes are scaled relative to either the "all taxpayers" income level (Table 1-2) or the average weekly wages and salaries, industrial composite index drawn from the labour force survey. This is also the source of total labour force data. Such general statistics are widely available; the best single source for data over several decades being the *Historical Statistics of Canada*, 2nd edition (F. H. Leacy, ed., Ottawa: Statistics Canada, 1983). More recent data are in the monthly *Canadian Statistical Review* published by Statistics Canada, or the monthly *Bank of Canada Review*, and many other places.

BIBLIOGRAPHY

Ableson, J.; Paddon, P.; and Strohmenger, C. 1983. *Perspectives on Health*. Statistics Canada Catalogue No. 82-540E. Health Division, Research and Analysis Section. Ottawa: Ministry of Supply and Services.

Aday, L.A., and Andersen, R. 1975. *Access to Medical Care*. Ann Arbor, Mich.: Health Administration Press.

Aday, L.A.; Andersen, R.; and Fleming, G.V. 1980. *Health Care in the U.S.: Equitable for Whom?* Beverly Hills, Cal.: Sage Publications.

Akerlof, G.A. 1970. "The Market for 'Lemons': Qualitative Uncertainty and the Market Mechanism." *Quarterly Journal of Economics* 84: 488-500.

American College of Surgeons and American Surgical Association. 1975. *Surgery in the United States: A Summary Report of the Study on Surgical Services for the United States*. Chicago: American College of Surgeons.

Andersen, R., and Anderson, O.W. 1967. *A Decade of Health Services*. Chicago: University of Chicago Press.

Archibald, G.C., and Donaldson, D.J. 1976. "Paternalism and Prices." In *Resource Allocation and Economic Policy*, eds. M. Allingham and M.L Burstein, pp. 26-34. London: MacMillan.

Arrow, K.J. 1963. "Uncertainty and the Welfare Economics of Medical Care." *American Economic Review* 53: 941-73. ✓

Bailey, R.M. 1970a. "Philosophy, Faith, Fact and Fiction in the Production of Medical Services." *Inquiry* 7: 37-53.

———. 1970b. "Economies of Scale in Medical Practice." In *Empirical Studies in Health Economics*, ed. H.E. Klarman, pp. 255-73. Baltimore: Johns Hopkins Press.

———. 1977. "From Professional Monopoly to Corporate Oligopoly: The Clinical Laboratory Industry in Transition." *Medical Care* 15: 129-46.

———. 1979. *Clinical Laboratories and the Practice of Medicine*. Berkeley, Cal.: McCutchan.

Banta, H.D.; Behney, C.; and Willems, J.S. 1981. *Toward Rational Technology in Medicine: Considerations for Health Policy*. New York: Springer.

Banta, H.D., and Thacker, S.B. 1979. *Costs and Benefits of Electronic Fetal Monitoring: A Review of the Literature*. National Center for Health Services Research, Research Report Series. Department of Health, Education and Welfare (PHS) 79-3245. Washington, D.C.: DHEW.

Barer, M.L. 1981. *Community Health Centres and Hospital Costs in Ontario*.

Ontario Economic Council Occasional Paper no. 13. Toronto: Ontario Economic Council.

―――. 1982. "Case Mix Adjustment in Hospital Cost Analysis: Information Theory Revisited." *Journal of Health Economics* 1: 53-80.

Barer, M.L.; Evans, R.G.; and Stoddart, G.L. 1979. *Controlling Health Care Costs by Direct Charges to Patients: Snare or Delusion?* Ontario Economic Council Occasional Paper no. 10. Toronto: Ontario Economic Council.

Barer, M.L., and Evans, R.G. 1983. "Prices, Proxies, and Productivity: An Historical Analysis of Hospital and Medical Prices in Canada." In *Price Level Measurement*, eds. E. Diewert and C. Montmarquette, pp. 705-77. Proceedings of a conference sponsored by Statistics Canada. Ottawa: Statistics Canada.

Beck, R.G., and Horne, J.M. 1978. *An Analytical Overview of the Saskatchewan Co-payment Experiment in Hospital and Ambulatory Care Settings.* Toronto: Ontario Council of Health.

Benham, L. 1972. "The Effects of Advertising on the Price of Eyeglasses." *Journal of Law and Economics* 15: 337-52.

Benham, L., and Benham, A. 1975. "Regulating Through the Professions: A Perspective on Information Control." *Journal of Law and Economics* 18: 421-47.

Berg, R.L., ed. 1973. *Health Status Indexes*. Proceedings of a Conference Conducted by Health Services Research. Chicago: Health Research and Educational Trust.

Berki, S.E. 1972. *Hospital Economics*. Lexington, Mass.: D.C. Heath.

Birnbaum, H. *et al.* 1977. *A National Profile of Catastrophic Illness*. Cambridge, Mass.: Abt Associates.

Boulding, K.E. 1968. "An Economist's View of the Manpower Concept." In *Beyond Economics: Essays on Society, Religion, and Ethics*, pp. 14-27. Ann Arbor: University of Michigan Press.

Boulet, J-A., and Grenier, G. 1978. "Health Expenditures in Canada and the Impact of Demographic Changes on Future Government Health Insurance Program Expenditures." Economic Council of Canada Discussion Paper no. 123. Ottawa: ECC.

Boulet, J-A., and Henderson, D.M. 1979. "Distributional and Redistributional Aspects of Government Health Insurance Programs in Canada." Economic Council of Canada Discussion Paper #146. Ottawa: ECC.

British Columbia, 1975. *Report of the Children's Dental Health Research Project*. Victoria, B.C.: The Queen's Printer.

―――. Ministry of Health. Annually from 1968. *Report on Day Care Surgery*. Hospital Programs, Research Division. Victoria, B.C.: Ministry of Health.

―――. Ministry of Health, n.d. (i.e. 1983). *Statistics of Hospital Cases Discharged During 1981/82*. Hospital Programs, Research Division. Victoria, B.C.: Ministry of Health.

Broyles, R.W., *et al.* 1983. "The Use of Physician Services Under a National Health Insurance Scheme." *Medical Care* 21: 1037-54.

Bunker, J.P. 1970. "Surgical Manpower: A Comparison of Operations and Surgeons in the United States and England and Wales." *New England Journal of Medicine* 282: 135-44.

Canada, Department of National Health and Welfare. 1954. *Voluntary Medical Care Insurance: A Study of Non-Profit Plans in Canada*. General Series, Memorandum #4. Research Division. Ottawa: DNHW (April).

———. Department of National Health and Welfare, 1963a. *Expenditures on Personal Health Care in Canada 1953-1961*. Health Care Series Memorandum #16. Research and Statistics Division. Ottawa: DNHW (March).

———. Department of National Health and Welfare. 1963b. *Voluntary Medical Insurance in Canada 1955-1961*. Health Care Series Memorandum #17. Research and Statistics Division. Ottawa: DNHW (May).

———. Department of National Health and Welfare, n.d. *Expenditure on Personal Health Care in Canada 1960-1971*. Health Programs Branch, Health Economics and Statistics Directorate. Ottawa: DNHW.

———. Department of National Health and Welfare and Dominion Bureau of Statistics. 1960. *Illness and Health Care in Canada: The Canadian Sickness Survey 1950-51*. Dominion Bureau of Statistics Catalogue No. 82-518. Ottawa: The Queen's Printer (July).

———. Health and Welfare Canada. 1979. *National Health Expenditures in Canada 1960-1975*. Information Systems Branch, Health Economics and Statistics Division. Ottawa: Ministry of Supply and Services (January).

———. Health and Welfare Canada. 1980. *Canada Health Manpower Inventory 1979*. Policy, Planning and Information Branch, Health Information Division. Ottawa: HWC (August).

———. Health and Welfare Canada. 1981. *Medical Care Annual Report '78-9*. Cat. No. H 75-9/1979. Ottawa: Ministry of Supply and Services.

———. Health and Welfare Canada. 1983a. *Medical Care Annual Report '80-81*. Cat. No. H75-9/1981. Ottawa: Ministry of Supply and Services.

———. Health and Welfare Canada, 1983b. *Canada Health Manpower Inventory 1982*. Policy, Planning and Information Branch, Health Information Division. Ottawa: HWC (March).

———. Health and Welfare Canada. n.d. (1984). *National Health Expenditures in Canada: 1970-1982*. Policy, Planning and Information Branch, Information Dissemination Unit. Ottawa: HWC.

———. Health and Welfare Canada and Statistics Canada. 1981. *The Health of Canadians: Report of the Canada Health Survey*. Statistics Canada Catalogue No. 82-538E. Ottawa: HWC (June).

———. House of Commons. 1981. "The Health System" (ch. 4). In *Fiscal Federalism in Canada: Report of the Parliamentary Task Force on Federal-Provincial Fiscal Arrangements* (Breau Committee). Ottawa: Ministry of Supply and Services (August).

————. National Committee on Physician Manpower. 1975. *Report of the Requirements Committee on Physician Manpower*. Ottawa: Health and Welfare Canada.

————. Royal Commission on Health Services (Hall Commission). 1964. *Report*, vol. I. Ottawa: The Queen's Printer.

————. Statistics Canada. 1982. *Hospital Statistics—Preliminary Annual Report, 1980-81*. Catalogue 83-217 Annual. Ottawa: Statistics Canada.

————. Statistics Canada. 1984. *Hospital Statistics Preliminary Annual Report 1982-83*. Catalogue 83-X-202. Ottawa: Ministry of Supply and Services (January).

————. Task Force on the Periodic Health Examination. 1980. *Periodic Health Examination Monograph: Report of a Task Force to the Conference of Deputy Ministers of Health* (Spitzer Report). Ottawa: Health and Welfare Canada.

Canadian Medical Association. 1981. *Evidence presented to the Special Committee on The Federal-Provincial Fiscal Arrangements*. House of Commons, Canada, Minutes of Proceedings and Evidence, Issue No. 10, pp. 10-3 to 10-54, and 10A-1 to 10A-44: Tuesday, May 12, 1981, First Session, Thirty-Second Parliament, 1980-81.

Collard, D. 1978. *Altruism and Economy: A Study in Non-Selfish Economics*. Oxford: Martin Robertson.

Conrad, D., and Marmor, T.R. 1980. "Patient Cost Sharing." In *National Health Insurance: Conflicting Goals and Policy Choices*, eds. J. Feder, J. Holahan, and T.R. Marmor, pp. 385-422. Washington, D.C.: The Urban Institute.

Cooter, R. 1982. "The Cost of Coase." *Journal of Legal Studies* 11: 1-33.

Culyer, A.J. 1971. "The Nature of the Commodity 'Health Care' and Its Efficient Allocation." *Oxford Economic Papers* 23: 189-211.

————. 1978. *Measuring Health: Lessons for Ontario*. Ontario Economic Council Research Study No. 14. Toronto: University of Toronto Press.

————. 1981. "Health, Economics, and Health Economics." In *Health, Economics, and Health Economics*, eds. J. Van der Gaag and M. Perlman. pp. 3-11. Amsterdam: North-Holland.

————. 1982. "The NHS and the Market: Images and Realities." In *The Public/ Private Mix for Health: The Relevance and Effects of Change*, eds. G. McLachlan and A. Maynard, pp. 23-56. London: Nuffield Provincial Hospitals Trust.

————. 1984. "The Quest for Efficiency in the Public Sector: Economists versus Dr. Pangloss (or, Why Conservative Economists are Not Nearly Conservative Enough)." In *Public Finance and the Quest for Efficiency*, ed. H. Hanusch. Detroit: Wayne State University Press (forthcoming).

Culyer, A.J., and Simpson, H. 1980. "Externality Models and Health: A Rückblick over the Last Twenty years." *Economic Record* 56: 222-30.

Deeble, J.S. 1982. "Unscrambling the Omelet: Public and Private Health Care

Financing in Australia." In *The Public/Private Mix for Health: The Relevance and Effects of Change*, eds. G. McLachlan and A. Maynard, pp. 424-63. London: Nuffield Provincial Hospitals Trust.

Denton, F.T., and Spencer, B.G. 1983. "Population Aging and Future Health Costs in Canada." *Canadian Public Policy* 9: 155-63.

Dionne, G. 1982. "Moral Hazard and State-Dependent Utility Function." *Journal of Risk and Insurance* 49: 405-22.

Dobell, A.R. 1983. "What's the B.C. Spirit? Recent Experience in the Management of Restraint." Unpublished manuscript. Victoria, B.C.: University of Victoria.

Donabedian, A. 1966. "Evaluating the Quality of Medical Care." *Milbank Memorial Fund Quarterly* 44: 166-203.

Drummond, M.F. 1980. *Principles of Economic Appraisal in Health Care*. Oxford: Oxford University Press.

————.1981. *Studies in Economic Appraisal in Health Care*. Oxford: Oxford University Press.

Dunlop, B. 1982. "Compensation for Personal Injuries." In *Lawyers and the Consumer Interest*, eds. R.G. Evans and M.J. Trebilcock, pp. 383-405. Toronto: Butterworths.

Dyck, F.J., *et al*. 1977. "Effect of Surveillance on the Number of Hysterectomies in the Province of Saskatchewan." *New England Journal of Medicine* 296: 1326-28.

Eisner, R., and Strotz, R.H. 1961. "Flight Insurance and the Theory of Choice." *Journal of Political Economy* 69: 355-68.

Enterline, P.E., *et al*. 1973. "The Distribution of Medical Services Before and After 'Free' Medical Care — The Quebec Experience." *New England Journal of Medicine* 289: 1174-78.

Enthoven, A.S. 1980. *Health Plan: The Only Practical Solution to the Soaring Cost of Medical Care*. Reading, Mass.: Addison-Wesley.

Evans, R.G. 1972. (i.e. 1973). *Price Formation in the Market for Physician Services in Canada 1957-1969*. Research Study for the Prices and Incomes Commission. Ottawa: Information Canada.

————. 1974. "Supplier-Induced Demand: Some Empirical Evidence and Implications." In *The Economics of Health and Medical Care*, ed: M. Perlman, pp. 162-73. Proceedings of a Conference of the International Economics Association, Tokyo, 1973. London: MacMillan.

————. 1976. "Modelling the Economic Objectives of the Physician." In *Health Economics Symposium: Proceedings of the First Canadian Conference*, September 4-6, 1974, ed. R.D. Fraser, pp. 33-46. Kingston, Ont.: Queen's University Industrial Relations Centre.

————. 1978. "Universal access: the Trojan horse." In *The Professions and Public Policy*, eds. P. Slayton and M.J. Trebilcock, pp. 191-208. Toronto: University of Toronto Press.

————. 1980. "Professionals and the Production Function: Can Competition

Policy Improve Efficiency in the Licensed Professions?'' In *Occupational Licensure and Regulation*, ed. S. Rottenberg, pp. 225-64. Washington, D.C.: American Enterprise Institute.

―――. 1981. ''Incomplete Vertical Integration: The Distinctive Structure of the Health-Care Industry.'' In *Health, Economics, and Health Economics*, eds. J. Van der Gaag and M. Perlman, pp. 329-54. Amsterdam: North-Holland.

―――. 1982*a*. ''A Retrospective on the 'New Perspective.' '' *Journal of Health Politics, Policy and Law*. 7: 325-44.

―――. 1982*b*. ''Slouching Toward Chicago: Regulatory Reform as Revealed Religion.'' *Osgoode Hall Law Journal* 20: 454-84. Regulatory Reform Symposium issue, Part I.

―――. 1983. ''The Welfare Economics of Public Health Insurance: Theory and Canadian Practice.'' In *Social Insurance*, ed. L. Söderström, pp. 71-103. Amsterdam: North-Holland.

―――. 1984. ''We Have Seen the Future, and They Is Us.'' In *Proceedings of the Commonwealth Fund Forum on the Health Care of the Aged*, eds. T.W. Moloney and S.A. Schroeder. London, England, 23-26 May 1983 (forthcoming).

Evans, R.G.; Kliewer, E.V.; and Robinson, G.C. 1983. *The Impact of Surgical Day Care on Surgical Utilization: An Analysis of Ten Years' Experience in B.C.* Final Report, National Health Grant #6610-1212-46. Department of Paediatrics, Division of Population Paediatrics. Vancouver, B.C.: University of British Columbia.

Evans, R.G., and Robinson, G.C. 1980. ''Surgical day care: measurements of the economic payoff.'' *Canadian Medical Association Journal* 123: 873-80.

Evans, R.G., and Robinson, G.C. 1983. ''An Economic Study of Cost Savings on a Care-by-Parent Ward.'' *Medical Care* 21: 768-82.

Evans, R.G., and Stanbury, W.T. 1981. ''Occupational Regulation in Canada.'' Law and Economics Workshop Series, #WS 111-17, Faculty of Law, University of Toronto.

Evans, R.G., and Williamson, M.F. 1978. *Extending Canadian National Health Insurance: Policy Options for Pharmacare and Denticare*. Ontario Economic Council Research Study #13. Toronto: University of Toronto Press.

Evans, R.G., and Wolfson, A.D. 1980. ''Faith, Hope, and Charity: Health Care in the Utility Function.'' Department of Economics Discussion Paper #80-46. Vancouver: University of British Columbia.

Feldstein, M.S. 1971. ''Hospital Cost Inflation: A Study of Nonprofit Price Dynamics.'' *American Economic Review* 61: 853-72.

―――. 1973. ''The Welfare Loss of Excess Health Insurance.'' *Journal of Political Economy*. 81: 251-80.

Fraser, R.D. 1983. ''Vital Statistics and Health.'' In *Historical Statistics of*

Canada. 2nd ed., ed. F.H. Leacy. Ottawa: Statistics Canada with the Social Science Federation of Canada.

Fraser, R.D.; Spasoff, R.A.; and Prime, M.G. 1976. *An estimate of the economic burden of ill-health*. Toronto: Ontario Council of Health.

Freeland, M.S.; Anderson, G.; and Schendler, C.E. 1979. "National Hospital Input Price Index." *Health Care Financing Review* 1: 37-61.

Freidson, E. 1970. *Professional Dominance: The Social Structure of Medical Care*. New York: Atherton.

Friedman, M. 1962. *Capitalism and Freedom*. Chicago: University of Chicago Press.

Fries, J.F. 1980. "Aging, Natural Death and the Compression of Morbidity." *New England Journal of Medicine* 303: 130-35.

Fuchs, V.R. 1978. "The Supply of Surgeons and the Demand for Operations." *Journal of Human Resources* 13: 35-56. Supplement: National Bureau of Economic Research Conference on the Economics of Physician and Patient Behavior.

Fulda, T.K., and Dickens, P.F. 1979. "Controlling the Cost of Drugs: the Canadian Experience." *Health Care Financing Review* 1: 55-64.

Gibson, R.M. 1979. "National Health Expenditures, 1978" *Health Care Financing Review* 1: 1-36.

Gibson, R.M.; Waldo, D.R.; and Levit, K.R. 1983. "National Health Expenditures, 1982." *Health Care Financing Review* 5: 1-32.

Goldberg, L.E., and Greenberg, W. 1977. "The Effect of Physician-Controlled Health Insurance: U.S. vs. Oregon State Medical Society." *Journal of Health Politics, Policy and Law* 2: 48-78.

Gordon, M.J., and Fowler, D.J. 1981. *The Drug Industry*. Canadian Institute for Economic Policy. Toronto: James Lorimer.

Gorecki, P.K. 1981. *Regulating the Price of Prescription Drugs in Canada: Compulsory Licensing, Product Selection, and Government Reimbursement Programmes*. Economic Council of Canada Technical Report No. 8. Ottawa: ECC (July).

Gray, B.H., ed. 1983. *The New Health Care for Profit: Doctors and Hospitals in a Competitive Environment*. Washington, D.C.: National Academy Press.

Grossman, M. 1970. *The Demand for Health: A Theoretical and Empirical Investigation*. National Bureau of Economic Research Occasional Paper #119. New York: Columbia University Press.

Grossman, R.M. 1983. "A Review of Physician Cost-Containment Strategies for Laboratory Testing." *Medical Care* 21: 783-802.

Hadley, J. 1974. "Research on Health Manpower Productivity: A General Overview." In *Health Manpower and Productivity*, ed. J. Rafferty, pp. 143-203. Lexington, Mass.: D.C. Heath.

Hall, K.W.; Behun, M.; Irving-Meek, J.; and Otten, N. 1981. "Use of Cimetidine in Hospital Patients." *Canadian Medical Association Journal* 124: 1579-84.

Hammond, P.J. 1982. "Utilitarianism, uncertainty and information." In *Utilitarianism and beyond*, eds. A. Sen and B. Williams, pp. 85-102. Cambridge: Cambridge University Press.

————. 1983. "Ex-post optimality as a dynamically consistent objective for collective choice under uncertainty." In *Social Choice and Welfare*, eds. P.K. Pattanaik and M. Salles, pp. 175-205. Amsterdam: North-Holland.

Hardwick, D.F., *et al.* 1982. "Structuring Complexity of Testing: A Process Oriented Approach to Limiting Unnecessary Laboratory Use." *American Journal of Medical Technology* 48: 605-608.

Harris, J.E. 1977. "The internal organization of hospitals: some economic implications." *The Bell Journal of Economics* 8: 467-82.

Hartle, D.G., and Trebilcock, M.J. 1983. "Regulatory Reform and the Political Process." *Osgoode Hall Law Journal* 20: 643-77. Regulatory Reform Symposium issue, Part II.

Haynes, R.B., *et al.* 1978. "Increased Absenteeism from Work after Detection and Labelling of Hypertensive Patients." *New England Journal of Medicine* 229: 741-44.

Hill, J.D.; Hampton, J.R.; and Mitchell, J.R. 1978. "A randomized trial of home versus hospital management for patients with suspected myocardial infarction." *Lancet* 1: 837-41.

Hornbrook, M.C., and Goldfarb, M.G. 1981. "Patterns of Obstetrical Care in Hospitals." *Medical Care* 19: 55-67.

Illich, I. 1975. *Medical Nemesis: The Expropriation of Health*. Toronto: McClelland and Stewart.

Irazuzta, J.O. 1979. *A Trend Analysis of Hospital Utilization in Canada*. M.Sc. thesis, Department of Health Administration, University of Toronto.

Jacobs, P. 1974. "A Survey of Economic Models of Hospitals." *Inquiry* 11: 83-97.

Jönsson, B. 1981. *The Costs of Health Care: Trends and Determining Factors*. THE Report 1981:3. Lund: The Swedish Institute for Health Economics.

Katz, S. 1952. "The High Cost of Being Sick." *Maclean's* June 15, 65: 7-15, 62, 64-67.

Kessel, R.A. 1958. "Price Discrimination in Medicine." *Journal of Law and Economics* 1: 20-53.

Kilpatrick, K.E.; Mackenzie, R.S.; and Delaney, A.G. 1972. "Expanded-Function Auxiliaries in General Dentistry: A Computer Simulation." *Health Services Research* 7: 288-300.

Klarman, H.E. 1965. *The Economics of Health*. New York: Columbia University Press.

Klass, A. 1975 *There's Gold in Them Thar Pills*. Harmondsworth, Middlesex: Penguin Books.

Lalonde, M. 1974. *A New Perspective on the Health of Canadians* (White Paper). Ottawa: Government of Canada (April).

Lave, J.R., and Lave, L.B. 1979. "Empirical Studies of Hospital Cost Functions." In *Health Handbook*, ed. G.K. Chacko, pp. 957-73. Amsterdam: North-Holland.

LeClair, M. 1975. "The Canadian Health Care System." In *National Health Insurance: Can We Learn from Canada?*, ed. S. Andreopoulos, pp. 11-93. New York: John Wiley.

Lerner, A.P. 1944. *The Economics of Control: Principles of Welfare Economics.* New York: MacMillan.

Lewin, L.S.; Derzon, R.A.; and Margulies, R. 1981. "Investor-owneds and nonprofits differ in economic performance." *Hospitals: Journal of the American Hospital Association* 55: 52-58.

Lichtner, S., and Pflanz, M. 1971. "Appendectomy in the Federal Republic of Germany: Epidemiology and Medical Care Patterns." *Medical Care* 9:311-30.

Lieberman, J.K. 1978. "Some reflections on self-regulation." In *The Professions and Public Policy*, eds. P. Slayton and M.J. Trebilcock, pp. 89-97. Toronto: University of Toronto Press.

Lubitz, J., and Deacon, R. 1982. "The Rise in the Incidence of Hospitalizations for the Aged, 1967 to 1979." *Health Care Financing Review* 3:21-40.

Luft, H.S. 1981. *Health Maintenance Organizations: Dimensions of Performance.* New York: Wiley-Interscience.

Luft, H.S.; Feder, J.; Holahan, J.; and Lennox, K.D. 1980. "Health Maintenance Organizations." In *National Health Insurance: Conflicting Goals and Policy Choices*, eds. J. Feder, J. Holahan, and T.R. Marmor, pp. 129-80. Washington, D.C.: The Urban Institute.

Lundman, S.B. 1982. *An Economic Investigation of the Quality of Hospital Care in British Columbia.* Doctoral dissertation, Department of Economics. Vancouver: University of British Columbia.

Marmor, T.R., and Bridges, A. 1980. "American Health Planning and the Lessons of Comparative Policy Analysis." *Journal of Health Politics, Policy and Law* 5: 419-30.

Marmor, T.R.; Wittman, D.A.; and Heagy, T.C. 1976. "The Politics of Medical Inflation." *Journal of Health Politics, Policy and Law* 1:69-84.

Martin, A.R., *et al.* 1980. "A Trial of Two Strategies to Modify the Test-Ordering Behavior of Medical Residents." *New England Journal of Medicine* 303: 1330-36.

Mather, H., *et al.* 1971. "Acute Myocardial Infarction: Home and Hospital Treatment." *British Medical Journal* 3: 334-38

McNeer, J.F., *et al.* 1978. "Hospital Discharge One Week after Acute Myocardial Infarction." *New England Journal of Medicine* 298: 229-32.

McNeil, B.J.; Weichselbaum, R.; and Pauker, S.G. 1978. "Fallacy of the Five-Year Survival in Lung Cancer." *New England Journal of Medicine* 299: 1397-1401.

McPherson, K.; Wennberg, J.E.; Hovind, O.B.; and Clifford, P. 1982. "Small-Area Variations in the Use of Common Surgical Procedures: An International Comparison of New England, England, and Norway." *New England Journal of Medicine* 307: 1310-14.

Meade, J.E. 1972. "The Theory of Labour-Managed Firms and of Profit Sharing." *Economic Journal* 82: 402-28.

———. 1974. "Labour-Managed Firms in Conditions of Imperfect Competition." *Economic Journal* 84: 817-24.

Migue, J.-L., and Belanger, G. 1974. *The Price of Health*. Toronto: Macmillan.

Mitchell, B.M., and Vogel, R.J. 1973. *Health and Taxes: An Assessment of the Medical Deduction*. RAND Publication R-1222-OEO. Santa Monica,: The RAND Corporation.

Morgan, R.W. 1977. *Prospects for Preventive Medicine: A Catalogue*. Ontario Economic Council Occasional Paper no. 2. Toronto: Ontario Economic Council.

Muzondo, T.R., and Pazderka, B. 1979. *Professional Licensing and Competition Policy: effects of licensing on earnings and rates of return differentials*. Research Monograph No. 5. Bureau of Competition Policy, Research Branch, Consumer and Corporate Affairs Canada. Ottawa: Ministry of Supply and Services (April).

Nelson, R.R. 1981. "Assessing private enterprise: an exegesis of tangled doctrine." *Bell Journal of Economics* 12: 93-111.

Neuhauser, D., and Lewicki, A.M. 1976. "National Health Insurance and the Sixth Stool Guaiac." *Policy Analysis* 2: 175-96.

Newhouse, J.P. 1970. "Toward a Theory of Non-profit Institutions: An Economic Model of a Hospital." *American Economic Review* 60: 64-74.

Newhouse, J.P., et al. 1982. *Some Interim Results from a Controlled Trial of Cost Sharing in Health Insurance*. RAND Publication R-2847-HHS. Santa Monica, Cal.: The RAND Corporation.

Ontario, Ministry of Treasury and Economics, 1981. *Expenditures of the Health Care System in Ontario 1970/71 to 1977/78*. Central Statistical Services. Toronto: MTE (May).

Pattison, R.V., and Katz, H.M. 1983. "Investor-Owned and Not-for-Profit Hospitals." *New England Journal of Medicine* 389: 347-53.

Pauly, M.V. 1969. "A Measure of the Welfare Cost of Health Insurance." *Health Services Research* 4:281-92.

Pauly, M.V., and Redisch, M. 1973. "The Not-for-Profit Hospital as a Physicians' Cooperative." *American Economic Review* 63:87-100.

Plain, R. 1982. "Charging the Sick: Observations on the Economic Aspects of Medical/Social Policy Reforms." Paper presented at the Canadian Centre for Policy Alternatives Conference. "Medicare: The Decisive Year." Montreal: McGill University (November).

Posner, R.M. 1974. "Theories of economic regulation." *Bell Journal of Economics* 5: 335-58.

Rafferty, J., ed. 1974. *Health Manpower and Productivity* Lexington Mass.: D.C. Heath.

Record, J.C., ed. 1981. *Staffing Primary Care in 1990: Physician Replacement and Cost Savings.* New York: Springer.

Reder, M. 1982. "Chicago Economics: Permanence and Change." *Journal of Economic Literature* 20: 1-38.

Reinhardt, U.E. 1972. "A Production Function for Physicians' Services." *Review of Economics and Statistics* 54: 55-66.

———. 1973. "Manpower Substitution and Productivity in Medical Practice: Review of Research." *Health Services Research* 8: 200-227.

———. 1975. *Physician Productivity and the Demand for Health Manpower.* Cambridge, Mass.: Ballinger.

———. 1978. "Comment." In *Competition in the Health Care Sector: Past, Present, and Future*, ed. W. Greenberg, pp. 156-90. Proceedings of a Conference sponsored by the Bureau of Economics, Federal Trade Commission. Washington, D.C.: U.S. Federal Trade Commission.

Robertson, W. 1976. "Merck Strains to Keep the Pots Aboiling." *Fortune* March: 134-39, 168, 170.

Robinson, G.C., and Clarke, H.F. 1980. *The Hospital Care of Children.* Oxford: Oxford University Press.

Roemer, M.I. 1961. "Bed Supply and Utilization: A Natural Experiment." *Hospitals: Journal of the American Hospital Association* 35: 35-42.

Roos, L.L. 1983. "Supply, Workload and Utilization: A Population-Based Analysis of Surgery in Rural Manitoba." *American Journal of Public Health* 73: 414-21.

Roos, N.P., and Roos, L.L. 1981. "High and Low Surgical Rates: Risk Factors for Area Residents." *American Journal of Public Health* 71: 591-600.

Rothschild, M., and Stiglitz, J.E. 1976. "Equilibrium in Competitive Insurance Markets: An Essay on the Economics of Imperfect Information." *Quarterly Journal of Economics* 90: 629-50.

Sackett, D.L. 1980. "Evaluation of Health Services." In *Public Health and Preventive Medicine (Maxcy-Rosenau)*, 11th ed., ed. J.M. Last, pp. 1800-1823. New York: Appleton-Century-Crofts.

Schelling, T.C. 1978. *Micromotives and Macrobehavior.* New York: Norton.

Scherer, F.M. 1964. *The Weapons Acquisition Process: Economic Incentives.* Boston: Harvard Graduate School of Business Administration.

Schneider, E.L., and Brody, J.A. 1983. "Aging, Natural Death, and the Compression of Morbidity: Another View." *New England Journal of Medicine* 309: 854-55.

Schoemaker, P.J.H. 1982. "The Expected Utility Model: Its Variants, Purposes, Evidence, and Limitations." *Journal of Economic Literature* 20: 529-63.

Schroeder, S.A.; Kenders, K.; Cooper, J.K.; and Piemme, T.E. 1973. "Use of Laboratory Tests and Pharmaceuticals: Variation Among Physicians and

Effects of Cost Audit on Subsequent Use.'' *Journal of the American Medical Association* 225: 969-73.

Shillington, C.H. 1972. *The Road to Medicare in Canada.* Toronto: Del Graphics.

Siemiatycki, J.; Richardson, L.; and Pless, I.B. 1980. ''Equality in Medical Care under National Health Insurance in Montreal.'' *New England Journal of Medicine.* 303: 10-15.

Silverman, M., and Lee, P.R. 1974. *Pills, Profits, and Politics.* Berkeley,: University of California Press.

Silverman, M.; Lee, P.R.; and Lydecker, M. 1981. *Pills and the Public Purse.* Berkeley,: University of California Press.

Slayton, P., and Trebilcock, M.J. 1978. *The Professions and Public Policy.* Toronto: University of Toronto Press.

Smith, H.L. 1958. ''Two Lines of Authority: The Hospital's Dilemma.'' In *Patients, Physicians and Illness*, ed. E.G. Jaco, pp. 468-77. New York: The Free Press.

Smith, K.R.; Miller, M.; and Golladay, F.L. 1972. ''An Analysis of the Optimal Use of Inputs in the Production of Medical Services.'' *Journal of Human Resources* 7:208-25.

Spitzer, W.O. 1978. ''Evidence that justifies the introduction of new health professionals.'' In *The Professions and Public Policy*, eds. P. Slayton and M.J. Trebilcock, pp. 211-36. Toronto: University of Toronto Press.

Starr, P. 1982. *The Social Transformation of American Medicine.* New York: Basic Books.

Stason, W.B., and Weinstein, M.C. 1977. ''Allocation of Resources to Manage Hypertension.'' *New England Journal of Medicine* 296: 732-39.

Stigler, G.J. 1971. ''The theory of economic regulation.'' *Bell Journal of Economics and Management Science* 2:3-21.

Stockwell, H., and Vayda, E. 1979. ''Variations in Surgery in Ontario.'' *Medical Care* 17: 390-96.

Stoddart, G.L., and Seldon, J.R. 1983. ''Publicly Financed Competition in Canadian Health Care Delivery: A Proposed Alternative to Increased Regulation.'' Paper read at the Second Canadian Conference on Health Economics, 9-11 September 1983, at Regina, Saskatchewan.

Stoddart, G.L., and Woodward, C.A. 1980. ''The Effect of Physician Extra-Billing on Patients' Access to Care and Attitudes Toward the Ontario Health System.'' Background Paper prepared for *Health Services Review '79.* (The Hon. Emmett M. Hall, Special Commissioner.) Ottawa: Health and Welfare Canada.

Stoddart, G.L., and Barer, M.L. 1981. ''Analyses of Demand and Utilization through Episodes of Medical Service.'' In *Health, Economics, and Health Economics*, eds. J. Van der Gaag and M. Perlman, pp. 149-70. Amsterdam: North-Holland.

Temin, P.B. 1979. "Technology, regulation, and market structure in the modern pharmaceutical industry." *Bell Journal of Economics* 10: 429-46.

Thomas, L. 1971. "The Technology of Medicine." *New England Journal of Medicine* 284: 1366-68.

Titmuss, R.M. 1970. *The Gift Relationship*. London: George Allen & Unwin.

Torrance, G.M. n.d. (i.e. 1972). *The Influence of the Drug Industry in Canada's Health System*. Paper Commissioned by the Community Health Centre Project. Dr. John Hastings, Director. Ottawa: Canadian Public Health Association.

Trauner, J.B. 1983. *Preferred Provider Organizations: The California Experiment*. Institute for Health Policy Studies Monograph. San Francisco: University of California San Francisco, Institute for Health Policy Studies.

Trebilcock, M.J., and Shaul, J. 1983. "Regulating the Quality of Psychotherapeutic Services." *Law and Human Behavior* 7:265-78.

Trebilcock, M.J.; Tuohy, C.J.; and Wolfson, A.D. 1979. *Professional Regulation. A Staff Study of Accountancy, Architecture, Engineering and Law in Ontario*. Prepared for the Professional Organizations Committee. Toronto: Ministry of the Attorney-General of Ontario (January).

Tuohy, C.J., and Wolfson, A.D. 1977. "The Political Economy of Professionalism: A Perspective." In *Four Aspects of Professionalism*, ed. M.J. Trebilcock, pp. 41-86. Ottawa: Consumer Research Council, Department of Consumer and Corporate Affairs.

———. 1978. "Self-regulation: who qualifies?" In *The Professions and Public Policy*, eds. P. Slayton and M.J. Trebilcock, pp. 111-22. Toronto: University of Toronto Press.

United States, Department of Health and Human Services 1980. *Health United States 1980*. DHHS Publication No. (PHS) 81-1232. Public Health Service, Office of Health Research, Statistics, and Technology. National Center for Health Statistics and National Center for Health Services Research. Hyattsville, Maryland: DHHS.

Vancouver Sun. 1983. "Drugs overpriced, study shows," and "Pharmacare's secret: customer aided by competition." — Thursday, 3 November.

Vanek, J. 1977. *The Labor-Managed Economy*. Ithaca, N.Y.: Cornell University Press.

Vayda, E. 1973. "A Comparison of Surgical Rates in Canada and in England and Wales" *New England Journal of Medicine* 289: 1224-29.

———. 1977. "Prepaid Group Practice under Universal Health Insurance in Canada." *Medical Care* 15: 382-89.

Vayda, E., and Anderson, G.D. 1975. "Comparison of Provincial Surgical Rates in 1968." *Canadian Journal of Surgery* 18: 18-26.

Vayda, E.; Morison, M.; and Anderson, G.D. 1976. "Surgical Rates in the Canadian Provinces, 1968 to 1972." *Canadian Journal of Surgery* 19: 235-42.

Walker, H.D. 1971. *Market Power and Price Levels in the Ethical Drug Industry.* Bloomington: Indiana University Press.

Warner, K.E. 1975. "A 'Desperation-Reaction' Model of Medical Diffusion." *Health Services Research* 10:369-83.

Warner, K.E., and Luce, B.R. 1982. *Cost-Benefit and Cost-Effectiveness Analysis in Health Care: Principles, Practice and Potential.* Ann Arbor, Mich.: Health Administration Press.

Weisbrod, B.A. 1971. "Costs and Benefits of Medical Research: A Case Study of Poliomyelitis." *Journal of Political Economy* 79:527-44.

Wennberg, J., and Gittelsohn, A. 1982. "Variations in Medical Care among Small Areas." *Scientific American* 246: 120-34 (April).

Williams, A. (1978). "Need: An Economic Exegesis." In *Economic Aspects of Health Services*, eds. A.J. Culyer and K.G. Wright, pp. 32-45. London: Martin Robertson.

Williamson, O.E. 1975. *Markets and Hierarchies: Analysis and Anti-Trust Implications.* New York: The Free Press.

Wilson, C. 1977. "A Model of Insurance Markets with Imperfect Information." *Journal of Economic Theory* 16:167-207.

Wilson, G.; Sheps, C.G.; and Oliver, T.R. 1982. "Effects of Hospital Revenue Bonds on Hospital Planning and Operations." *New England Journal of Medicine* 307:1426-30.

Wolfson, A.D. 1976. "The Supply of Physicians' Services." *In Health Economics Symposium: Proceedings of the First Canadian Conference*, September 4-6, 1974, ed. R.D. Fraser pp. 140-50. Kingston, Ont.: Queen's University Industrial Relations Centre.

Wolfson, A.D.; Evans, R.G.; and Lomas, J.1980. "Physician Incomes in Canada." Background Paper prepared for *Health Services Review '79.* The Hon. Emmett M. Hall, Special Commissioner. Ottawa: Health and Welfare Canada.

Wolfson, A.D., and Tuohy, C.J. 1980. *Opting Out of Medicare: Private Medical Markets in Ontario.* Ontario Economic Council Research Study #19. Toronto: University of Toronto Press.

GLOSSARY

ADVERSE SELECTION: Insurance is a process of *risk-pooling*. Transactors each facing possible large loses agree to contribute a small premium payment to a common pool, to be used to compensate whichever of them actually suffers the loss. Contributions must cover losses plus administration costs. If potential purchasers face different risks, which are not matched by different premiums, then high risk people will tend to join, and low risk people, whose premiums would exceed their expected losses, may not. Such *adverse selection* raises the premiums of those in the plan, which must be sufficient to cover the losses of the insured group. The risk-pooling process may break down entirely if the lowest risks in the insured group continue to withdraw.

AGENCY: In an *agency* relationship the seller of a commodity acts not in a strictly self-interested manner but rather to direct the buyer's decisions on the buyer's behalf. Such a relationship may respond to ASSYMETRY OF IN-FORMATION, which would otherwise permit the seller to exploit an informational advantage. Professional institutions are intended to induce and protect provider agency behaviour which will (usually) resolve the inevitable conflict of (economic) interest between provider and consumer in favour of consumer/patients.

ALLOCATIVE EFFICIENCY: *See* EFFICIENCY.

ASYMMETRY OF INFORMATION: A particular class of transactions displays *asymmetry of information* if sellers normally have more information about the value of commodities to buyers than buyers have or can reasonably hope to get.

CAPITATION REIMBURSEMENT: *See* REIMBURSEMENT.

CARTEL: Suppliers of similar products may co-ordinate their behaviour by fixing common prices, sharing markets, cross-licensing patents, or otherwise behaving like a single organization to raise overall prices and profits. Such co-ordination ranges from "conscious parallelism"—behaviour recognizing mutual interdependence—through formal agreements, to outright merger. Cartel activities by professional organizations may include collective fee setting, regulation or suppression of advertising, and controls on practice structure and organization.

369

COMMUNITY RATING: An insurance program charging each enrollee in a region the same premium for a particular level of coverage, regardless of individual characteristics affecting probability of loss, is *community rated*.

CONSUMER SOVEREIGNTY: As a NORMATIVE postulate, *consumer sovereignty* implies that the proper aim of economic activity is the satisfaction of consumer wants, as interpreted by themselves rather than external observers, bureaucrats, or experts. As a POSITIVE statement, consumer sovereignty describes the extent to which consumers' preferences do in fact determine how much of what commodities get produced in a particular economy or society.

COST-BENEFIT, COST-EFFECTIVENESS, COST-UTILITY ANALYSIS: Program evaluation asks whether the consequences of a particular activity are suficiently valuable to justify its costs. It requires the assembly of information on all the costs and consequences of the activity in a comparable form. *Cost-benefit analysis* consists of identifying all costs and consequences across the whole society and valuing each in terms of a common unit such a dollars. The activity is worth doing if its net present value (dollar benefits less dollar costs, each appropriately discounted), is positive. *Cost-effectiveness analysis* measures outcomes in terms of some natural unit, such as numbers of children immunized or numbers of fatal accidents averted, and calculates costs *per* this natural unit. The value of the natural unit of outcome remains a political judgement. *Cost-utility analysis* extends cost-effectiveness by converting the units of output to a common measure, their relative value to those experiencing the outcome (*see* LIFE YEARS).

CREAM-SKIMMING or CREAMING OFF: A rational transactor will try to select the most favourable cases out of a set of options. Insurance companies try to cover the "best" or lowest risks from a population, and avoid the high risks. For-profit hospitals in the U.S. are alleged to encourage their physicians to admit relatively healthy patients with private insurance and uncomplicated medical or surgical diagnoses. *Cream-skimming* therefore depends on a structure of prices or reimbursements which are not proportional to costs, as well as on the objectives of the organization, which define what constitutes "cream". Non-profit organizations might select cases by interest rather than profitability.

DEMAND, SUPPLY: The quantity of a commodity that buyers want to purchase, at given prices (to themselves), is the quantity *demanded*. It need not equal UTILIZATION, which measures the amount of the commodity actually used up. SUPPLY refers to the amount of a commodity that present or potential sellers want to put on the market, in response to the price offered by (or on behalf of) buyers. Both supply and demand are behavioural concepts, describing the way particular transactors are expected to respond to prices offered or charged, assuming other factors are held constant.

DIAGNOSIS-RELATED GROUPS (DRGS): *See* REIMBURSEMENT.

EFFECTIVENESS: *See* EFFICACY.

EFFICACY, EFFECTIVENESS: The *efficacy* of a diagnostic or therapeutic intervention refers to its capacity to achieve a desired result under ideal circumstances. An efficacious intervention ''works,'' if properly applied. *Effectiveness* refers to the impact of the intervention in actual practice. Patients may not comply with a prescription for an efficacious drug, because of complexity, side-effects, or simple lack of understanding. Practitioners may lack the ability to carry out an intervention properly. Or other circumstances may intervene.

EFFICIENCY, ALLOCATIVE and TECHNICAL: The production of particular commodities is *technically efficient* if it uses up the least costly quantity and mix of INPUTS consistent with the desired outcome. Technical efficiency depends on the relative prices of inputs, as well as on management; labour-intensive production may be wasteful in a high-wage economy, not in a low-wage one. *Allocative efficiency* refers to the mix of goods and services produced; an economy is allocatively efficient if a reallocation of resources from one type of production to another could not be found which could make anyone better off without making someone else worse off. An economy that produced goods and services that no one wanted, but at the lowest possible cost, would be allocatively very inefficient, though technically efficient. People could be made better off by reallocating resources to other forms of production.

EPISODE-BASED REIMBURSEMENT: *See* REIMBURSEMENT.

EXTERNALITIES or EXTERNAL EFFECTS: One person or organization's behaviour may affect others, independent of any voluntary transaction. My playing of loud music at night disturbs your sleep; my refusal to be immunized increases your chance of getting polio, my failure to wear seatbelts increases your taxes to pay my hospital bills. Conversely my beautiful garden not only gives you pleasure, but raises your property value. Insofar as my behaviour fails to take account of such effects, because others have no way to induce me to respond to their preferences, I will (from a society-wide perspective) over-(under-)indulge in activities with negative (positive) externalities.

FALSE POSITIVE, FALSE NEGATIVE: Few diagnostic tests are absolutely accurate; most will yield a proportion of erroneous results. A *false positive* is a test result which is erroneously interpreted as showing a particular condition, when in fact the patient tested does not have the condition. A *false negative* wrongly identifies the patient as free of the condition.

FEE-FOR-SERVICE REIMBURSEMENT: *See* REIMBURSEMENT.

FIRM, FOR-PROFIT, NOT-FOR-PROFIT: The *firm* in economic analysis is a conceptual construct which directs the process of PRODUCTION. Its real-world counterpart might be a small owner-managed business, a partnership, or a giant multinational enterprise. Whatever its scale, the firm is a single transactor, a coherent decision-maker or management, focussing its attention on a well-defined objective or set of objectives. Most firms in industry or commerce are *for-profit*, their behaviour and responses to the external environment being determined by perceived profit opportunities. In a *not-for-profit* firm the legal owners are not entitled to remove resources for their own use. They act as trustees, carrying on production, to serve other objectives, such as community service somehow defined. In *not-only-for-profit* firms such as professional practices the owner has clear title to all profits. But the owner is also manager and principal worker in the firm, and as such has an interest in the quality of the work environment and in her own earnings as worker which compete directly with the interest in profits. A professional interest in practice style and in the outcomes experienced by patients also competes with the profit motive. These considerations are not merely means to an end, as they are for the for-profit firm, they are ends in themselves.

FOR-PROFIT FIRM: *See* FIRM.

HUMAN CAPITAL: Investment is a PRODUCTION process, using up resources to create capital which will yield a stream of services as *inputs* to future production. Capital may be physical (machinery, factories, rail lines and roads), or intangible (new software). *Human capital* is increased productive capacity embodied in more highly trained and productive human beings. Such training requires the investment of the time and energy of the trainee, as well as the direct training costs. It thus uses up resources to increase productivity, just as if a physical machine had been created for that person to work with.

IGNORANCE: *See* UNCERTAINTY.

INCENTIVE REIMBURSEMENT: *See* REIMBURSEMENT.

INCOME OR WEALTH TRANSFERS: All public policies, and even price changes, generate *income or wealth transfers*—shifts of purchasing power from one person to another without any corresponding transfer of goods or services. In principle it is possible to use price changes to redirect economic activity while compensating people for the wealth changes involved; in practice this almost never happens.

INCOMPLETE VERTICAL INTEGRATION OF PRODUCTION: *See* VERTICAL INTEGRATION OF PRODUCTION, INCOMPLETE.

INPUT: *See* PRODUCTION.

INTENSITY OF SERVICING: Measures of the activity of health care institutions are often at an aggregated level, such as a patient-day in hospital or a visit to a physician's office or clinic. Yet these measures are themselves bundles of services, whose content will differ across patients, institutions, regions, and time. *Intensity of servicing* describes the amount of activity associated with a particular measure of health care output such as patient-days or office visits.

LIFE AND LIMB VALUATION: Programs for expanding (or contracting) health care services are usually expected to have consequences measured in terms of mortality and morbidity. Particular people will have their life expectancies lengthened or shortened, or will spend greater or lesser periods of time in states of disability or discomfort, as a result of the program activities. *Life and limb valuation* refers to the process of trying to place values on these morbid or mortal consequences, or their avoidance, in such a way that the programs which generate them can be evaluated (*see* LIFE YEARS).

LIFE YEARS: One can measure the consequences of "lifesaving" programs in terms of *life years* gained, by adding the estimated increases in life expectancy resulting from the program across all potential beneficiaries. A further refinement takes account of the fact that not all time is equally valuable. Thus one may attach weights to the extra life years yielded by a program, adding them up by counting each year spent in a state of normal function as one, but each year spent in a state of particular disability or discomfort as somewhat less than one. The result is a measure of program consequences in terms of *quality-adjusted life years* (QALYS), which can then be balanced against program costs.

MONOPOLY MODEL: Professions are sometimes viewed as simply a group of suppliers of a particular product who have acquired the political privilege of self-regulation which can then be used to limit the numbers of their members and the supply of their services. The profession as monopoly drives up the prices of its members' services, and thereby their incomes, at the consumer's expense.

MONOPOLY, MONOPSONY, OLIGOPOLY, MONOPOLISTIC COMPETITION: Literally, a *monopoly* is the sole supplier of a particular commodity in a particular market. Similarly a *monopsonist* is the sole buyer of a given product. An *oligopoly* is a small group of sellers, each taking direct account of the pricing and output behaviour of its rivals in setting its own strategy. A market is characterized by *monopolistic competition* if there are a large number of sellers, each supplying a product only slightly differentiated from the others. The common feature of all these situations is that the seller has a degree of monopoly power, power over the price at which a commodity is sold.

MORAL HAZARD: This describes a tendency for losses to be greater or more frequent when covered by insurance. Those insured may fail to take due care or may over-estimate their losses. It must be distinguished from ADVERSE SELECTION, which arises if the insurance pool draws in the higher risk members of the group of potential insurance buyers. In that case observed losses will be higher among the insured than among the uninsured even though no behavioural change, and no increase in overall loss, has occurred. *Moral hazard* refers to the risk of loss and/or the size of losses (actual or reported) increasing as a result of their being insured.

MÜNCHAUSEN'S SYNDROME: A form of mental illness whose sufferers derive satisfaction from undergoing medical interventions, and who become adept at counterfeiting symptoms so as to gain access to clinics and hospitals and to induce providers to carry out diagnostic and therapeutic manoeuvres on them.

NAIVE MODELS, MEDICO-TECHNICAL and ECONOMIC: A simplified description of the behaviour of an individual or organization, or of the systematic interactions among such transactors, is a model. Any prediction about behaviour rests on some implicit model of the "behaver." The "naive" models represent alternative descriptions of the health care system and the transactors in it. The *naive medico-technical model* begins from a normative judgement that the health system should use resources so as to improve the health status of the people in a community to the fullest extent possible. It then makes the positive assumptions that providers control the use of health care resources, and direct them solely to the improvement of patients' health. The "right" level of resources to devote to health care is that which providers say is necessary. The model is silent on how to assure that resources are used efficiently, or how provider remuneration is to be determined; apparently responsible providers look after these issues too. The *naive economic model* posits that the proper function of a health care system is to allocate resources so that consumers get the services which they are willing and able to pay for, when those services are priced at their true (opportunity) costs of production. The positive assumptions are that consumers determine all utilization of health care, reacting to their own information and to the prices they must pay. Providers merely offer services; consumers decide what to use and are not influenced by providers in this process. The level of remuneration of providers is determined, and the technical efficiency of production is assured, by competition (including most importantly price competition) among providers, and institutions which inhibit this competition should be removed.

NET ADVANTAGES: The decision to enter an occupation represents a choice among future patterns of training costs and income streams, but also among degrees of risk of success, and general lifestyles. The *net advantages* model of occupational choice suggests that (in the absence of restrictions on entry) choices by new entrants will lead to the equalization across occupations of the present value of all the monetary and non-monetary aspects of each occupation, principally by the adjustment of relative earnings levels.

NORMATIVE AND POSITIVE PROPOSITIONS: A *normative* statement or proposition asserts an obligation; it either does or could contain the word "ought." Policy recommendations are usually normative. A *positive* statement by contrast seeks to describe a situation or a cause-and-effect relationship; it asserts, rightly or wrongly, what "is." It can have an apparently normative form: if you want to achieve X you should do A. But this is an assertion of a causal link between X and A. The normative statement would be that you should seek to achieve X.

NOT-FOR-PROFIT FIRM: *See* FIRM.

NOT-ONLY-FOR-PROFIT FIRM: *See* FIRM.

OLIGOPOLY: *See* MONOPOLY.

OPPORTUNITY or RESOURCE COST: The true cost of any commodity, viewed from the perspective of a whole society, is the *resource cost*, the amounts of different types of productive inputs which had to be used up to produce that commodity (*see* PRODUCTION). But the resources themselves are valuable only insofar as they have alternative uses for which they will not be available if used to produce the commodity in question. Thus the *oppor-*

tunity cost of a commodity is the value of the best alternative use to which those resources could have been put, the value of the productive opportunities foregone by the decision to use them in produing that commodity.

ORGANIC AND TRANSACTION MODELS OF HOSPITALS: Some attempts to provide an explanation of the economic behaviour of hospitals have treated them as single entities, transactors, with a well-defined set of objectives and a management structure which pursues those objectives in a coherent way. *Organic* models of hospitals view them as striving, subject to the constraints imposed by the outside environment and the limitations of organization and technique, to achieve their objectives, in the same way that a private firm tries to maximize its profits. The not-for-profit hospital just has different objectives. *Transaction models*, on the other hand, suggest that despite its apparent coherence as a legal, organizational, and physical entity, the hospital is not a single transactor and has no clear set of objectives of its own. It is rather a framework within which other transactors seek their objectives through a complex set of interactions, sometimes co-operative and sometimes competitive.

OUTPUT: *See* PRODUCTION.

OVERUTILIZATION: *See* UTILIZATION.

PANGLOSS: The character in Voltaire's *Candide* whose common expression was, "All is for the best in the best of all possible worlds." As a believer in the omnipotence and unfailing beneficence of Divine Providence, he drew the inevitable conclusion that whatever happened in the world, no matter how awful it appeared, was nonetheless the best thing that could have happened.

PHYSICIANS' CO-OPERATIVE MODEL OF HOSPITALS: The *physicians' co-operative* view of hospitals sees them as managed by a group of physicians whose objective is postulated to be the maximization of their own net incomes. The result might appear to be an intermediate case between the ORGANIC and TRANSACTION models of hospitals, since it envisions a group of physicians with objectives defined independently of the hospital coming together to seek those objectives through the hospital, and yet assumes a single well-defined objective—maximum average net income per physician—for the group as a whole. In fact, however, the physicians' co-operative is not a model of hospital behaviour at all, because the hospital has disappeared as an institution. Rather it is a model of a medical clinic, completely owned and managed by a physician partnership, which has overnight beds and more extensive facilities.

POSITIVE PROPOSITION: *See* NORMATIVE.

PRODUCER SOVEREIGNTY: This concept, like that of CONSUMER SOVEREIGNTY, has both NORMATIVE and POSITIVE versions. As a positive proposition, *producer sovereignty* asserts that in a particular economy or sector, producers' preferences and decisions determine what will be produced, and how, and what consumers will use. This might be because producers control consumers' perceptions through advertising or because professional expertise backed up by legal restrictions on consumer behaviour and/or consumers' deference to expertise enables producers to control actual decisions. As a normative proposition, the idea that producers' objectives *ought* to govern resource allocation processes has no obvious relation to any more general system of political or ethical values. But in professionalized industries like health care, the argument can be advanced that producer sovereignty yields a better outcome for consumers, who are unable to know their own needs.

PRODUCTION, INPUT, OUTPUT, PRODUCTION FUNCTION: *Production* is the process of transforming *inputs* into *outputs*. Inputs are productive resources: human time, energy, and skills, the services of capital equipment such as buildings and machinery, raw materials, intermediate products which are themselves the outputs of prior production processes, and "knowhow" to combine all these. The outputs are commodities, goods and services, which are valued by some end user or some other producer who will use them in a subsequent stage of production. The *production function* is an expression summarizing, for each type and amount of output, the range of different combinations of inputs which could be combined to yield that output. This "function" might be a mathematical expression, or a computer algorithm, or a set of blueprints, or simply a description of the "knowhow" of an experienced producer.

PROSPECTIVE REIMBURSEMENT: *See* REIMBURSEMENT.

QUALITY OF CARE: The adequate definition of this concept is extremely difficult. But it is generally agreed that *quality of care* must refer to the nature of the effects produced on patients' health status by particular forms of health care. Higher quality interventions produce better and/or more reliable results. In some analyses, quality of care is confused with INTENSITY OF SERVICING, but these are quite distinct concepts. In health care, more is not in general better.

QUALITY-ADJUSTED LIFE YEARS (QALYS): *See* LIFE YEARS.

REIMBURSEMENT—CAPITATION, EPISODE-BASED, FEE-FOR-SERVICE, INCENTIVE, PROSPECTIVE: Hospitals or physicians may be "reimbursed" for the service they provide to patients, by either a government or a private insurance agency, or the patients themselves, or a private charity or public agency.

But the form which this reimbursement takes, and the way it responds to the activity of the provider, can vary. *Capitation* reimbursement pays the provider a fixed sum per time period for each patient on a specified list. The provider accepts responsibility for providing services to that population, either all "necessary" services or some defined subset. *Fee-for-service*, by contrast, pays the provider a certain amount for each act performed. Total reimbursement depends on activity level. The fee level may be determined by the provider, or set by negotiation with the reimburser. *Episode-based* reimbursement applies to some forms of physicians' services, obstetrical confinements for example, and has been recommended for hospital care. In this form, a particular illness is regarded as requiring a "package" of treatment, and a level of reimbursement is determined for that "package." A hospital might be paid a fixed amount for each appendectomy, for example, regardless of the length of stay of each individual case or the number of services provided during the episode. Such a system obviously requires a large number of categories in which to classify patients for reimbursement purposes. One such is the set of *diagnosis-related groups* (DRGs) developed in the U.S., which are mutually exclusive and collectively exhaustive, and define a reimbursement category for every hospital patient. Without some such system, episode-based reimbursement is obviously impossible. *Prospective reimbursement* refers to determination of the level of reimbursement at the beginning of the period of activity. *Incentive reimbursement* refers to systems of reimbursement which attempt to induce providers to be more efficient, to control costs, by enabling them to retain some share of savings as discretionary funds. In fact, all forms of reimbursement embody incentives to some forms of behaviour, and disincentives to others. Fee-for-service, for example encourages servicing and fast throughput; capitation and fixed budgets do not.

RESOURCE COST: *See* OPPORTUNITY.

RISK: *See* UNCERTAINTY.

RISK-POOLING: *See* ADVERSE SELECTION.

ROEMER'S LAW: The proposition that the utilization of hospital beds is causally linked to the availability of beds, independently of the morbidity of the population served or the point of service charges to users, is known as Roemer's Law. This effect is not just a capacity constraint; bed availability is asserted to affect physicians' predisposition to hospitalize as well as the number of people they can actually put in beds.

SENSITIVITY ANALYSIS: The costs and consequences of a program being evaluated will rarely if ever all be known with certainty. In many cases, best estimates of the magnitude of particular factors will have to be made. Once the evaluation has been done, the robustness of the conclusion may be tested by *sensitivity analysis*. This involves inserting alternative values (over a plausible range) for uncertain factors in the analysis to see if the overall evaluation conclusion is reversed. If the conclusion is sensitive to such variations, then more effort should be devoted to determining the values of the uncertain factors. In the meantime, no decision should be based upon the evaluation.

SHADOW PRICES: To compare the costs and consequences of an activity, it is necessary to value them in common units such as dollars. The unit value of inputs to or outputs from the activity which have a well-defined market price can be measured by that price. Some activities, however, have inputs or outputs which are not traded on markets, or alternatively are traded at prices which do not reflect their true OPPORTUNITY OR RESOURCE COSTS. The analyst may then try to estimate *shadow prices* which reflect the opportunity costs of the inputs or outputs concerned. The alternative is to abandon the approach of valuing all costs and consequences in dollars, and to meaure some aspects in physical units (*See* LIFE YEARS).

SUPPLY: *See* DEMAND.

TECHNICAL EFFICIENCY: *See* EFFICIENCY.

TIME DISCOUNT RATE: The costs and consequences of a program usually arrive as a flow through time over a more or less extended planning horizon. But costs or benefits which accrue in the future cannot be valued on the same basis as those available today. Even abstracting from inflation, dollars next year are worth less than dollars of the same purchasing power now because the resources they represent could be used productively in the meantime. Thus costs and consequences which occur in the future must be discounted back to a common present value. The *time discount rate* is the percentage by which a value is reduced for each year it is deferred into the future.

TRANSACTION MODEL, HOSPITAL: *See* ORGANIC.

UNCERTAINTY, RISK, IGNORANCE: All three are aspects of incomplete information. *Uncertainty* and *risk* both refer to the future, incomplete information as to what is going to happen. The transactor facing risk has a reasonably clear perception of the possible outcomes, and has information as to the probability of occurrence of each outcome. Uncertainty describes a future in which neither outcomes nor probabilities are clear. Risk can be managed by *risk-pooling* through insurance; but more general forms of uncertainty may or may not be insurable. *Ignorance* by contrast refers to lack of knowledge about present circumstances—what is wrong with me, and what should I do about it, for example. This form of incomplete information is not insurable, and in the case of professional services is remedied by the creation of an AGENCY relationship between the uninformed consumer and a better informed provider.

UNDERUTILIZATION: *See* UTILIZATION.

UTILIZATION, OVER- and UNDER-: *Over-* and *underutilization* of health care can be judged against two quite different standards. From a health care perspective, provision and utilization of care past the point where it can be expected to have a positive impact on health status is "too much." Failure to provide or use care which could be expected to have a significant (positive) effect on the user's health status is underutilization. From the perspective of conventional economic analysis, however, overutilization occurs when people use care for which they would not be willing to pay the full OPPORTUNITY COST; underutilization when they are unable to get care for which they would be prepared to pay the cost. No account is taken of their "needs," or level of wealth or information. The choice between reference standards is ultimately a social value judgement about what standards ought to govern health care provision; it cannot be derived from either economics or the health disciplines.

VERTICAL INTEGRATION OF PRODUCTION, INCOMPLETE: PRODUCTION is as noted the conversion of *inputs* into *outputs*. Among these inputs will be intermediate products, which are themselves the outputs of a prior stage of production. The farmer's output of grain is an input to the miller or maltster; their outputs of flour or malt are inputs to the baker or brewer. Production is more or less *vertically integrated*, according to the extent to which stages of production are combined under a single management. In a vertically integrated system, production is organized and controlled by administrative mechanisms—"central planning" within the firm—while non-integrated industries co-ordinate production through arm's-length market transactions. *Incomplete vertical integration* is a mixed form. The private physician, for example, is not an employee or owner of the hospital where she admits patients. Yet she does not deal with the hospital as an independent, arm's-length contractor either. Physicians exercise management rights in hospitals, although they are not part of the administrative hierarchy.

WEALTH TRANSFERS: *See* INCOME.

INDEX